PHARMACOLOGY - RESEARCH, SAFETY TESTING AND REGULATION

PHARMACOGENOMICS IN LATIN AMERICA

CHALLENGES AND OPPORTUNITIES

PHARMACOLOGY - RESEARCH, SAFETY TESTING AND REGULATION

Additional books in this series can be found on Nova's website
under the Series tab.

Additional e-books in this series can be found on Nova's website
under the eBooks tab.

LATIN AMERICAN POLITICAL, ECONOMIC, AND SECURITY ISSUES

Additional books in this series can be found on Nova's website
under the Series tab.

Additional e-books in this series can be found on Nova's website
under the eBooks tab.

PHARMACOLOGY - RESEARCH, SAFETY TESTING AND REGULATION

PHARMACOGENOMICS IN LATIN AMERICA

CHALLENGES AND OPPORTUNITIES

LUIS A. QUIÑONES
EDITOR

nova biomedical
New York

Additional color graphics may be available in the e-book version of this book.

Library of Congress Cataloging-in-Publication Data

ISBN: 978-1-53611-031-9
Library of Congress Control Number: 2017934375

Published by Nova Science Publishers, Inc. † New York

CONTENTS

FOREWORD

José A. G. Agúndez*, MD, PhD
Professor of Pharmacology
University of Extremadura. Avda. de la Universidad s/n, 10071, Cáceres, Spain.

Pharmacogenomics constitutes an important part of what we now know as precision medicine. Pharmacological therapy has always had a problem with predicting drug response, because the events that take place between drug administration and drug response very often go unchecked. Pharmacokinetics monitorization is often too time-consuming and costly to be readily applicable to all patients, and therefore is limited today to a handful of highly toxic drugs. Pharmacodynamics monitorization is even more difficult, and often we do not have any means of predicting drug response. Therefore, the most common situation in drug therapy is that in which we prescribe a drug and then we observe whether the treatment is efficient or not, disregarding what is actually happening in the background. As a consequence, when adverse drug reactions occur, it is too late.

One of the most important promises of precision medicine is the avoidance of adverse drug reactions by adjusting drugs and doses to every single patient and to determined diseases and determined situations, which may vary along time. To this end, it is crucial to gather information about the patient, the disease and the situation that can be used to tailor the treatment accordingly. The items of information (measurements that can be collected) which indicate biological processes, and which can be used in clinical practice for disease diagnosis, prognosis, therapy selection, dose adjustment, and monitoring outcomes, are known as biomarkers.

Previous to the use of these biomarkers, drug therapy was a sort of Procrustean bed, that is, a standard to which exact conformity was forced. Procrustes, also known as "the Stretcher", was a mythological character who forced his victims to fit the exact size of an iron bed, either by stretching them or cutting their legs to size. The Procrustean equivalent in drug therapy is to administrate the same dose to all patients, regardless of any additional considerations.

With the advent of pharmacogenomics, the situation improved. Nowadays many genetic biomarkers of drug response are well known, and several clinical practice guidelines are now

* Email: jagundez@unex.es.

available. These guidelines make recommendations such as "No action required; select an alternative drug; reduce the dose by a determined percentage; or monitor plasma concentration". What we have now is a handful of varying sizes of Procrustean beds from which the best is selected for each patient, but this situation is far from satisfactory because a fine-tuning of therapy for every patient in every situation it is still not possible.

Pharmacogenomics, as a science, is still young. We know some genes and mutations which have an effect on drug response, but we are ignorant of many factors that may modify drug response in individuals with identical genetic backgrounds. Further refinement in pharmacogenomics biomarkers is expected from the use of next generation sequencing technologies but, in my opinion, it is much more important to analyze a wide variety of human populations, not only because genetic factors are expected to be different in diverse human groups, but also because a close relationship exists between genetics and environment. Environmental factors can shape the genetic background of a human population by means of selection pressure (for example individuals who, because of their genetic background, are able to bioinactivate determined dietary or environmental compounds would have an evolutionary advantage). Furthermore, if we take into consideration that drug response is the result of the interaction of genetics and environment, it becomes evident that to refine the power of pharmacogenomics, different human populations and different environments must be analyzed in detail. Most of the knowledge of pharmacogenomics we currently possess has been obtained in Europe or North-America. Now it is imperative to analyze in detail the role of genetics/environment interplay in drug response in other human populations.

Pharmacogenomics research in Latin-America constitutes a unique opportunity to gain ground in this discipline because of the large variety of human populations present there (several autochthonous populations, several immigrant populations and diverse admixed populations) and because of the immensely rich ecosystem that might interact with genetics and with drug response, either by inducing or inhibiting drug metabolism, causing interactions, etc. This book reflects the joint effort of a group of Latin-American scientists to deal with several aspects of Pharmacogenomics. It is important to stress the relevance of research done on the ground, since local researchers are aware of therapy habits, usual dosages, dietary habits and health policies, which foreign researchers may not be aware of. All these factors underlie local particularities that might be involved in differences in biomarker-based prediction of drug response. The 13 chapters in this book cover a wide range of topics all linked to Pharmacogenomics in Latin-America and, hopefully, will be the seed of a fruitful interaction among Latin-American research groups interested in Pharmacogenomics. I am sure that this book will be an important benchmark, as we follow the development and refinement of the predictive power of human Pharmacogenomics, and that crucial scientific information will emerge from this joint effort.

In: Pharmacogenomics in Latin America
Editor: Luis A. Quiñones

ISBN: 978-1-53611-031-9

Chapter 1

THE INCORPORATION OF CLINICAL GUIDELINES OF PHARMACOGENOMICS IN LATIN AMERICA

Luis A. Quiñones[1,*], PhD and Ismael Lares-Asseff[2,†], MD, PhD
[1]Laboratory of Chemical Carcinogenesis and Pharmacogenetics,
Department of Basic-Clinical Oncology (DOBC),
Faculty of Medicine, University of Chile, Chile
[2]National Polytechnic Institute-CIIDIR, Durango, Mexico

ABSTRACT

In Latin America the Pharmacogenetics and Pharmacogenomics areas are recently emerging fields and the main focus of the research is to evaluate ethnic differences to apply adapted guidelines to manage personalized pharmacotherapy. Large differences between countries in the awareness and in the use of pharmacogenomic testing are presumed, but are not well assessed to date. In this chapter, we present the efforts to investigate variability in drug response in the region, using molecular approaches, and we discuss the limitations to apply pharmacogenomics test in clinical centers and hospitals.

Keywords: pharmacogenomics, pharmacogenetics, guidelines, Latin America, ethnicity

INTRODUCTION

Pharmacogenomics is an emergent field and currently this discipline is addressed to personalization of the patient pharmacotherapy, being an important tool of the personalized medicine. In this respect, it´s a well known fact that patients respond differently to drug therapy and no drug is completely effective in all patients. This variability in response, largely due to genetic, epigenetic, biological, physiological, physiopatological and environmental factors affecting proteins that metabolize or transport drugs, their therapeutic targets

* Corresponding Author E-mail: lquinone@med.uchile.cl.
† ismaelares@yahoo.com.

(receptors) or both, influence its effectiveness and safety (Ma et al., 2011). The contribution of each factor varies among drugs (Evans & McLeod, 2003; Wijnen et al., 2007; Zhou et al., 2008; EMA, 2015; Quiñones et al., 2016). Table 1 summarizes the factors influencing the interindividual variation in drug response.

On the other hand, the development of non-invasive techniques of genetic engineering and the necessity to find explanations for the variations in response to the action of drugs have posed pharmacogenomics as a very important area in drug research. Important substrates for pharmacogenomic development have been several genomic projects as for example the human Genome project (HUGO, 2016), the International HapMap project (2016), 1000 Genomes project (2016), the SNP consortium (2016) and the GWAS (Genome-Wide Association studies) (2016). Together, the results of this initiatives have significantly contributed to our understanding of human genetic variation (Deenen et al., 2011; Innocenti et al., 2011; Simon & Roychowdhury, 2013). Thus, it is now known that there are 20,296 coding genes, 148,892,479 SNPs (single nucleotide polymorphisms) and 4,363,564 structural variants (insertions, deletions, duplications, translocations, complex chromosomal rearrangements, etc.) (Ensembl, 2016). Therefore, their results have been important inputs for customization of drug therapy and for the development of the first 35 pharmacogenomic clinical guidelines (CPIC, 2016).

Table 1. Factors conditioning interindividual variation in response to drugs (Adapted from Quiñones et al., 2016, Rev Med Chile, in press)

Drug
Quality Physicochemical, pharmacokinetic and pharmacodynamic properties Type of excipients used Posology Route of administration Interaction with other drugs
Patient
Genetic factors: Transporters efficacy, metabolic activity enzyme, receptor sensitivity. Epigenetic factors: CpG islands methylation, histone acetylation, expression of miRNAs and others. Physiological factors: Pregnancy-lactation age, sex, renal and hepatic function: Pathological factors: kidney disease, liver or another. Psychological factors: placebo effect
Environment
Diet: caffeine, meat, vegetables. Alcohol intake Cigarette smoke Pollutants

CpG: Citosine and Guanine rich sites. miRNA: micro RNA.

GENETIC POLYMORPHISMS

Genetic polymorphisms can modify expression and function of enzymes and proteins involved in drug metabolism, affecting absorption, distribution, biotransformation and excretion as well as the drug-target interaction. Therefore, the presence of allelic variants will define to people as poor, extensive, intermediate or rapid/ultrarapid metabolizers, giving rise to differences in efficacy and safety.

Accordingly, the current practices for the dosing of therapeutic agents should be improved through the understanding of gene variation associated with "drug life" inside the human body. Therefore, in order to be able to predict patient's predispositions to treatment complications and poor outcome it is essential to examine all candidate loci influencing response to drugs. We should also investigate metabolic pathways for activation or inactivation of drugs, the interaction between drugs, age and gender sensitivities, the impact of ethnicity and environmental factors to understand the individual and population variability in drug response. This is particularly important in Latin America, where there is a very heterogeneous profile of ethnicity and also different environmental conditions.

As we mention before, it is well known that the efficacy and safety of drug therapy show substantial inter-individual variability which is based on genetic variations affecting pharmacokinetic and/or pharmacodynamic factors (Evans, 2003). However, it is also known that there are non-genetic factors affecting drug response, for example age, sex, organ function, concomitant therapies, drug interactions, evolution of disease, nutritional factors, smoking habit, alcohol consumption, the presence of virus, among others. Therefore failure in efficacy or toxicity of drug therapy is due to the interaction of genes with environmental factors. A drug that is well tolerated and causes a strong response in some patients may be ineffective, toxic or may cause adverse drug reactions in other patients. In fact, it has been reported that 1 in 15 hospital admissions in the United Kingdom are due to adverse drug reactions (Pirmohamed et al., 2004) and that adverse drug effects in hospitalized patients are the fifth leading cause of death in the United States (Mancinelli et al., 2000). It has been reported that approximately 2 millions adverse drug reactions lead to spending of U$100 billion annually (Ross et al., 2011).

THE PHARMACOGENOMICS/PHARMACOGENETICS DEVELOPMENT IN LATIN AMERICA

From the academic point of view, there has been an increase in the number of research articles and clinical trials of pharmacogenomics/pharmacogenetics studies since 1961, just after the German pharmacologist Friedrich Vogel (1959) coined the term pharmacogenetics. As it is observed in Figure 1 from Vogel's definition, the number of publications has constantly increased, especially in the last 15 years, concomitantly the development of pharmacogenomics has evolved. Moreover an important number of Journal addressed to the pharmacogenomic field has appeared.

While the most conservative use of pharmacogenomics aims to stratify patient populations into poor, extensive, intermediate and rapid/ultrarapid metabolizer testing could be more useful in outlier patients.

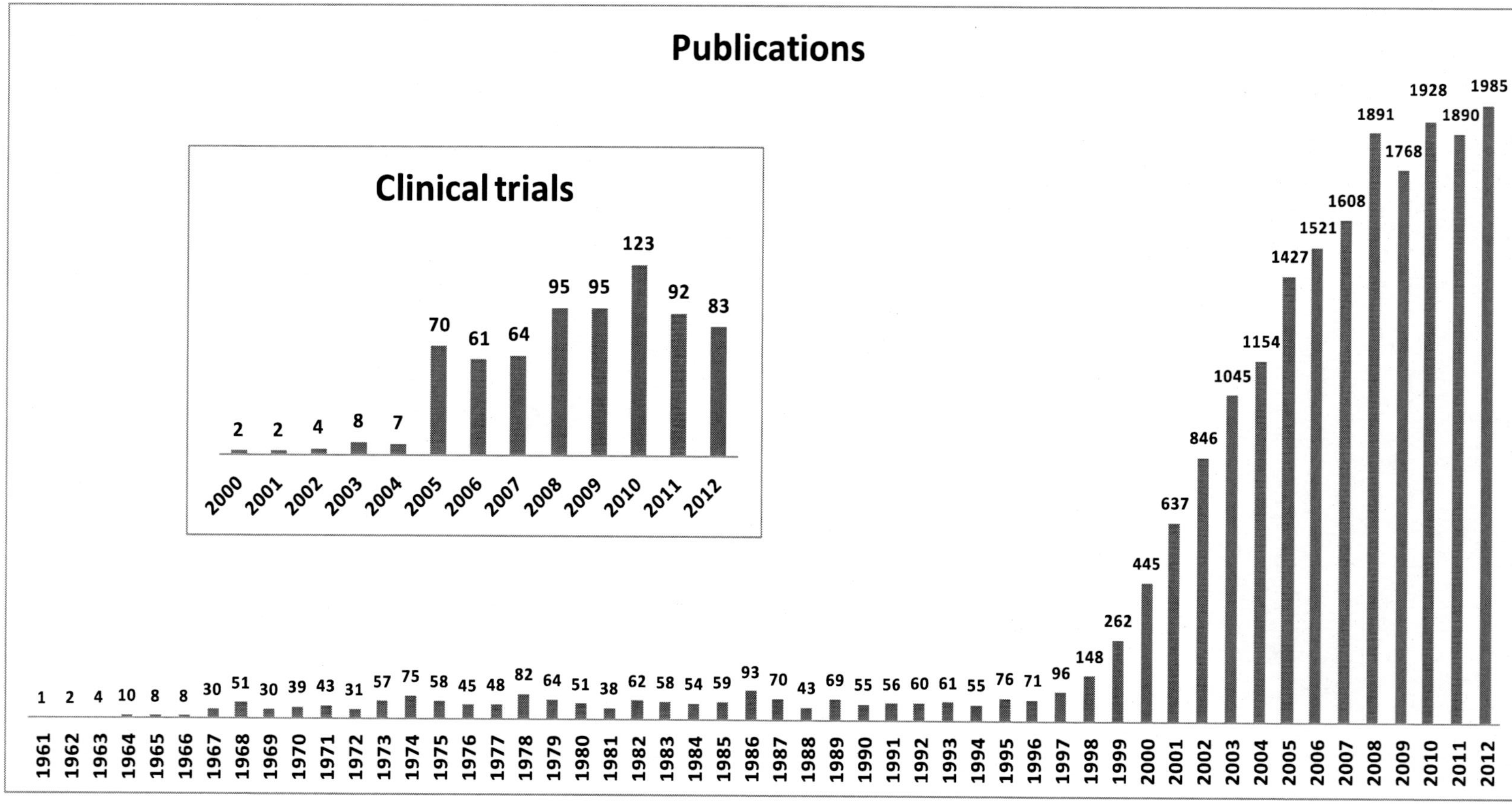

Figure 1. Variation in number of publications [Scopus] and clinical trials including pharmacogenomics/pharmacogenetics studies from 1961 (extracted from Curr Drug Metab, 15(2): 202-8).

In Latin America efforts to address pharmacogenetics/pharmacogenomics discipline starting from 1988 in Mexico and 1995 in Chile, together with the first study of genetic polymorphisms in CYP enzymes. In 1998 the frequencies of genetic variants of CYP1A1, GSTM1 and CYP2E1 were published in the Amerindian "Mapuche" population (Muñoz et al., 1998) and later, in Chilean general population, frequencies were reported comparatively in relation to other populations (Quinones et al., 1999). Lares Asseff et al. performed clinical pharmacokinetic studies in pediatric Mexican patients, showing a great interindividual variability which should be explained by pharmacogenetics and environmental factors as a modifier factor. In a study conducted by the same group (Lares-Asseff et al., 2005) included 55 Tepehuano Amerindian subjects, all were extensive metabolizers (metabolic ratio MR <0.3). Moreover, they found a monoexponential relationship between the metabolic ratio of DM and DX (Dextrometorphan/Dextrorphan), and their oncentrations respectively, which can have clinical applications, since metabolic ratio can be predicted from a known DM or DX concentration.

In parallel, a number of studies on the ethnic distribution of these genetic polymorphisms were developed by a joint effort of several Latin American researchers supported by Spanish leading researchers in this field, so in 2006, borned the Latin American Network of pharmacogenetics and Pharmacogenomics (RIBEF), which originates from a call of the Ibero-American Science and Technology CYTED, a Project with great Impact on Public Health, leaded by Dr. Adrián Llerena. This entity celebrated in 2008 its first conference in Cartagena de Indias on "Pharmacogenetics, Pharmacovigilance and Clinical Trials" with a broad representation of the Latin American Scientific Community and Professionals. This conference lead to the "Declaration of Cartagena" which set out the principles of the network. Currently, the RIBEF is a scientific society comprised of professionals whose regular work pharmacogenetics and pharmacogenomics is a main tool. The "Mission" of the RIBEF is the promotion of teaching, research and clinical care implementation of pharmacogenetics and pharmacogenomics in humans.

Recently, in 2014, begins the creation of a new Latin American network that brings together the highlights of the pharmacogenomic researchers and the study of the limitations of pharmacogenomics to be included in clinical (Quinones et al., 2014). This network is consolidated in the "I Latin American Congress of Pharmacogenomics and personalized Medicine" in Viña del Mar, Chile (May 21 to 23), which was carried out with participation of the majority of the Latin American pharmacogenomics researchers, one of the main world exponent of the discipline Dr. Magnus Ingelman-Sundberg and the Coordinator of Clinical Pharmacogenetics Implementation Consortium (CPIC), Mrs. Kelly Caudle. From that conference it was created the Latin American Society of Pharmacogenomics and Personalized Medicine (SOLFAGEM) entity that aims to strengthen the development of pharmacogenomics scientific research, both theoretical and experimental, in order to lead to progress and dissemination of creating discipline, clinical tools search and find products or biomarkers that can improve current treatments of diseases that afflict humans, as well as any other initiative aimed at maximum utilization of this scientific discipline for the benefit of the Latin American and global public health. In August of 2015 the president of SOLFAGEM (Dr. L. Quiñones) is included to CPIC as the first representative of a Latin American countries. Nowadays SOLFAGEM is looking for the adaptation of more than 30 clinical guidelines already implemented by the CPIC (2016) to the Latin American ethnic and socioeconomic reality.

Table 2. Dosing Guidelines - CPIC (Available in https://www.pharmgkb.org/view/dosing-guidelines.do?source=CPIC)

	Drug	Guidelines	Updated
1	abacavir	CPIC *CPIC Guideline for abacavir and HLA-B*	10/18/2016
2	allopurinol	CPIC *CPIC Guideline for allopurinol and HLA-B*	10/18/2016
3	amitriptyline	CPIC *CPIC Guideline for amitriptyline and CYP2C19,CYP2D6*	10/18/2016
4	atazanavir	CPIC *CPIC Guideline for atazanavir and UGT1A1*	10/18/2016
5	azathioprine	CPIC *CPIC Guideline for azathioprine and TPMT*	10/18/2016
6	capecitabine	CPIC *CPIC Guideline for capecitabine and DPYD*	10/18/2016
7	carbamazepine	CPIC *CPIC Guideline for carbamazepine and HLA-B*	10/18/2016
8	citalopram	CPIC *CPIC Guideline for citalopram,escitalopram and CYP2C19*	10/18/2016
9	clomipramine	CPIC *CPIC Guideline for clomipramine and CYP2C19,CYP2D6*	02/07/2014
10	clopidogrel	CPIC *CPIC Guideline for clopidogrel and CYP2C19*	10/18/2016
11	codeine	CPIC *CPIC Guideline for codeine and CYP2D6*	10/18/2016
12	desipramine	CPIC *CPIC Guideline for desipramine and CYP2D6*	09/15/2016
13	doxepin	CPIC *CPIC Guideline for doxepin and CYP2C19,CYP2D6*	09/15/2016
14	escitalopram	CPIC *CPIC Guideline for citalopram,escitalopram and CYP2C19*	10/18/2016
15	fluorouracil	CPIC *CPIC Guideline for fluorouracil and DPYD*	10/18/2016
16	fluvoxamine	CPIC *CPIC Guideline for fluvoxamine and CYP2D6*	10/18/2016
17	imipramine	CPIC *CPIC Guideline for imipramine and CYP2C19,CYP2D6*	09/15/2016
18	ivacaftor	CPIC *CPIC Guideline for ivacaftor and CFTR*	10/18/2016
19	mercaptopurine	CPIC *CPIC Guideline for mercaptopurine and TPMT*	10/18/2016
20	nortriptyline	CPIC *CPIC Guideline for nortriptyline and CYP2D6*	10/18/2016
21	paroxetine	CPIC *CPIC Guideline for paroxetine and CYP2D6*	10/18/2016
22	Peginterferon alfa-2a	CPIC *CPIC Guideline for peginterferon alfa-2a,peginterferon alfa-2b,ribavirin and IFNL3*	10/18/2016
23	peginterferon alfa-2b	CPIC *CPIC Guideline for peginterferon alfa-2a,peginterferon alfa-2b,ribavirin and IFNL3*	10/18/2016
24	phenytoin	CPIC *CPIC Guideline for phenytoin and CYP2C9,HLA-B*	10/18/2016
25	rasburicase	CPIC *CPIC Guideline for rasburicase and G6PD*	10/18/2016
26	ribavirin	CPIC *CPIC Guideline for peginterferon alfa-2a,peginterferon alfa-2b,ribavirin and IFNL3*	10/18/2016
27	sertraline	CPIC *CPIC Guideline for sertraline and CYP2C19*	10/18/2016
28	simvastatin	CPIC *CPIC Guideline for simvastatin and SLCO1B1*	10/18/2016
29	tacrolimus	CPIC *CPIC Guideline for tacrolimus and CYP3A5*	10/18/2016
30	tegafur	CPIC *CPIC Guideline for tegafur and DPYD*	10/18/2016
31	thioguanine	CPIC *CPIC Guideline for thioguanine and TPMT*	10/18/2016
32	trimipramine	CPIC *CPIC Guideline for trimipramine and CYP2C19,CYP2D6*	09/15/2016
33	warfarin	CPIC *CPIC Guideline for warfarin and CYP2C9,VKORC1*	06/19/2014

In the work of the Quiñones et al. (2014) there was reported the perceived importance of barriers for implementing the use of pharmacogenomics testing in clinical practice for Latin American countries, showing three major closely related groups of barriers: a) the necessity of clear guidelines for the use of pharmacogenomics in clinical practice, b) the insufficient awareness about pharmacogenomics among clinicians and c) the absence of a regulatory institution that facilitates the use of pharmacogenetic tests. Moreover, in this work it was included a survey for the analysis of the perceived relevance of the usefulness for 51 gene/drug pairs. As a result the Latin American health professionals considered relevant the TPMT/thioguanine, TPMT/azathioprine, CYP2C9/warfarin, UGT1A1/irinotecan, CYP2D6/ amitriptiline, CYP2C19/citalopram and CYP2D6/clozapine pairs, however none pair received a higher than 50% of importance. The higher ranks for psychiatric drugs give rise to the idea that in the Latin American countries the variability in the response to these drugs (e.g., antidepressants) is fairly important. These results were considered as preliminary because the pharmacogenomic is poor developed in the region and due to that the importance of the gene/drug pairings in different countries could be evaluated differently because of the absence of some drugs in each market according to drug acquisition policies of each Ministry of Health.

Conclusion

In Latin America the Pharmacogenetics and Pharmacogenomics areas are recently emerging fields. The main focus of the research in these disciplines is to evaluate ethnic differences to adapt proposed CPIC guidelines to manage personalized pharmacotherapy in mestizo and amerindians populations. Large differences between countries in the awareness and in the use of pharmacogenomic testing are presumed, but are not well assessed to date.

References

1000 genomes, IGSR: The International Genome Sample Resource. Available in http://www.internationalgenome.org (accessed on October 24, 2016).

CPIC, Clinical Pharmacogenetics Implementation Consortium. PharmGkb [Internet]. Available in: https://www.pharmgkb.org/page/cpic.

Deenen MJ, Cats A, Beijnen JH, Schellens JHM. Part 1: background, methodology, and clinical adoption of pharmacogenetics. *Oncologist.* 2011;16(6):811–9.

EMA, Guideline on key aspects for the use of pharmacogenomics in the pharmacovigilance of medicinal products, *European Medicines Agency.* WC500196800. p15. (2015).

Ensembl [Internet]. EMBL-EBI. [c2016; citado 20 de Mayo de 2016]. Available in: http://www.ensembl.org/Homo_sapiens/Location/Genome.

Evans WE, McLeod HL. Pharmacogenomics, drug disposition, drug targets, and side effects. *N Engl J Med.* 2003 Feb 6;348(6):538–49.

Evans WE. Pharmacogenomics: marshalling the human genome to individualise drug therapy. *Gut* 2003, 52 Suppl 2, 10-8.

Green ED, Guyer MS. Charting a course for genomic medicine from base pairs to bedside. *Nature* 2011, 10, 470 (7333):204-213.

GWAS Catalog [Internet]. EMBL-EBI. Available in: http://www.ebi.ac.uk/gwas/>.

HUGO. The Human Genome project [Internet]. *National Human Genome Research Institute.* Available in: http://www.genome.gov/10001772.

Innocenti F, Cox NJ, Dolan ME. The use of genomic information to optimize cancer chemotherapy. *Semin Oncol.* 2011 Apr;38(2):186–95.

International HapMap Project [Internet]. [citado 20 de Mayo de 2016]. Available in: http://hapmap.ncbi.nlm.nih.gov/index.html.

Lares-Asseff I., Sosa-Macías M., Elizondo-Azuela G., Flores-Pérez C., Flores-Pérez J. and Bradley-Alvarez F.. Phenotypical Expression of CYP2D6 in Amerindians of Tepehuano Origin from Durango, Mexico. *Proc West Pharmacol Soc* 2005 Feb; 48: 102-107.

Ma Q, Lu AYH. Pharmacogenetics, pharmacogenomics, and individualized medicine. *Pharmacol Rev.* 2011 Jun;63(2):437–59.

Mancinelli L, Cronin M, Sadee W. Pharmacogenomics: the promise of personalized medicine. *AAPS Pharm. Sci.* 2000, 2: E4.

Muñoz S, Vollrath V, Vallejos MP, Miquel JF, Covarrubias C, Raddatz A, Chianale J. Genetic polymorphisms of CYP2D6, CYP1A1 and CYP2E1 in the South-Amerindian population of Chile. *Pharmacogenetics.* 1998 Aug; 8(4): 343-51.

Pirmohamed M, James S, Meakin S, Green C, Scott AK, Walley TJ, Farrar K, Park BK, Breckenridge AM. Adverse drug reactions as cause of admission to hospital: prospective analysis of 18 820 patients. *BMJ* 2004, 329(7456), 15-9.

Quiñones L, Berthou F, Varela N, Simon B, Gil L, Lucas D. Ethnic susceptibility to lung cancer: differences in CYP2E1, CYP1A1 and GSTM1 genetic polymorphisms between French Caucasian and Chilean populations. *Cancer Lett.* 1999 Jul 1;141(1-2):167-71.

Quinones LA, Lavanderos MA, Cayun JP, Garcia-Martin E, Agundez JA, Caceres DD, Roco AM, Morales JE, Herrera L, Encina G, Isaza CA, Redal MA, Larovere L, Soria NW, Eslava-Schmalbach J, Castaneda-Hernandez G, Lopez-Cortes A, Magno LA, Lopez M, Chiurillo MA, Rodeiro I, Castro de Guerra D, Teran E, Estevez-Carrizo F, Lares-Assef I. Perception of the usefulness of drug/gene pairs and barriers for pharmacogenomics in Latin America. *Curr Drug Metab.* 2014 Feb;15(2):202-8.

Quiñones LA., Roco AM., Cayún JP., Escalante P., Miranda C., Varela N., Meneses F., Gallegos B., Zaruma-Torres F., Lares-Asseff I. Pharmacogenomics, personalized Medicine and the clinical practice. *Rev Med Chile,* 2016 (in press).

Ross CJ, Visscher H, Rassekh SR, Castro-Pastrana LI, Shereck E, Carleton B, Hayden MR. “Pharmacogenomics of serious adverse drug reactions in pediatric oncology”, *J. Popul. Ther. Clin. Pharmacol.* 2011, 18: 134-151.

Simon R, Roychowdhury S. Implementing personalized cancer genomics in clinical trials. *Nat Rev Drug Discov.* 2013 May;12(5):358–69.

SNP Consortium. Thorisson GA, Stein LD. The SNP Consortium website: past, present and future. *Nucleic Acids Res.* 2003 Jan 1;31(1):124–7.

Swen JJ, Nijenhuis M, de Boer A, Grandia L, Maitland-van der Zee AH, Mulder H, Rongen GA, van Schaik RH, Schalekamp T, Touw DJ, van der Weide J, Wilffert B, Deneer VH, Guchelaar HJ. Pharmacogenetics: from bench to byte--an update of guidelines. *Clin. Pharmacol. Ther.* 2011, 89(5), 662-73.

Vogel F. Moderne Problem der humangenetik. *Ergebn. Inn. Med. Kinderheilkd* 1959, 12, 52 – 125.

Wijnen PAHM, Op den Buijsch RAM, Drent M, Kuijpers PMJC, Kuipers PMJC, Neef C, et al. Review article: The prevalence and clinical relevance of cytochrome P450 polymorphisms. *Aliment Pharmacol Ther.* 2007 Dec;26 Suppl 2:211–9.

Zhou S-F, Di YM, Chan E, Du Y-M, Chow VD-W, Xue CC, et al. Clinical pharmacogenetics and potential application in personalized medicine. *Curr Drug Metab* 2008 Oct;9(8): 738–84.

In: Pharmacogenomics in Latin America
Editor: Luis A. Quiñones
ISBN: 978-1-53611-031-9

Chapter 2

GENETIC VARIABILITY AND RESPONSE TO DRUGS IN LATIN AMERICAN POPULATIONS: ETHNICITY AND ANCESTRY

Idania Rodeiro Guerra*[1,*], *PhD and
José Alfredo Herrera Isidrón*[2,†], *PhD
[2]Pharmacology Department, Center of Marine Bioproducts, CEBIMAR, Environmental Agency, Havana, Cuba
[2]Havana University, Havana, Cuba

ABSTRACT

Differences among patients in the therapeutic response to many drugs can be explained in part from the knowledge of individual genetic variations associated to the disease. Genetic factors are important in the clinical manifestation of these variations, but other non-genetic factors may also influence although. Therefore, to find out why some patient does not respond to the drug treatment as it is expected involves a complex problem, which is not limited to individual genetics. Patient age, sex, physiological and pathological state and toxic habits plus drug interactions, among others are non-genetic factors which influence in response variability. Thus, one of the great challenges pharmacology and therapeutics currently deal with is how to explain inter-individual variability in response to drugs, in the attempt to maximize drug efficacy and to reduce adverse effects.

In this sense, Latin American countries exhibit high genetic heterogeneity, the diversity of their populations is complex. More than 500 million people live in Latin American and the Caribbean. Meanwhile, many differences exist between these peoples, where are present the human development index, the historical conditions of their origins, ethnicity, and culture among others. As people resulted from a history of miscegenation and population mix, the development of genetic studies in the region face complex and serious challenges. However, this heterogeneity of their populations provides a powerful resource for analyzing the genetic basis of complex diseases in the region. Thus, the

* Corresponding Author E-mail: autoridania.rodeiro@infomed.sld.cu.
† jose@imre.uh.cu.

development of personalized medicine in the region requires the identification of pharmacogenomic biomarkers in these populations.

Keywords: pharmacogenetics, pharmacogenomics, Latin America, ethnicity, ancestry

Introduction

A new era is opening in the response to drugs, role of pharmacogenetics and pharmacogenomics.

Despite of the advances in the biomedical sciences, one of main problems pharmacology and therapeutics still face is the great variability among individuals in the response to drugs. In the twentieth century, Sir William Osler revolutionized the diagnosis and treatment of diseases when he stated "if variability among individuals was not so grate, medicine would be a science and not an art". Today, the development achieved by molecular biology, opens new opportunities for integrating information derived from study of the human genome. The application of this information into clinical pharmacology has been recognized as a step in the way for establishing personalized therapies and a positive impact is expected over drug response to diseases (HUGO, 1992; Jorgensen, 2011).

Differences among patients in the therapeutic response to certain drugs in clinically uniform diseases can be explained in part from the knowledge of individual genetic variations associated to the disease (Cabaleiro et al., 2011). Genetic factors are important in the clinical manifestation of these variations, but other non-genetic factors may also influence although. Therefore, to find out why some patient does not respond to the drug treatment as it is expected involves a complex problem, which is not limited to individual genetics. Patient age, sex, physiological and pathological state and toxic habits plus drug interactions, among others are non-genetic factors which influence in response variability (Cabaleiro et al., 2011, Ingelman-Sundberg & Sim, 2010) (Figure 1). Thus, one of the great challenges pharmacology and therapeutics currently deal with is how to explain inter-individual variability in response to drugs, in the attempt to maximize drug efficacy and to reduce adverse effects (HUGO, 1992; Ingelman-Sundberg & Sim, 2010). The development in recent decades of the omics and the deep knowledge of the human genome has contributed to develop two new disciplines within the pharmacology. These are pharmacogenetics and pharmacogenomics, which are able to address and to explain the sources of variability (Del Llano et al., 2004).

Pharmacogenomics is concerning to the study of the genome and of the entirety of expressed and non-expressed genes. These two fields of study are concerned with a comprehensive, genome-wide assessment of the effects of certain interventions, mainly drugs or toxicants. Pharmacogenomics is related with the systematic assessment of how chemical compounds modify the overall expression pattern in a tissue. Pharmacogenomics does not focus on differences from one person to the next with regard to the drug's effects, but rather focuses on differences among several drugs or compounds with regard to a "generic" set of expressed or non-expressed genes.

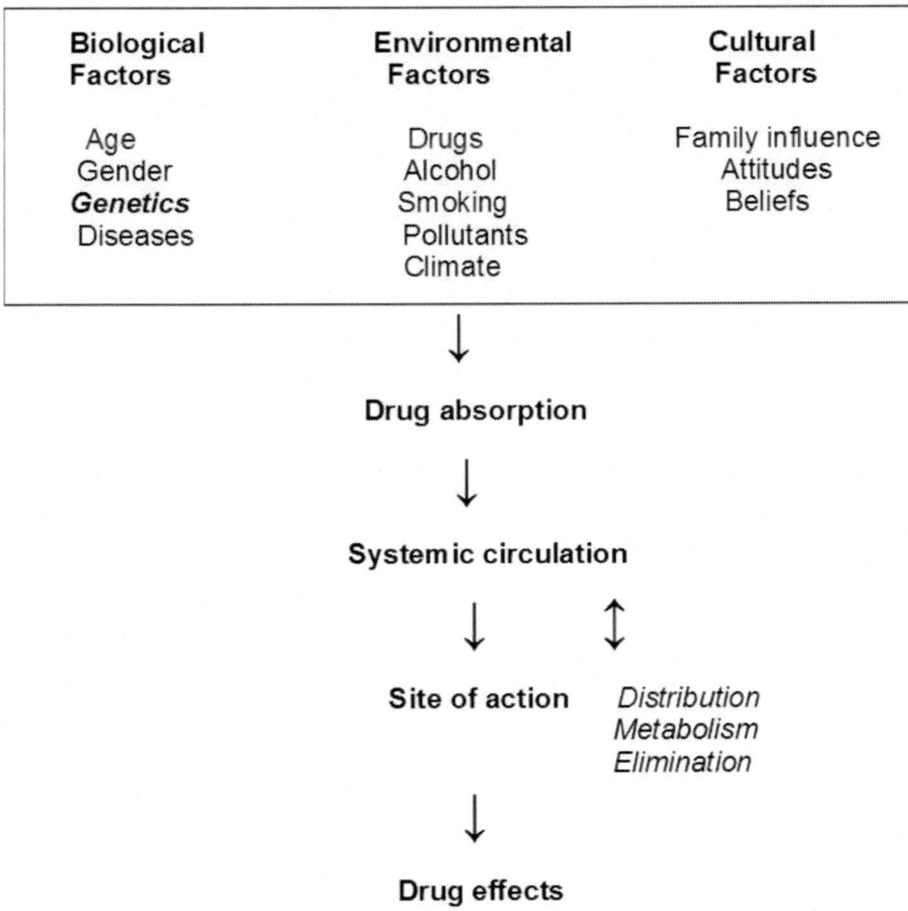

Figure 1. Factors contributing to variability in drug response. Adapted from Poolsup et al. (2000).

In contrast, the term "-genetics" relates etymologically to the presence of individual properties as a consequence of having inherited them. Thus, pharmacogenetic describes the interaction between the drug and the individual characteristics. Pharmacogenetics, therefore, is based on observations of clinical efficacy and/or the safety and tolerability profile of a drug in individuals – the phenotype – and tests the hypothesis that inter-individual differences in the observed response may be associated with the presence or absence of individual-specific biological markers that may allow prediction of individual drug response. Although, both branches refer to the evaluation of drug effects using nucleic acid technology, the directionalities of their approaches are distinctly different: pharmacogenetics represents the study of differences among a number of individuals with regard to clinical response to a particular drug, whereas pharmacogenomics represents the study of differences among a number of compounds with regard to gene expression response in a single genome (Del Llano et al., 2004; Shastry, 2013). Pharmacogenetic scope expands to all processes involved in medicines pharmacokinetics (absorption, distribution, metabolism and excretion) and also pharmacodynamics (receptors, transporters, enzymes, ion channels). Its main goal relates to the individualization or personalization of treatments because it studies individual variability in the expression of genes related to drug response (Del Llano et al., 2004).

Genetic Polymorphisms

Genetic polymorphisms have been identified in more than 30 human metabolizing enzymes. Allelic distribution varies widely among different ethnic groups. For instance, differences in base sequence have been reported for multiple genes encoding enzymes related to intermediary metabolism of drugs, like some isoforms of the P450 system and conjugating enzymes. Polymorphisms associated to genetic variability in the response of other systems like drug transporters and drug receptors have also been described (Zanger et al., 2013; Llerena & Peñas-Lledó, 2015; Ingelman-Sundberg, 2005; Daly, 2003). But, polymorphic variants in the genes coding for these enzymes and proteins introduces also the possibility of affecting the biotransformation and elimination of endogenous compounds, which in turn has been associated to the prognosis and development of high morbidity/mortality diseases (Zanger, 2013). However, single genes are not usually responsible for the risk of a disease. The genetic risk in an individual is usually depends on the combination of several polymorphisms in the code of involved proteins (Millan & Arenas, 2004).

Xenobiotic biotransformation increases solubility of compounds in aqueous medium thereby facilitating excretion from the body through urine or bile. When a drug enters the body, several biotransformation processes occurs. Among them, drug absorption and distribution until it reaches the pharmacological action site, afterward drug interaction with targets (receptors and enzymes), drug metabolism and finally disposal (ADME) (Gonzalez et al., 1993). Drug metabolism occurs primarily in liver but it is also carried out in other tissues, such as lung, skin, intestine and kidneys. Metabolizing enzymes are expressed in almost all human tissues. Except for a few drugs which suffer no transformation and are excreted unchanged, most of them do are metabolized and every ADME processes may involve genetic variations (Gonzalez et al., 1993; Guengerich et al., 1982).

There are plenty of different reactions involved in the biotransformation of drugs. It is accepted that they mainly involve two phases: Phase I and II. Phase I reactions included chemical processes of different nature: oxidation, oxygenation, reduction, hydrolysis, alquilations and halogenations. As a result, molecules suffer chemical modifications and new functional groups are added to them. These modifications generally increase polarity of the molecules, which facilitates their excretion (Guengerich et al., 2003). Metabolites generated as a result of Phase I reactions often are covalently bound to cell endogenous molecules. These reactions are called Phase II and they produce molecules conjugated to glucuronic acid, glutathione, sulfate and different amino acids. The combined effect of both processes facilitates renal or biliar elimination of metabolites, frequently called Phase III metabolism (Guengerich et al., 2003). Not all xenobiotics biotransformation combines phase I plus phase II reactions. Sometimes only phase I or II reactions are necessary to achieve polarity enough for allowing transport and disposal of the xenobiotic. From a cellular perspective, it is more common than drugs just suffer conjugation reactions because conjugation facilitates removal.

Phase I reactions are catalyzed by a group of enzymes found in the endoplasmic reticulum of cells, specially the P450 enzyme system (Guengerich et al., 1982). Cytochrome P450 system is a super family of enzymes responsible for drug metabolism of endogenous compounds and xenobiotics, including medicines. This family has been extensively studied and is considered responsible for metabolizing more drugs than any other family of enzymes

(Donato, 2004). CYP2D6, 3A4, 2C9, 2C19, 1A1 and 2E1 isoforms are the most important ones regarding drug metabolism (Table 1). Several P450 isoforms expressed polymorphisms among individuals within a population. CYP2D6 was the first P450 enzyme identified as polymorphic and it is the most polymorphic gene within P450 family. This characteristic gives 2D6 high phenotypic variability and makes it possibly the most popular one in the therapeutic (Kirchheiner & Seeringer, 2007). More than 100 allelic variants of this gene been identified and characterized so far, which affect its enzymatic activity.

Table 1. Polymorphic P450 isoforms found in the human liver involved in the biotransformation of several drugs

CYP450	Liver (%) *	Inter-individual Variability **	Drugs metabolized by the enzyme (%) ***
1A2	10	30	3 (1A1/2)
2A6	5	100	3
2B6	3-5	50	3
2C8	<1	30	12 (2C8/9)
2C9	15	30	
2C19	4	30	8
2D6	2-5	200	19-25
2E1	7-10	50	1
3A4	30-40	80	> 50
3A5	10-30	>10	1

*Relative percentage of each enzyme respect to total P450 system.
**Variability of each enzyme in the liver between individuals.
***Estimation of the participation of each enzyme in drug metabolism in humans.

Genetic polymorphisms in the genes coding for the expression of conjugating enzymes like glutathione-S transferase, N-acetyltransferase, UDP-glucuronyl transferase and thiopurine S-transferase have also been described (Olivera & Vega, 2010; Honmaa et al., 2008). Genes encoding for proteins of the drug transport systems are not exempt of polymorphism, either (Leschziner et al., 2007, Teh et al., 2007). Among these, the ones coding for the expression of ABC transporters family stand out. These transporters are energy dependent proteins responsible for extruding numerous drugs out of cells. P-glycoprotein, encoded by the ABCB1 gene and influx transporters is responsible for the uptake of organic and inorganic cations such as OATP and SLCO.

ETHNIC DIFFERENCES

Important differences between different ethnic groups within populations across the world have been established in terms of the prevalence of polymorphisms of genes involved in drug metabolism. In addition to the clinical relevance these polymorphisms may have over individual therapeutic response to drugs, it must be taking into account the effects at population level and the impact on health policies (Llerena, 2015). The study of the clinical implications of genetic polymorphisms has been favored with today international achievements in pharmacogenetics. This discipline undoubtedly offers new opportunities to prescribe, identify and make recommendations on the safest and most effective drugs and doses based on the knowledge of patient genotype. Adverse drug reactions are a major cause of morbidity and mortality, they affect between 10% and 20% hospitalized patients and more than 7% from the general population (Sim et al., 2012). Consequently, by knowing about individual and population response capabilities should substantially reduce the need for hospitalization and the associated costs. So, it is important to develop pharmacogenetic studies as part of the national pharmacovigilance programs in order to reduce adverse reactions and therapeutic failures. Health services and regulatory agencies in different countries should take interest in understanding the behavior of population pharmacogenetics to improve the cost-benefit balance (Rodriguez et al., 2010).

Risk factors have been identified among different ethnic groups within some populations for a significant number of drugs; the strategy is to identifying groups with vulnerability to adverse reactions or therapeutic failures. Accordingly, it has been possible to develop treatments focused to groups of individuals who share common genetic characteristics, which is known as stratified medicine. The capability to deliver individual treatment has not been reached yet, but stratified medicine is an approach on the way to personalized medicine (Jorgensen, 2011).

In this context, regulatory agencies such as the Food and Drug Administration (FDA) and the European Medical Agency (EMA) point out the need to incorporate pharmacogenetic analysis as biomarkers of the therapeutic response and safety in clinical trials. Said approach will produce future increases in the efficacy and the safety use of drugs (Llerena, 2013, Maliepaard et al., 2013). At present, different analysis have been recommended as genomic markers, they need to be labeled according to the drug used and consequently customize their use according to the individual genetic polymorphisms identified in the patient.

The implementation of these strategies takes on a different dimension in countries with histories linked to intense processes of miscegenation. As a consequence of the large multi-ethnicity and genetic heterogeneity, it is advisable to determine how frequently each genetic variant is represented within the population. In this way, countries which mixed population would establish their own population patterns and treatment guidelines. The use of pharmacogenetic biomarkers in clinical practice should take ethnic, cultural and socio-economic variations into consideration. Genetic heterogeneity and inter-ethnic frequency variability of biomarkers revealed by population studies should be taken into consideration among nations (Llerena, 2013; Martin & Eichelbaum, 2002; Burroughs et al., 2002), but also between different regions of the same country (HapMap, 2005). This is the case of Latin American peoples, where mixing processes have occurred differently across the continent. However, drug regulatory agencies from Latin America countries have not yet assimilated this information.

The development of genomic population-level maps is allowing the integration of genetic markers which are informative of ancestry (Seldin, 2007). These maps are being used in population studies conducted to identify variations in the risk of suffering common diseases. Ancestry markers allow taking into account differences in the ancestral components of the samples under study. This is important because it generates more accurate results when studying populations with great miscegenation, like the Latin America one.

LATIN AMERICAN POPULATIONS, CHALLENGES AND PECULIARITIES

Latin American countries exhibit high genetic heterogeneity, the diversity of their populations is complex. More than 500 million people live in Latin American and the Caribbean. Meanwhile, many differences exist between these peoples, where are present the human development index, the historical conditions of their origins, ethnicity, and culture among others (HapMap, 2005). As people resulted from a history of miscegenation and population mix, the development of genetic studies in the region face complex and serious challenges (Gonzalez-Burchard et al., 2005). However, this heterogeneity of their populations provides a powerful resource for analyzing the genetic basis of complex diseases in the region (Wang et al., 2008). Thus, the development of personalized medicine in the region requires the identification of pharmacogenomic biomarkers in these populations.

The mixing process favored the formation of a population with new genetic patterns derived from the crossing of genetically divergent parental populations and followed by the free mix among their descendants. During this process, individuals from the hybrid population develop the "linkage disequilibrium by mixing", which is the appearance of large haplotype blocks and not random associations like single nucleotide polymorphisms (SNPs) (Gonzalez-Burchard et al., 2005; Wang et al., 2008).

Different genetic and anthropological studies address miscegenation in Latin American countries. These studies show that almost the whole population of the continent is di-hybrid or tri-hybrid and it shows great heterogeneity between populations (Sans, 2000) as a result of the conquest and colonization process. The presence of sub-structures has been reported in this population. Said approach has suggested the identification and quantification of the ethnic mixture by associative mapping studies. However, despite the recognition of this problem, there is currently not enough genetic information about Latin American countries to determine the possible differentiation between population subgroups in each particular region (Price et al., 2007).

Mestizos are recognized as a newly formed population group as a result of the mixture the American continent has suffered over the past centuries. The ancient origins of this miscegenation product come from Amerindian, European and African people (Wang et al., 2008; Sans et al., 2000). Some studies have associated the appearance of miscegenation patterns in this population with the predisposition and susceptibility to certain diseases, with the ability to respond to drug therapy and with the occurrence of adverse effects related to drug therapy. By taking into consideration these findings, investigations have been developed and coordinated in different countries of the region with the aim of characterizing the pharmacogenetic and pharmacogenomic patterns of Latin American (De Andrés et al., 2013; Sosa-Macías & Llerena, 2013; Llerena et al., 2013; Llerena et al., 2014; Isaza et al., 2007; Cerda et al., 2014; Chiurillo, 2015; Céspedes-Garro, 2015; Bravo-Villalta et al., 2005; Quiñones et al., 2001). It should be highlighted the role played by the Ibero-Latin American Network of Pharmacogenetics and Pharmacogenomics (RIBEF, http://www.ribef.com) and the recent creation of the Latin American Society for pharmacogenetics and Personalized Medicine. Both initiatives have been made available pharmacogenetic data on populations from Latin America and the Caribbean.

On the other hand, the identification of genes associated with complex diseases has been successfully addressed by associative studies of the whole genome and miscegenation mapping studies. The former method is based on the efficient capture of (SNPs) (WTCCC, 2007; McCarthy et al., 2008) and the later one relay on the availability of markers panels distributed throughout the genome, markers with different frequencies among ancestral populations (Smith & O'Brien, 2005; Seldin, 2007). However, populations without full representation in the Haplotype Map of the Human genome (HapMap) (2005), i.e., Latin American population, have drawbacks to evaluate the genetic diversity through capture strategies. In these populations it is necessary to use more pharmacogenetic markers than in Asian or European populations in order to achieve similar statistical power (De Bakker, 2006). The lack of information about specific patterns of linkage disequilibrium found in this population also influence in the analysis (Huang et al., 2009). The high proportion of mestizo individuals should be taken into consideration when the analysis is performed in populations having individuals with significant differences in the ancestral constitutions. Available information about the genomic diversity of population in the region is still insufficient (Jakobsson et al., 2008). Meanwhile, some studies in the population of Latin American countries have demonstrated the existence of different patterns of ancestral contribution among groups and within groups of people.

The mapping according to imbalances of linking mixture is a genetic epidemiology tool suitable to be applied in populations recently mixed as the America one does. This technique has been useful in the identification and study of susceptibility genes associated with diseases where ethnicity may introduce variability in the pharmacological response. The development of these tools is favored as long as availability of databases describing gene variants for each ethnic group increases. Other favorable influences are the development of new methods for large-scale genotyping and the design of statistical algorithms and bioinformatics programs for managing databases. The application of this strategy in a whole population may be useful for identifying genetic risk factors associated with complex diseases.

The vast surface of the American continent, with numerous natural barriers has led throughout history that geographically distant regions show different population dynamics. This fact has been related not only to the great ancestral diversity of the continent but also with the specific demographic conditions presented in each particular region. Several Latin American civilizations used to have a rich history long before the pre-Columbian era, history in continuous development after the conquest. The current population of these countries is the result of a complex process of miscegenation derived from the particular development of each civilization throughout history and the contribution of different ethnic origins to their formation process. However, policies and public health programs in most of these countries do not take into account the genetic diversity when health standards are set. It should be noted that some countries within the region have recently initiated projects aimed to characterize the genetic composition of the population by using ancestry informative markers. The outcomes from these projects should contribute to the future development of pharmacogenomic studies and to the introduction of genetic diversity in the orientation of new public health policies for these populations.

Advances in the field of molecular biology and the study of the Human Genome Project, facilitate the search for disease-susceptibility genes. The cases and controls method employs population and family approaches, Latin America and the Caribbean can not remain oblivious to this reality. This method is one of the most used in association studies because it facilitates the recruitment of volunteers (Hincapié et al., 2009). The following facilities can be mentioned: the analysis of the determinants of human mutations, the assessment of the role played by non-specific genetic markers in the etiology of the disease and that it takes into account the value of the etiological role of genetic traits. Associative mapping studies have been useful for linking some diseases to DNA markers located near a gene of interest or a candidate gene.

Genetic associations between unlinked markers frequently appear in populations who have suffered a recent mix. This phenomenon is often associated with the sub-structured populations and with groups sharing inheritance relationships. Associations are also favored by the presence of consanguinity and demographic, cultural, religious and geographical factors. Said factors could be mistakenly associated with a disease and should be considered potential factors responsible for the detection of "false associations". Associations occur as the result of the mixing, stratification or subdivision process (Hincapié et al., 2009), therefore it reveals information about the underlying genetic structure of a population.

The ability of the researchers responsible for the studies is a factor of interest when the subjects of a population are chosen, selected subject should be the most suitable for inclusion in molecular epidemiological studies. It is necessary to know about the origins of the population under study because it allows establishing selection criteria which led to robust and objective interpretation of the results to be achieved. For example, the verification of alleles associations with a disease must be taken into account when cases and controls from mixed populations are investigated. The difficulty for assigning individuals to groups based on one or more markers justifies verification. Accordingly, association studies are widely used to investigate heterogeneous populations, thus reducing the negative impact of confounding variables (Jakobsson et al., 2008).

Subsequent research in these populations should introduce the study of other markers, for example SNPs analysis. This would allow more precise allocations despite diversity and the inheritable genetic conditions involved in susceptibility and disease development. In addition, it would let to asses how much impact produce the population components from a particular geographic region. Therefore, the design of panel with specific molecular markers for each population would be justified. Panels should make possible to verify ancestry, to confirm analyzes of the genetic structure in mixed populations and to validate conclusions derived from case-control studies.

Conclusion

The new lines of research should take into account the genetic origin and its relation to the protection or predisposition to certain diseases. In genetic studies where groups of cases and controls are compared it will be necessary to make adjustments according to the population stratification and variations of the genetic mixture should be considered during the experimental design of the study. This approach goes toward the development of personalized or precision medicine and it should be also valid to study different regions within the same country, especially in populations where the behavior of the proportions of the mixture are different, as is in many Latin American countries.

The great heterogeneity in the distribution of ethnic components at the genetic level found in Latin American peoples leads to use specific statistical methods in processing data from the studies conducted in the region. Otherwise erroneous conclusions would be achieved in the diagnosis of patients and in predicting population health.

In summary, as it was mentioned, genes are not fully responsible for the susceptibility or progression of a disease. Genes are in constant interaction with the environment where human live and social health determinants are also important. Demographic variables like educational level and other risk factors should be included when the development, prognosis and treatment of diseases is analyzed. All these factors in association to ancestral origins should be studied starting from individual genetic information. Coming years should gradually incorporate the results of the genome projects to routine medical practice and research results will include data obtained from studies in the Latin American peoples. Public policies of Latin American countries must assimilate this information, which undoubtedly will contribute to the application of genomic information in the regional medical practice.

REFERENCES

Bravo-Villalta H, Yamamoto K, Nakamura K, Baya A, Okada Y, Horiuchi R. (2005). Genetic polymorphism of CYP2C9 and CYP2C19 in a Bolivian population: an investigative and comparative study. *Eur J Clin Pharmacol.;* 61: 179–184.

Burroughs V., Maxey R., Levy R. Racial and ethnic differences in response to medicines: towards individualized pharmaceutical treatment. *J Natl Med Assoc.* 2002, 94:1–26.

Cabaleiro T, Abad Santos F. Farmacogenética: presente y futuro. *Farmacoterapia.* 2011; 9: 13-19.

Cerda A, Hirata MH, Hirata RD. Pharmacogenetics of drug metabolizing enzymes in Brazilian populations. *Drug Metabol Drug Interact* 2014, 29:153–77.

Céspedes-Garro C, Naranjo M-E, Ramírez R, Serrano V, Farinas H, Barrantes R. Pharmacogenetics in Central American healthy volunteers: interethnic variability. *Drug Metabol Pers Ther* 2015, 30:19–31.

Chiurillo MA. Genomic biomarkers related to drug response in Venezuelan populations. *Drug Metab Pers Ther* 2015, 30:33–41.

Daly AK. Pharmacogenetics of the major polymorphic metabolizing enzymes. *Fundam Clin Pharmacol.;* 17(1):27-41, 2003.

De Andrés F, Sosa-Macías M, Lazalde-Ramos BP, Naranjo ME, Tarazona-Santos E, Llerena A. (Evaluation of drug-metabolizing enzyme hydroxylation phenotypes in Hispanic populations: the CEIBA cocktail. *Drug Metabol Drug Interact* 2013, 28: 135–46.

de Bakker PI, Burtt NP, Graham RR, Guiducci C, Yelensky R, Drake JA, Bersaglieri T, Penney KL, Butler J, Young S, Onofrio RC, Lyon HN, Stram DO, Haiman CA, Freedman ML, Zhu X, Cooper R, Groop L, Kolonel LN, Henderson BE, Daly MJ, Hirschhorn JN, Altshuler D. *Nat Genet.* 2006 Nov, 38(11):1298-303.

Del Llano J, Jorcano JL, Nuñez JM et al. (2004). In: *Genomic and Medicin.* Nov. 2004 ISBM 84-609-3002-5. Spain Info SA. Copyright. Spain Fundation for Development of Genomic and Proteomic Research.

Donato MT. Que es el citocromo P-450 y cómo funciona? En: Citocromo P-450. (Editoras Angosto MC. Y Gomez-Lechón MJ.) Instituto de España, Real Academia Nacional de Farmacia; 23-68, 2004.

Gonzalez-Burchard E, Borrell LN, Choudhry S, Naqvi M, Tsai HJ, Rodriguez-Santana JR, Chapela R, Rogers SD, Mei R, Rodriguez-Cintron W, Arena JF, Kittles R, Perez-Stable EJ, Ziv E, Risch N. Latino populations: a unique opportunity for the study of race, genetics, and social environment in epidemiological research. *Am J Public Health* 2005, 95, 2161-2168.

Gonzalez, F.J., Liu, S.Y., Yano, M., 1993. Regulation of cytochrome P450 genes: molecular mechanisms. *Pharmacogenetics* 3, 51-57.

Guengerich, F. P., Wang, P., Davidson, N. K., 1982. Estimation of isozymes of microsomal cytochrome P-450 in rats, rabbits, and humans using immunochemical staining coupled with sodium dodecyl sulfate-polyacrylamide gel electrophoresis. *Biochemistry.* 21, 1698-706.

Guengerich, F.P., 2003. Cytochrome P450 oxidations in the generation of reactive electrophiles: epoxidation and related reactions. *Arch. Biochem.* Biophys. 409, 59-71.

HapMap. The International HapMap Consortium. A haplotype map of the human genome. *Nature* 2005, 437, 1299-1320.

Hincapié M., Gil M., Pico A., Gusmão L., Rondón F., Vargas C., Castillo A. Análisis de la estructura genética en una muestra poblacional de Bucaramanga. *Colombia Médica* 2009, Vol 40, No 4: 362-373.

Honmaa H., De Capitania E., Perroud M., Barbeiroa A., Torob I., Costac D., Lima C., Zambon L. (2008). Influence of *p53* codon 72 exon 4, GSTM1, GSTT1 and GSTP1*B polymorphisms in lung cancer risk in a Brazilian population. *Lung Cancer* 61, 152—162.

Huang L, Li Y, Singleton AB, Hardy JA, Abecasis G, Rosenberg NA, Scheet P. Genotype-imputation accuracy across worldwide human populations. *Am J Hum Genet* 2009, 84, 235-250.

HUGO, The human Genome Project where did it come from, where is it going? *Am J Hum Genet.* 1992; 51: 1-6.

Ingelman-Sundberg M, Sim SC. Pharmacogenetic biomarkers as tools for improved drug therapy; emphasis on the cytochrome P450 system. *Biochem. Biophys. Res. Commun.* 2010; 396: 90–4.

Ingelman-Sundberg M. Genetic polymorphisms of cytochrome (2005). P450 2D6 (CYP2D6): Clinical consequences, evolutionary aspects and functional diversity. *Pharmacogenomics* J; 5: 6–13.

Isaza C., Henao J., Isaza J., Sepúlveda J., Beltrán L. Phenotype-genotype analysis of CYP2C19 in Colombian mestizo individuals. *BMC Clinical Pharmacology* 2007, 7:6.

Jakobsson M, Scholz SW, Scheet P, Gibbs JR, VanLiere JM, Fung HC, Szpiech ZA, Degnan JH, Wang K, Guerreiro R, Bras JM, Schymick JC, Hernandez DG, Traynor BJ, Simon-Sanchez J, Matarin M, Britton A, van de Leemput J, Rafferty I, Bucan M, Cann HM, Hardy JA, Rosenberg NA, Singleton AB. Genotype, haplotype and copy-number variation in worldwide human populations. *Nature* 2008, 451, 998-1003.

Jorgensen JT. A challenging drug development process in the era of personalized medicine. Drug Discov Today. 2011; 16(19-20):891-7.

Kirchheiner J, Seeringer A. Clinical implications of pharmacogenetics of cytochrome P450 drug metabolizing enzymes. *Biochimica et Biophysica Acta;* 1770:489–494, 2007.

Leschziner GD, T Andrew, M Pirmohamed, MR Johnson. ABCB1 genotype and PGP expression, function and therapeutic drug response: a critical review and recommendations for future research. *The Pharmacogenomics Journal,* 2007, 7, 154–179.

LLerena A, Naranjo ME, Rodrigues F, Penas EM, Fariñas H, Tarazona E. Interethnic variability of CYP2D6 alleles and of predicted and measured metabolic phenotypes across world populations. *Expert Opin Drug Metab Toxicol* 2014, 10:1569–83.

Llerena A. (Population pharmacogenetics and global health. *Drug Metabol Pers Ther* 2015, DOI 10.1515/dmdi-2015-0014.

Llerena A. Clinical pharmacology of drug metabolism and drug interactions: clinical, inter-ethnical and regulatory aspects. *Drug Metabol Drug Interact* 2013, 28:1–3.

LLerena A., Dorado P., Ramírez R., Calzadilla L., Peñas- LLedó E., Álvarez M., Naranjo M., González I., Pérez B., CEIBA Consortium of the Ibero–American Network of Pharmacogenetics & Pharmacogenomics RIBEF. CYP2D6-1584C>G promoter polymorphism and debrisoquine ultrarapid hydroxylation in healthy volunteers. *Pharmacogenomics* 2013, 14(16), 1973–1977.

Llerena A., Peñas-Lledó E. (2015). Metabolic phenotype prediction from genotyping data: a bottleneck for the implementation of pharmacogenetics in drug development and clinical practice. *Drug Metabol Pers Ther.,* DOI 10.1515/dmdi-2015-0014.

Maliepaard M., Nofziger C., Papaluca M., Zineh I., Uyama Y., Prasad K., Grimstein C., Pacanowski M., Ehmann P., Dossena S., Paulmichl M. Pharmacogenetics in the evaluation of new drugs: a multiregional regulatory perspective. *Nature reviews, drug discovery* 2013, vol 12, 103.

Martin F. From and Michel Eichelbaum. *Pharmacogenomics of Human P-Glycoprotein, in Pharmacogenomics: The Search for Individualized Therapies.* Edited by J. Licinio and M.L. Wong Copyright © 2002 Wiley-VCH Verlag GmbH & Co. KGaA ISBNs: 3-527-30380-4, 3-527-60075-2.

McCarthy MI, Abecasis GR, Cardon LR, Goldstein DB, Little J, Ioannidis JP, Hirschhorn JN. Genome-wide association studies for complex traits: consensus, uncertainty and challenges. *Nat Rev Genet* 2008, 9, 356-369.

Millan J and Arenas J. (2004). *Impacto del conocimiento genético en la clínica.* In: Genoma y Medicina. Cap. II, Pág. 17, Nov. 2004 ISBM 84-609-3002-5. Span Info SA. Copyright. Fundación española para el desarrollo de la investigación en genómica proteómica.

Olivera A. and Vega L. Role of glutathione s-transferase enzymes in toxicology, pharmacology and human disease. In: *Xenobiotic metabolizing enzymes and xenobiotics receptors. Pharmacological and toxicological aspects.* 2010. Cap 3., Ed. Elizondo G. Transworld Res. Network, Kerala, India.

Price AL, Patterson N, Yu F, Cox DR, Waliszewska A, McDonald GJ. A genome wide admixture map for Latino populations. *Am J Hum Genet,* 2007, 80(6):1024-36.

Quiñones, L., Berthou, F., Godoy, J., Caceres, D., Berthou, F., Varela, N., Lee, K., Acevedo, C., Martinez, L., Aguilera, A.M., Gil, L. CYP1A1, CYP2E1, and GSTM1 genetic polymorphisms. The effect of single and combined genotypes on lung cancer susceptibility in Chilean people. *Cancer Lett.* 2001, 174, 35-44.

Rodriguez C., Gomez A., Karlgren M., Sim S., Ingelman M. (2010).*Hum. Gen,* 127, 1-17.

Sans M. Admixture studies in Latin America: From the 20th to the 21st Century. *Hum Biol.* 2000, 72:155-177.

Seldin MF Admixture mapping as a tool in gene discovery. *Curr Opin Genet Dev* 2007, 17, 177-181.

Seldin MF. Admixture mapping as a tool in gene discovery. *Curr Opin Genet Dev* 2007, 17, 177-181.

Shastry BS. Pharmacogenetics and the concept of individualized medicine. *The Pharmacogenomics Journal* 6, 16–21, 2006.

Sim, SC, Kacevska, M, Ingelman-Sundberg, M. *The pharmacogenomics J.*, 2012, 13, 1-11.

Smith MW & O'Brien SJ. Mapping by admixture linkage disequilibrium: advances, limitations and guidelines. *Nat Rev Genet* 2005, 6, 623-632.

Sosa-Macías M, Llerena A. Cytochrome P450 genetic polymorphisms of Mexican indigenous populations. *Drug Metabol Drug Interact* 2013, 28:193–208.

Teh L., W., Lee L., Amir J., Salleh. M., Ismail R. Single step PCR for detection of allelic variation of MDR1 gene (P-glycoprotein) among three ethnic groups in Malaysia. *Journal of Clinical Pharmacy and Therapeutics,* 2007, 32, 313–319.

Wang S, Ray N, Rojas W, Parra MV, Bedoya G, Gallo C, Poletti G, Mazzotti G, Hill K, Hurtado AM, Camrena B, Nicolini H, Klitz W, Barrantes R, Molina JA, Freimer NB, Bortolini MC, Salzano FM, Petzl-Erler ML, Tsuneto LT, Dipierri JE, Alfaro EL, Bailliet G, Bianchi NO, Llop E, Rothhammer F, Excoffier L, Ruiz-Linares A. Geographic patterns of genome admixture in Latin American Mestizos. *PLoS Genet* 2008, 4, e1000037.

WTCCC. The Wellcome Trust Case Control Consortium Genome-wide association study of 14,000 cases of seven common diseases and 3,000 shared controls. *Nature* 2007, 447, 661-678.

Zanger UM, Schwab M. Cytochrome P450 enzymes in drug metabolism: regulation of gene expression, enzyme activities, and impact of genetic variation. *Pharmacol. Ther.* 2013; 138: 103–41.

In: Pharmacogenomics in Latin America
Editor: Luis A. Quiñones

ISBN: 978-1-53611-031-9

Chapter 3

PHARMACOGENOMIC STUDIES IN MEXICO, CENTRAL AMERICA AND CUBA IN AMERINDIANS GROUPS: CLINICAL APPLICATIONS AND TOXICOLOGY

Ismael Lares-Asseff*[1,*], *MD, PhD,
Fausto Zaruma Torres*[1,2,†], *PhD
and Claudia E. Bailón-Soto*[1,‡], *PhD(c),
[1]National Polytechnic Institute-CIIDIR, Durango, Mexico
[2]School of Biochemistry and Pharmacy,
University of Cuenca, Cuenca, Ecuador

ABSTRACT

In Latin America, the first study focused on the pharmacogenetics of CYP2D6 was developed in 1986 by the team headed by Arias TD et al., with Cuna Amerindians from Panama. Since that date up to 2015 there have been published 29 studies about CYP2D6 in Latin American countries; from which 17 were developed in Mexico, 3 in Cuba, and 9 in Central America (2 from Nicaragua, 2 from Costa Rica and 5 from Panama). Moreover, 23 studies were undertaken in Amerindian and Mestizo populations and finally, 6 with clinical application. Therefore, it is important to accurately spread the hard work of research being carried out in this part of the globe with crucial implications for improvement of regional personalized therapy.

Keywords: pharmacogenomics, pharmacogenetics, Latin America, clinician toxicology, clinical pharmacology

[*] Corresponding Author E-mails: ismaelares@yahoo.com.
[†] fausto.zaruma@ucuenca.edu.ec.
[‡] claudbay@yahoo.com.mx.

Latin American Studies of Genetic Polymorphisms in Phase I Enzymes

CYP2D6 Research in Amerindian and Mestizo Populations

In the past century, in 1986 Arias TD et al. (Arias, Jorge, and Inaba 1986) reported the absence of sparteine poor metabolizers (PM), this alkaloid is an antiarrhythmic, oxytocic agent studied in Cuna Amerindians from Panama. Subsequent studies realized in Panama by Petersen et al. (Petersen et al., 1991) claimed they had found the BamHI polymorphism which had not been described before that time. This was a very important finding three decades ago, since this polymorphism correlated with the PM phenotype in Ngawbé-Guayamí Amerindians under study.

Also, Jorge FL et al. (Jorge et al., 1993) stated that the CYP2D6B mutant allele is responsible of the enzyme deficiency in PM individuals. The presence of the mutant allele in Amerindians suggested an evolutive history older, by far, than it was previously thought. All the Restriction Fragment Polymorphism (RFLP) and Polimerase Chain Reaction (PCR) analyses demonstrated a diminishing pattern in the genetic diversity of the Ngabwe subjects, in concordance with their demographic history.

In addition to this finding, the results obtained in another research by Jorge LF et al. (Jorge et al., 1999) allowed them to propose the conversion of CYP2D6 into a vestigial, non restricted characteristic driven by dietetic and stress factors as a result of cultural strategies of survival in early human beings and hominids. Human evolution of CYP2D6 was primarly affected by random genetic drift, and not by adaptive selection. Another study guided by Jorge FL and Arias TD (Jorge and Arias 1995) in Embera and Ngabwe Amerindians from Panama made clear that both groups posess a low CYP2D6 genotypic and phenotypic diversity. On the other hand, Agúndez JA et al. (Agúndez et al., 1997) reported that 34% of Nicaraguan individuals were poor metabolizers (PM), instead of 33 to 37% PM individuals reported in Asian population.

Furthermore, López M et al. (López et al., 2005) performed an study on healthy Mexican Mestizo population to determine their genotype and phenotype. They found that 10% were PM individuals and their values were similar to Caucasian Spanish; while the allelic frequencies of CYP2D6 *2,*3,*4,*5,*10 and *17 sampled and tested in Mexican Mestizo population under study, matched to a mixture of Caucasian, Asian and African races.

Moreover, another study carried out by Sosa Macias M et al. (Martha Sosa-Macías et al., 2006), were CYP2D6 alleles were phenotyped to the metabolic rate (MR) of Dextromethorphan/dextrorphan (DM/DX) of 58 Tepehuano indigenous individuals and 88 Mestizo individuals from Durango, Mexico; also, 195 individuals were genotyped including 85 Tepehuano indigenous individuals and 110 Mestizo individuals). The association between genotype-phenotype resulted statistically significant (r^2= 0.45; p=0.005) in Mestizo individuals. Additionally, the Tepehuano indigenous individuals did not present the PM phenotype, while the Mestizo individuals presented a PM phenotype frequency of 6.8%. Moreover, the Tepehuano indigenous subjects showed a low genotypic and phenotypic diversity in contrast to other Amerindian groups. But, the frequencies of the allele variants in Mestizos were similar to those reported in white population. Similarly, Lares-Asseff I et al. (Ismael Lares-Asseff et al., 2005) L reported that 55 Tepehuano indigenous individuals under study resulted to be rapid metabolizers (RM). Their metabolic rate was DM/DX <0.3. No association between age, gender or nutritional condition and RM was found.

González I et al. (González et al., 2007) analized the interethnic differences based on the polymorphic hydroxylation of debrisoquine between a Cuban and Mexican population. They found that the frequency of the debrisoquine between a Cuban and a Spanish population was similar. The frequency of the PM phenotype was almost identical to the reported in Spanish metabolizers, 4.6% and 4.9% respectively; while the ultrarapid metabolizers (UM) were less present in Cubans than in Spanish, 3.8% and 5.2%, respectively. Therefore, the clinical implications in the therapeutic response dependent on the inter-ethnic differences are conclusive. Likewise, the study undertaken by Rodeiro I et al. (Rodeiro et al., 2009) reported the in vitro inhibitory effects of herbal products over the enzyme system of CYP450 used during decades from Cuban and Mexican individuals to improve traditional medicine. The results from their study suggest that the so called herbs inhibit the main CYP450 enzymes involved in drug metabolism, which might induce potential interactions between herbs and drugs.

The aim of the study conducted by Sosa-Macías M et al. (Martha Sosa-Macías et al., 2010) was to explain the variability in the activity of CYP2D6 for the identification, deletion and multiplication of CYP2D6 single nucleotide polymorphisms (SNP) -1584 C→G, 31 G→A and 2988 G→A in Mexican Mestizo and Tepehuano individuals. The polymorphisms studied had different frequencies between Tepehuanos and Mestizos (p <0,001). However, the Tepehuano group presented a low influence in their phenotypic expression which help in the understanding of genotype-phenotype of CYP2D6 in the studied Mexican populations.

It is noticeable that Contreras AV et al., (Contreras et al., 2011) reported the first exhaustive resequencing analysis of CYP2D6 in Mexicans and other Latin American population, that yielded information concerning to the relevant genetic diversity for the development of Pharmacogenomics in the aforementioned region. There, 64 polymorphisms were identified, including (Salazar-Flores et al., 2012) 14 new variants: 13 SNPs and a conversion in exon 2 of CYP2D7 that was renamed as CYP2D6*82 by the human P450 Cytochrome (CYP450), the Allele Nomenclature Committee. According to these findings, it is foreseen that 3 new SNPs may have functional effects. In the specific case of CYP2D6*82 it is postulated its Amerindian origin supported in the correspondent identification in three Mexican Amerindian groups (Mayas, Tepehuanos and Mixtecas).

In the same matter, Salazar-Flores J et al. (Salazar-Flores et al., 2012) after analysis of SNPs found a poor metabolizer´s phenotype in Amerindian groups and Mestizo groups that had not been previously studied. They found the predominant wild-type *1 allele in Mexican populations, plotting a relative homogenous distribution of CYP2C19 and CYP2D6. The exception to the rule is the Tarahumara Amerindian group that shows a marked possible risk to adverse reactions mediated by the CYP2C19 metabolyzing drugs.

Llerena A et al. (Llerena et al., 2012) analyzed the CYP2D6 genotype and the debrisoquine metabolic ratio (MR) in 133 Mestizo Nicaraguan (MsN) and 260 Cuban divided in Mestizo Cuban (MC) and White Cuban (WC) and found that phenotype variability of CYP2D6 might be related to differences in allele frequency among groups. The CYP2D6*10 allele was greater in the MsN (3.1%) than the MC (0.8%, p<0.05), and the CB (0.4%, p<0.05). The CYP2D6*17 allele resulted to be greater in the MC (10.2%) than the CB (2.7%, p<0.005), and the MsN (0%). Therefore, the variability found in the CYP2D6 phenotype might be related to the differences in allele frequency between groups; meaning that

CYP2D6*10 and *17 are higher in the MsN and the MC). However, the influence of environmental factors or different non studied alleles cannot be discarded.

The Amerindian groups studied by Sosa M and Llerena A (2013) showed a low CYP2D6 phenotypic activity and low genotypic activity of CYP2D6 and CYP2C9 in comparison to Mexican Mestizo groups. Additionally, the frequency of polymorphisms in genes CYP1A1, CYP2C19, CYP2E1 and CYP3A4 was similar between Mexican Amerindian and Mestizo groups, with exception of CYP1A2 gene which presented the highest frequency described to date for the variant *1F in Mexican Amerindian groups.

Besides, Cespedes-Garro C et al. (2014) developed a study in three groups from Costa Rica. They recruited 385 subjects (139 Mestizo, 197 Amerindian and 49 Afro-Caribbean volunteers). The aim of their study was to determine the frequency of ultrarapid metabolizers (UMs) and poor metabolizers (PM) concluding that UMs and PM frequencies for CYP2D6 presented an amply variation between Costa Rica populations composed by Mestizo, Amerindian and Afro-Caribbean people. The highest UMs frequencies reported were 10.1% and, 10.2% for PM, found in Mestizo and Amerindian groups respectively. While the overall Costa Rica population yielded a frequency of UMs of 6.5% and PM of 6.0%.

In this regard, results obtained by López- López M et al. (2014) in Lacandon Amerindian population and Mestizo population from southern Mexico supported the very low frequency of CYP2D6 PM previously reported in Mexican Amerindian groups. The UMs phenotype found in Lacandon and Mestizo groups was the lowest ever reported for most of Mexican populations. Accordingly, the PM frequency was 0% for Lacandon people and 1% for Mestizo individuals; while the UMs frequency was 2.6% for Lacandon and 3.0% for Mestizo groups in that region of the country.

Later, Bonifaz-Peña V et al. (2014) characterized the distribution of polymorphisms of pharmacogenetic and pharmacogenomic relevance in two population samples from Brazil and Mexico, the two most populated countries in Latin America. In such study, admixture proportion was evaluated in samples of both populations, using a panel of ancestry informative markers extracted from the DMET matrix and then validated, later, with data from the whole genome. Therefore, they demonstrated the huge impact of differences found in the admixture history over the distribution of allelic and genotypic frequencies at population level.

Interestingly, Lazalde Ramos BP et al. (2014) assisted by postgraduate students achieved the genotyping of the large amount of 508 Amerindian subjects. The analysis of CYP2D6*5 and the allele multiplication was performed by long-range PCR, while the CYP2D6*2, *3, *4, *6, *10, *17, *29, *35, *41 and copy number were evaluated by real-time PCR. After analysis, results demonstrated a lower frequency of CYP2D6 inactive alleles and a higher frequency of duplication/multiplication of CYP2D6 active alleles in Amerindian indigenous populations compared to Amerindian Mestizo groups.

More importantly, the research leaded by Cespedes-Garro et al. (Céspedes-Garro, Naranjo et al. 2015) yielded information about genetic markers tested in Central America populations. The polymorphisms evaluated included CYP2C19, LDLR, CYP2E1, MDR1, G6PD, TP53, CYP1A2, CYP3A4 and CYP3A5; unfortunately, data from other 91 biomarkers evaluated in Central America populations are unavailable. Neither was found differences in the frequency of some biomarkers of pharmacogenetics and metabolic phenotyping importance that show the inter-ethnic variability in Central America and other Latin America populations.

Concerning to CYP2D6 variants, Pérez-Páramo et al. (.2015) after analyzing their distribution in Mexican natives and Mestizo population from Chiapas, two populations ethnically related cohabiting the same econiche, and their relationship with a distant Mestizo community found that sharing of CYP2D6 alleles in both Chiapanecan populations suggests an ongoing gene-flow. According to this, another study from Pérez-Paramo YX et al. (2015) focused in the diversity and interpopulation relationships of CYP2D6 variants in Mexican southern natives to define the predicted phenotypes, they found that the functional CYP2D6 variants are frequent in Mexican natives which may predict specifically the drug extended metabolizers. Besides, they found that allele frequencies are related to the Amerindian groups´ geographic distribution and display important population stratification.

CYP2D6 Studies with Clinical Application

In this crucial matter, Lares-Asseff I and Trujillo Jiménez F (2001) affirmed in their research that therapeutic efficacy and pharmacologic security are important aspects that must be considered and achieved in the clinical use of drugs or medicines in individuals under pharmacological treatment. Due to the presence of drug metabolizing enzymes, drugs may participate as enzyme inhibitors or inductors; and moreover, their activity may vary among individuals. Therefore, the aim of this study was to make the scientific community aware of the importance of knowledge and comprehension of drug metabolism in order to improve patient´s therapeutic management.

Further, research done by Aceves Avila FJ (2004) et al. focused on the evaluation of cyclophosphamide (CYC) and the influence of CYP2D6 on micronuclei expression (MN) in patients with systemic lupus erythematosus (SLE). They found that genotoxicity assessed by the MN assay, is increased in patients with SLE after CYC boluses. The CYP2D6 allele expressed in SLE patients showed no correlation with CYC induced chromosomal injury.

In addition to, González et al. (2008) had previously demonstrated in a Spanish population that interindividual variability in CYP2D6 hydroxylation capacity was related to personality differences in cognitive social anxiety. Therefore, they decided to analyze the relationship between personality and CYP2D6 phenotype and genotype in a population of healthy volunteers from different latitude and culture like a Cuban population. For such study they recruited 253 university students and personnel from the "Hospital Psiquiátrico de la Habana." And they found that the differences in cognitive social anxiety-related personality traits involved in the four CYP2D6 hydroxylation capacity groups were noteworthy similar to the results found in Spanish volunteers.

It is noticeable that Alcazar-Gonzalez et al. (2013) did a pharmacogenetics research in breast cancer (BC) to predict the tamoxifen efficacy and paclitaxel toxicity and capecitabine. They determined the frequency of CYP2D6 polymorphisms due to the association with the tamoxifen activation. They also evaluated CYP2C8, CYP3A5 and DPYD genes associated to toxicity of placlitaxel and capecitabine. Moreover, they included the IL-10 gene polymorphism associated to a diagnosis of advanced tumor. After the corresponding analysis they found out that CYP2D6 genotyping predicted that 90.8% of patients treated with tamoxifen were normal metabolizers, 4.2% ultrarapid, 2.1% intermediate and 2.9% poor metabolizers. For paclitaxel and the CYP2C8 gene, 75.3% were normal, 23.4% intermediate and 1.3% poor metabolizers. In reference to the DPYD gene, only one patient was a poor metabolizer. For the IL-10 gene, 47.1% were poor metabolizers.

Concerning to depression, Peñas-Lledó EM et al. (2013) made evident that early interruption of therapy with antidepressant drugs (ADPs) is frequent and approximately occurs during the 6th week. Among the main reasons for these ADPs interruptions are adverse reactions and lack of improvement; which only can be explained by the interindividual variability in drug metabolism. Interestingly, interruption of amitriptylene or fluoxetine, two of the most frequently used antipressants all over the world, which are metabolized by CYP2D6 might be related to CYP2D6 genetic polymorphisms. The UM metabolism is associated to risk factors of mental illness and antidepressant treatment failure in different populations; thereby, it is highly justified the need to implement their evaluation during clinical practice.

Summarizing, the aim of the study undertaken by Cuautle-Rodriguez et al. (2014) was to provide an accurate insight of the existing situation of the pharmacogenetics research in Mexico. They focused on drug metabolizing enzymes with clinical implications that have not been phenotype yet, in order to develop a phenotyping cocktail to specifically evaluate Mexican population. This Mexican specific cocktail may significantly contribute to a better and deep understanding on variability in drug response to a lower price and less time. It is worth mention that, there are currently validated phenotyping cocktails with some practical advantages like security and reliability at low cost. These are valuable tools because such cocktails require a single experiment to provide information referent to the Cytochrome different activities.

CYP2C9 Studies in Latin America

The first studies realized in Latin America concerning to CYP2C9 pharmacogenetics initiated in 2008 by the research group leaded by Aguilar B et al. (Aguilar, Rojas, and Collados 2008) focused on Mexican population. Lately to year 2015, there have been published 19 research studies about CYP2C9 issues in Latin American countries; from which 14 have been developed in Mexico, 2 in Cuba and 3 in Central America. To narrow it down, 8 studies are centered in Amerindian and Mestizo populations and 11 have clinical application.

CYP2C9 in Amerindian and Mestizo Populations

In reference to a study developed by Aguilar B et al. (2008) in 100 volunteers in Mexico, they found that the allele frequencies of CYP2C9*2 and *3 of 0.1 and 0.03 respectively, were not significantly different to the reported in Mexican Mestizo population (Mexican Mestizo and Mexican American). However, the CYP2C9*2 allele was significantly higher in them than in Tepehuano indigenous groups from Mexico.

Afterwards, Dorado et al. (2011) analyzed the existence of possible differences in CYP2C9 allelic frequencies between Mexican-Tepehuanos (MT) and Mexican-Mestizos (MM) living in northwestern Mexico and Spain (SP) they expected to find lower CYP2C9*2 frequencies in indigenous MT than in the other two groups, and lower in MM than in SP as they stated in a previous report. Moreover, the CYP2C9 genotypes among the studied populations were in equilibrium. The frequencies of CYP2C9*2 were 0.01, 0.07, 0.08, and 0.16 for MT, MM, MA, and SP subjects, respectively. In agreement with their hypothesis, CYP2C9*2 was significantly lower in the Mexican populations than in the SP (P<0.05), and among Mexicans in the MT than in the MM and MA groups (P<0.05), who presented similar frequencies. Moreover, the frequency of CYP2C9*3 was found to be lower (P<0.05) in MM (0.015) and MT (0.015) than in MA (0.06) and SP (0.08). Finally, the CYP2C9*6 allele was present just in one MM subject, and CYP2C9*4 and *5 were not found in the studied populations. Thus, their findings added further evidence about CYP2C9 genetic diversity within Hispanic populations with regard to their ancestry. Considering that CYP2C9*2 and CYP2C9*3 alleles have altered catalytic activities relative to CYP2C9*1, their exposed data suggested the need for more pharmacogenetic studies in order to optimize drug dosages in different populations.

Later, Mendieta-Wejebe et al. (2011) emphasized that the metabolism of drugs by CYP2C9 can yield either safe or toxic products, which may be related to the recognition and binding modes of the substrates to this isoform. And they propose that such interactions can be studied using in silico methods such as quantum chemistry, molecular dynamics and docking simulations, which can also be useful for predicting the structure of metabolites. In these study types of studies, the ligand and the protein must be tridimensional models; thus, the protein can be built by homology modeling or retrieved from the Protein Data Bank. Therefore, they stated that these computational tools allowed them to describe the principal characteristics of the active site of the CYP2C9 isoform at the molecular level and the chemical properties of its ligands.

In virtue of the lack of applicability of extrapoled pharmacogenetics data in most indigenous populations, Sosa-Macías & LLerena (2013) have stated that studies directed at indigenous populations need to be developed. The Amerindians analyzed in their study showed a low phenotypic (CYP2D6) and genotypic (CYP2D6, CYP2C9) diversity, unlike Mexican Mestizos. The frequency of polymorphisms in the CYP1A1, CYP2C19, CYP2E1, and CYP3A4 genes was more similar among the Amerindians and Mexican Mestizos, with the exception of the CYP1A2 gene, which *1F variant frequency in Mexican Amerindians was the highest described until that date. Later, in another study Sosa-Macías M et al. (2013) determined the influence of ethnic admixture components on the CYP2C9 allele distribution in 505 Amerindian from eight indigenous populations through genotyping CYP2C9*2, *3 and *6 alleles by real-time PCR and molecular evaluation of ancestry. The frequencies for CYP2C9*2 were 0.026 in Seris, and 0.057 in Mayos, being higher than in Asians (P<0.001). CYP2C9*3 was found in Tarahumaras (0.104), Mayos (0.091), Tepehuanos (0.075), Guarijíos (0.067), Huicholes (0.033) and Coras (0.037), with East Asians having lower frequencies than the former three groups (P<0.001). CYP2C9*6 was not found. The frequency of CYP2C9*2 was lower in Amerindians than in European populations, and higher than their Asian ancestors. Therefore, the presence of this allele in ethnic groups in Mexico can be explained by European admixture.

Then, in a research developed by Castelán-Martínez et al. (2013) their objective was to analyze the most relevant CYP2C9 functional variants which are CYP2C9*2 (rs1799853) and CYP2C9*3 (rs1057910). These polymorphisms show variation in allele frequencies among different population groups. Therefore, they analyzed these polymorphisms in 947 Mexican-Mestizo from Mexico City and 483 individuals from five indigenous Mexican populations: Nahua, Teenek, Tarahumara, Purepecha and Huichol. The CYP2C9*2 allele frequencies in the Mestizo, Nahua and Teenek populations were 0.051, 0.007 and 0.005, respectively. As for CYP2C9*3, the allelic frequencies in the Mestizo, Nahua and Teenek populations were 0.04, 0.005 and 0.005, respectively. The CYP2C9*2 and CYP2C9*3 alleles were not observed in the Tarahumara, Purepecha and Huichol populations. These findings are in agreement with previous studies reporting very low allele frequencies for these polymorphisms in American Indigenous populations.

More importantly, Céspedes-Garro C et al. (2015) identified seventy-eight original research articles that included a total of 31,978 subjects. In their expert opinion they said that CYP2C9*2 allele is the most frequent in Caucasian populations (average 14%), with the lowest frequencies in Africans (0.46%), East Asians (0.56%) and Native Americans (1.25%) were in agreement with the hypothesis about the low prevalence in Amerindians. CYP2C9*3 showed the highest frequency among South Asians (11.7%), while CYP2C9*5 (1.56%) and *8 (4.70%) showed that frequencies in African Americans. The predicted poor metabolizers (PM's) were entirely found in a low frequency, with the highest frequency detected in South Asians, in accordance with the CYP2C9*3 frequency in these populations. Their study showed the worldwide variability in the CYP2C9 allele frequencies across different ethnic and geographic groups. Finally, data about CYP2C9 measured metabolic phenotypes is still limited, according to them.

CYP2C9 Studies with Clinical Applications

In this regard, Rojas et al. (2005) make evident that the use of oral anticoagulants (OA) is problematic due to its association with hemorrhagic complications. OA metabolism relies on the CYP2C9 complex. Genetic variations compromising metabolic competence of this complex may explain the risk of excessive and hazardous anticoagulation. A pharmacogenetics-based approach to this issue could be beneficial for choosing adequate dose and duration of treatment, in addition to having a better understanding of pharmacological interactions to which OA are susceptible. However, evidence from several basic and clinical studies indicates that both a complicated system of regulation of expression of multiple genes and the influence of a wide variety of epigenetic factors could be responsible for adverse drug reactions associated with the use of OA. Emphasis on understanding the gene-environment interactions could attain new paths to facilitate the use of these important drugs in the daily clinical practice.

According to different strategies, Garcia DA (2008) has pointed out that a genotype that suggests for the need of a patient of a drug low dose may lead to an initial underdose with resulting subtherapeutical levels, which may expose the patient to a great and inevitable risk of thrombosis. Any of these undesirable adverse effects originated from the pharmacogenetics testing, should be subtracted from the hypothetical benefits based on the appropriate cost-effectiveness. He also marked off the need of finding the critical pathway of warfarin dosage, through the search of an optimal dosage strategy based on pharmacogenetics.

In reference to epilepsy, the research conducted by López et al. (2011) contributed to the knowledge of patients treated with antiepileptic drugs that can exhibit large interindividual variability in clinical efficacy or adverse effects. This could be partially due to genetic variants in genes coding for proteins that function as drug metabolizing enzymes, drug transporters or drug targets. Therefore, they explained the pharmacogenetics of two commonly prescribed antiepileptic drugs with similar mechanisms of action; phenytoin (PHT) and lamotrigine (LTG). These two drugs were selected in order to model the pharmacogenetics of Phase I and Phase II metabolism for PHT and LTG, respectively. In light of their found evidence, patients treated with PHT could benefit from CYP2C9 and CYP2C19 genotyping/phenotyping. For those under treatment with LTG, UGT1A4 and UGT2B7 genotyping might be of clinical use and could contribute to the interindividual variability in LTG concentration to dose ratio in epileptic patients.

In virtue of the clinical usefulness of genetic polymorphisms coding for proteins implicated in the metabolism of some antiepilectic drugs (AED), the research conducted by Saldaña-Cruz et al. (2013) made evident the importance of describing the genetic polymorphisms coding for CYP450 proteins involved in the metabolism of some of the main AED. Knowledge of interindividual variability in response to AED may allow a personalized treatment focused on efficiency maximization and toxicity risk diminishing, without considering the clinical variability and adverse effects of treatment, which could be manifested in a minority of patients.

In the study realized by Nastasi-Catanese et al. (2013) the objective was to determine the contribution of CYP2C9, CYP2C19, and APOE polymorphisms to the variations in response to the doses of acenocoumarol, which is the main anticoagulant prescribed to the Mexican population. The polymerase chain reaction-restriction fragment length polymorphism method (RFLP) was applied to identify 2 and 3 of CYP2C9, 2 of CYP2C19, and APOE variants. They claimed to show the first report in Mexico searching for the relationship between CYP450 and APOE polymorphisms and the dose requirements of acenocoumarol. Their results suggested that CYP2C19 is more involved in acenocoumarol metabolism than CYP2C9 and APOE in the Mexican population. Besides considering the age factor, pharmacogenetic testing for CYP2C19 2 before initiating acenocoumarol treatment could lead to a safer anticoagulation therapy in Mexican patients.

As previously stated, due to the importance of CYP2C9 and CYP2C19 genetic polymorphisms in the metabolism of antiepilectic drugs (AED), López-García et al. (2014) searched for these key words in public databases worldwide of genetic polymorphisms like PubMed, Medscape, RxList and Pharmgkb, among others and from the NCBI website for CYP450 Allele nomenclature. They found out that CYP2D6, CYP2C9, CYP3A4 and CYP2D19 were involved in the metabolism of most AED, depending on the allele frequency in populations and as function of the variability associated to the clinical response.

It is noticeable that in the work developed by Bello et al. (2014) two simulation computing methods were combined (docking and molecular dynamics (MD), in order to get knowledge related to the protein substrate orientation inside the active sites. Such methods allow the identification of the binding mechanisms for prediction of regioselectivity in the binding mode of valproic acid (VPA) on three cytochrome P-450 (CYP) isoforms CYP2C9, CYP2C11, and CYP2E1, which are involved in the biotransformation of VPA yielding reactive hepatotoxic intermediate 2-n-propyl-4-pentenoic acid (4nVPA). There are experimental data about hydrogen atom abstraction of the C4-position of VPA to yield 4nVPA; however, there are not structural evidence about the binding mode of VPA and 4nVPA on CYPs. Therefore, the complexes between these CYP isoforms and VPA or 4nVPA were studied to explore their differences in binding and energetic stabilization. Docking results showed that VPA and 4nVPA are coupled into CYPs binding site in a similar conformation, but it did not explain the VPA hydrogen atom abstraction. On the other hand,

MD simulations showed a set of energetic states that reorient VPA at the first ns, then making it susceptible to a dehydrogenation reaction. For 4nVPA, multiple binding modes were observed in which the different states could favor either undergo other reaction mechanism or ligand expulsion from the binding site. Otherwise, the energetic and entropic contribution pointed out a similar behavior for the three CYP complexes, showing, as expected, a more energetically favorable binding free energy for the complexes between CYPs and VPA than with 4nVPA.

Later, the team leaded by Llerena (Llerena et al., 2014), evaluated the diclofenac metabolism in Hispanics from Cuba and Spain, and its relation to ethnicity, CYP2C9 genotypes and environmental factors. Diclofenac hydroxylation capacity (concentration ratios of diclofenac/metabolites in 8-h urine) was studied in 160 Cuban (classified as 76 Cuban-Whites-CWs and 84 Cuban-Mestizos-CMs) and 148 Spaniard (SPs) healthy volunteers. Diclofenac and its main metabolites, 4'-hydroxy (OH), 3'-OH and 5-OH diclofenac, and CYP2C9*2 to *6 and *8 alleles were also determined in 132 and 128 CWs and CMs, respectively. Gender, tobacco, caffeine and ethanol consumption were also evaluated. Their findings demonstrated for the first time interethnic differences between Hispanic groups measured in urinary diclofenac/4'-OH diclofenac ratios, and the relevance of CYP2C9*3 and CYP2C9*8 alleles.

Since the collection of pharmacogenetic variants in Mexican populations remains incomplete, research by Villegas-Torres et al. (2015) aimed to characterize the genotype frequency of eleven SNPs on CYP2C9 and VKORC1 in more than one-thousand individuals, and to explore their potential impact on coumarin dosing. In natives, genotype frequencies indicated that over 92% would reflect an extensive metabolism. Concerning to Mestizo populations, the proportion of CYP2C9 extensive (79%), intermediate (20.0%) and poor metabolizers (1.0%) was significantly different from native´s proportion, and varied among the different states of Mexico. Genotype frequencies of 7 SNP on VKORC1, were more homogenously distributed among natives and Mestizos. VKORC1 haplotype analysis revealed that most natives can be grouped into haplotypes H1 or H7-H8, while Mestizos showed a wider frequency distribution for other haplotypes. Their observations were in concordance with previous reports on the genotype distribution of major CYP2C9 alleles, and made a significant contribution to the of genotype frequencies collection on relevant VKORC1 variants.

Concerning to the metabolizing type and epilepsy, Ortega- Vazquez et al. (2016) explored the possible influence of CYP2C9 (*2, *3 and IVS8-109 A>T), CYP2C19 (*2, *3 and *17) and ABCB1 (1236C>T, 2677G>A/T and 3435C>T) on phenytoin (PHT) plasma concentrations in 64 Mexican Mestizo (MM) patients with epilepsy currently treated with PHT in mono- (n=25) and polytherapy (n=39). Genotype and allele frequencies of these variants were also estimated in 300 MM healthy volunteers. In their multivariate models, CYP2C9 IVS8-109 T was significantly associated with higher PHT plasma concentrations (t(64)=2.27; P=0.03). Moreover, this allele was more frequent in the supratherapeutic group as compared with the subtherapeutic group (0.13 versus 0.03, respectively; P=0.05, Fisher's exact test). Their findings suggested that CYP2C9 IVS8-109 T allele may decrease CYP2C9 enzymatic activity on PHT. But they stated that further research is necessary to confirm their findings.

To summarize, results published by Fricke-Galindo et al. (2015), showed the existence of adverse reactions to drugs (ARD) including a pharmacogenetics basis and a high interethnic variability which leads to the need for further research in different populations, in order to choose more useful and reliable results in the biggest number of patients included. Accurate search for biomarkers which may predict those adverse reactions to drugs, specifically to AED might improve greatly the epilepsy pharmacotherapy in days to come.

CYP2C19 Research in Latin America

Over the past years until 2015, a total of 16 studies focused on CYP2C19 pharmacogenetics have been realized. More specifically, nine research studies had clinical application; and seven were developed in Amerindian ethnic groups. On this topic, the very first study with clinical application was performed in 2002.

Studies on CYP2C19 in Amerindian Ethnic Groups

It is noteworthy that Salazar-Flores et al. (2012) analyzed the poor metabolizing phenotype (PM) in Amerindian and Mestizo groups from Mexico, including different polymorphisms located in CYP2D6 (*3, *4, *6, *7, and *8) and CYP2C19 (*2, *3, *4 and *5) in western Mestizos (n=145) and five Amerindian groups from Mexico: Tarahumaras from the North (n=88); Purépechas from the Center (n=101); and Tojolabales (n=68), Tzotziles (n=88), and Tzeltales (n=20) from the Southeast.. They found that the wild-type allele (*1) of both genes was predominant in the Mexican populations studied. The most widely observed alleles were CYP2C19*2 (range, 0%–31%) and CYP2D6*4 (range, 1.2%–7.3%), whereas CYP2D6*3 was exclusively detected in Mestizos. Conversely, CYP2C19*4 and *5, as well as CYP2D6*3, *6, *7, and *8, were not observed in the majority of the Mexican populations. The Tarahumara group presented a high frequency of the allele CYP2C19*2 (31%) and of homozygotes *2/*2 (10.7%), which represent a high frequency of potentially PM phenotypes in this Amerindian group. The genetic distances showed high differentiation of Tarahumaras (principally for CYP2C19 gene). In general, a relative proximity was observed between most of the Amerindian, Mexican-Mestizo, and Latin-American populations. Thus, they concluded that, in general, the wild-type allele (*1) is predominant in Mexican populations, outlining a relatively homogeneous distribution for CYP2C19 and CYP2D6. The exception turned out to be the Tarahumara group that displayed a potentially increased risk for adverse reactions to CYP2C19-metabolized drugs.

Interestingly, Sosa-Macías & Llerena (2013) analyzed the prevalence of CYP polymorphisms in Mexican indigenous groups and compared their findings with studies in Mexican Mestizo groups. Due to the lack of applicability of the extrapolation of pharmacogenetics data in most of the analyzed indigenous groups, the Amerindians studied showed a reduced phenotypic diversity of CYP2D6, and genotypic of CYP2D6 and CYP2C9, in comparison to Mexican Mestizo groups. The allele frequency in polymorphisms of CYP1A1, CYP2C19, CYP2E1 and CYP3A4 genes was similar between Mexican Amerindian and Mestizo groups, with exception of *1F variant of the CYP1A2 gene, which showed a variable frequency in Mexican Amerindians, being the latter, the highest described to date.

In a more comprehensive way, Vargas-Alarcón et al. (2014) determined to establish the gene frequency of six polymorphisms of the ABCB1, CYP3A5, CYP2C19, and P2RY12 genes in a population resident of Mexico City. The proteins encoded by these genes have been associated with the absorption, and biotransformation of clopidogrel. The ABCB1 T3435C, CYP3A5 V3 A6986G, P2RY12 G52T, P2RY12 C34T, CYP2C19 V2 (G681A) and V3 (G636A) polymorphisms were analyzed in a group of 269 healthy unrelated Mexican Mestizo individuals. The CYP2C19 V3 G636A polymorphism was not detected in the Mexican Mestizos population. However, the studied population presented significant differences ($P < 0.05$) in the distribution of the T3435C, A6986G, G681A, G52T and C34T polymorphisms when compared to reported frequencies of Amerindian of South America, Caucasian, Asian, and African populations. In summary, the distribution of the ABCB1, CYP3A5, CYP2C19, and P2RY12 gene polymorphisms make the Mexican Mestizo population distinguishable from other ethnic groups.

Since Central and South America remain largely uncategorized in the context of pharmacogenomics Marsh et al. (2015) decided to evaluate 15 polymorphisms from 12 genes (ABCB1 3435C>T, ABCG2 Q141K, CYP1B1*3, CYP2C19*2, CYP3A4*1B, CYP3A5*3C, ERCC1 N118N, ERCC2 K751Q, GSTP1 I105V, TPMT 238G>C, TPMT 460G>A, TPMT 719A>G, TYMS TSER, UGT1A1*28 and UGT1A1 -3156G>A) in 81 Peruvian and 95 Mexican individuals. Their findings reported that six polymorphism frequencies differed significantly between the two populations: ABCB1 3435C>T, CYP1B1*3, GSTP1 I105V, TPMT 460G>A, UGT1A1*28 and UGT1A1 -3156G>A. The pattern of observed allele frequencies for all polymorphisms could not be accurately estimated from any single previously studied population. Therefore, they concluded that it was highlighted the need to expand the scope of geographic data to be used in pharmacogenomics studies.

Due to the fact that ethnicity is one of the major factors involved in interindividual variability to drug response, Céspedes-Garro et al. (2015) described the frequency of the most relevant pharmacogenetic biomarkers and metabolic phenotypes in Central American healthy volunteers to determine its interethnic variability. Twenty-six original research articles on allelic, genotypes or metabolic phenotype frequencies were analyzed, in which a total number of 7611 Central American healthy volunteers were included (6118 were analyzed for genotype and 1799 for metabolic phenotype). No reports were available for population from Belize and Honduras. The CYP2D6*4 and *5 frequencies in Amerindian populations from Costa Rica have shown to be among the highest frequencies so far reported in the world. Furthermore, NAT2*5 and *6 presented higher frequencies in admixed populations than in Amerindians, but, inversely, the NAT2*7 was more frequent in Amerindians compared to an admixed population. Likewise, different patterns of distribution have been shown in HLA-A*02, *03 and HLA-B*07 among Native populations from Latin America. Reports on Central American populations were also found for the CYP2C19, LDLR, CYP2E1, MDR1, G6PD, TP53, CYP1A2, CYP3A4 and CYP3A5 biomarkers, but no data was available for the other 91 pharmacogenetic biomarkers revised in Central American populations. Interestingly, differences in the frequency of some pharmacogenetic biomarkers and metabolic phenotypes were found, showing interethnic variability within Central American and with other Latin American populations.

According to data of Mexican population, Favela-Mendoza et al. (2015) analyzed the CYP2C19*2, CYP2C19*3, CYP2C19*4 and CYP2C19*5 alleles related to the poor metabolizer (PM) phenotype in a Mexican population sample ($n = 238$), as well as CYP2C19*17, unique allele related to ultrarapid metabolizer phenotype (UMs). In addition to the wild-type CYP2C19*1 allele (77.1%), they only found CYP2C19*17 (14.3%) and

CYP2C19*2 (8.6%). Comparison with previous population reports demonstrated that these two SNPs are homogeneously distributed in Latin America ($P > 0.05$). Based on comparison with a previous pharmacokinetic study that determined the frequency of CYP2C19 phenotypes in the same population (western Mexican), they obtained the following findings: (i) based on the difference between the frequency of genotypes CYP2C19*2/*2 (presumably PM) versus the observed prevalence of PM phenotypes (0.4 versus 6.3%; $X(2) = 9.58$, $P = 0.00196$). Therefore, they inferred the plausible presence of novel CYP2C19 alleles related to the PM phenotype; (ii) the prevalence of UMs was in disagreement with the dominant inheritance pattern suggested for CYP2C19*17 (23.1 versus 4%; $P < 0.00001$); (iii) the apparent recessive inheritance pattern of CYP2C19*17, based on the agreement between homozygous CYP2C19*17/*17 (presumably UMs) and the observed prevalence of UMs (2.1 versus 4%; ($X(2) = 1.048$; $P = 0.306$).

Afterwards, Fricke-Galindo et al. (2015) evaluated the worldwide frequency distribution of CYP2C19 alleles and CYP2C19 metabolic phenotypes ('predicted' from genotypes and 'measured' with a probe drug) among healthy volunteers from different ethnic groups and geographic regions, as well as the relationship between the 'predicted' and 'measured' CYP2C19 metabolic phenotypes. A total of 52 181 healthy volunteers were studied within 138 selected original research papers. CYP2C19*17 was 42- and 24-fold more frequent in Mediterranean-South Europeans and Middle Easterns than in East Asians ($P<0.001$, in both cases). Conversely, CYP2C19*2 and CYP2C19*3 alleles were more frequent in East Asians (30.26% and 6.89%, respectively), and even a twofold higher frequency of these alleles was found in Native populations from Oceania (61.30% and 14.42%, respectively; $P<0.001$, in all cases), which may be a consequence of genetic drift process in the Pacific Islands. Regarding CYP2C19 metabolic phenotype, poor metabolizers (PMs) were more frequent among Asians than in Europeans, opposedly to the phenomenon reported for CYP2D6. Thus, they found a correlation between the frequencies of CYP2C19 poor metabolism 'predicted' from CYP2C19 genotypes (gPMs) and the poor metabolic phenotype 'measured' with a probe drug (mPMs) when subjects were either classified by ethnicity ($r=0.94$, $P<0.001$) or geographic region ($r=0.99$, $P=0.002$). Nevertheless, they strongly stated that further research is needed in African and Asian populations, which are under-represented, and additional CYP2C19 variants and the 'measured' phenotype should be studied.

CY2C19 Research with Clinical Application

In virtue of omeprazole (OM) usage as a testing drug for CYP2C19, González et al. (2002) developed a novel and reliable HPLC method for measuring omeprazole and its two main metabolites in plasma. This can be used for studying CYP2C19 and CYP3A4 genetic polymorphisms using omeprazole as the probe drug. This useful method is stable, reproducible, improves resolution and has practical advantages such as low cost for calculating metabolic index for CYP2C19 and CYP3A4 in adults and children. Moreover, in another study developed by González et al. (2003) the purpose was to evaluate the phenotype frequencies of the CYP2C19 polymorphism in West Mexicans. Besides omeprazole, sulfone was measured to evaluate CYP3A4 after administration of the 20-mg dose to 127 healthy volunteers. Logarithms of metabolic indexes of omeprazole/hydroxyomeprazole for CYP2C19 and omeprazole/omeprazole sulfone for CYP3A4 had trimodal distributions. Five subjects (4%) had a log CYP2C19 metabolic index below -0.9, suggesting an ultra-extensive phenotype. Poor metabolizers (log metabolic index > 0.6) were 6%. For CYP3A4, 11 subjects (9%) were below -0.3 of the log metabolic index. The log metabolic index of omeprazole/omeprazole sulfone was above the antimode of 0.6 for 11% of this population. The mean log metabolic index of CYP3A4 extensive metabolizers (80%) was 0.166, which seems to be higher than the data described for Caucasians and lower than that for Asians.

Besides, the pharmacokinetics of proton pump inhibitors (PPIs) have not been studied in children less than two years old. Therefore, Hoyo-Vadillo et al. (2005) determined the frequency of the main phenotypes of the metabolizing enzymes CYP2C19 and CYP3A4 in Mexican infants. Their results showed no significant differences between the 0.5 and the 1.5 mg/kg doses. The percentage of CYP2C19-poor metabolizers was 17% in babies below 4 months and was not detected in children above 3 months. When a combined CYP2C19- and CYP3A4- phenotype was estimated, omeprazole levels were significantly higher in poor metabolizers than in extended metabolizers. The percentage of ultra-extensive metabolizers in children older than 3 months were 20% and 33% for CYP2C19 and CYP3A4 respectively, compared to only 6% and 9% respectively, in babies between 1 and 3 months old. In general, children under 4 months had higher omeprazole levels and an immature metabolism. Studies in children older than 2 years old have showed similar pharmacokinetics to adults. For children between 1 month old and up to 9 months, they suggest the use of the 0.5 mg/kg dose, since it prevents accumulation in poor metabolizers. Nonetheless, caution is recommended to identify ultra-fast metabolizers, but this would require new studies.

It is important to state that Castillejos-López et al. (2008) have been describing an increase of the frequency of Directly Observed Therapy Short-course (DOTS) failure in countries with high rates of mycobacterial drug resistance. This increase could be due to the standardized doses of DOTS results in low or insufficient dosage of drugs in plasma. Several members of cytochrome P450 enzymes superfamily could explain the variations on acetylation velocity and in drug disposition. A population with slow acetylation has a higher toxicity risk, as that potent inhibition of cytochrome P450 (CYP450) isoforms by isoniazid (CYP2C19 and CYP3A) are dependent of INH plasmatic concentration. This inhibitory effect has been described also for CYP12, CYP2C9 and CYP2E1. INH is metabolized by N-acetyltransferase 2 (NAT2). The wide interethnic and intraethnic variability in acetylation velocity is associated to NAT2 polymorphisms. Patients with rapid acetylation have plasmatic concentration of INH low or insufficient which induces treatment failure. Therefore, they claimed that the study of genotypes of P450 and NAT2 would allow them to predict therapeutic and individualized dosages.

In a more sensitive view, López et al. (2011) provide a more general vision of current knowledge regarding pharmacogenetics of two commonly prescribed antiepileptic drugs with similar mechanisms of action; phenytoin (PHT) and lamotrigine (LTG). These two drugs have been selected in order to model the pharmacogenetics of Phase I and Phase II metabolism for PHT and LTG, respectively. In light of the evidence they have presented, patients treated with PHT could benefit from CYP2C9 and CYP2C19 genotyping/ phenotyping. For those under treatment with LTG, UGT1A4 and UGT2B7 genotyping might be of clinical use and could contribute to the interindividual variability in LTG concentration to dose ratio in epileptic patients. In addition to the previous findings, Nastasi-Catanese et al. (2013) determined the contribution of CYP2C9, CYP2C19, and APOE polymorphisms to the variations in response to the doses of acenocoumarol, which is the main anticoagulant prescribed to the Mexican population. The genetic distribution of every polymorphism tested showed high variability when compared to other populations worldwide. Their results showed statistical differences only in the CYP2C19 gene between the 1 1 and 1 2 groups, with effective acenocoumarol doses of 2.56 ± 1.34 mg/day vs 1.35 ± 0.84 mg/day (P = 0.005), respectively. Multiple regression analysis, including patient age and both the CYP2C9 and CYP2C19 genes, showed that these variables explained more than 20% of the dose variations. This was the first report in Mexico searching for the relationship between CYP450 and APOE polymorphisms and acenocoumarol dose requirements. Their results strongly suggested that, in the Mexican population, CYP2C19 is more involved in acenocoumarol metabolism than CYP2C9 and APOE. Besides considering the age factor, pharmacogenetic testing for CYP2C19 2 before initiating acenocoumarol treatment could lead to a safer anticoagulation therapy in Mexican patients.

In reference to genes coding for CYP450 isozymes and epilepsy, Lopez-Garcia et al. (2014) made an exhaustive revision related to pharmacogenetics, due to the fact that many antiepileptic drugs (AEDs) are metabolized by a variety of enzymatic reactions, and the cytochrome P450 (CYP) family has attracted considerable attention. Some of the CYPs exist as genetic (allelic) variants, which may also affect the plasma concentrations or drug exposure. Regarding the metabolism of AEDs, the polymorphic CYP2C9 and CYP2C19 are of particular interest. There have been recent advances in discovering factors such as these, especially those underlying the risk of medication toxicity. The review they wrote summarized the evidence about whether such polymorphisms affect the clinical action of AEDs to facilitate future studies on epilepsy pharmacogenetics. They performed Key Words searches in the public databases PubMed, Medscape, and Rxlisty, Pharm GKB for genetic polymorphisms and the NCBI website for the nomenclature of alleles of CYP450, finding that CYP2D6, CYP2C9, CYP3A4, and CYP2D19 were involved in the metabolism of most antiepileptic drugs, given the allele frequency in the population and the associated variability in clinical response.

In regard to drug clinical response to clopidogrel, Garcés-Eisele et al. (2014) studied the effect of selection of volunteers homozygous for the CYP2C19*1 haplotype on the bioavailability of clopidogrel. Its clinical response varies widely due to under-dosing, drug interactions and intrinsic interindividual differences resulting from genetic polymorphisms, in this case, due P450-2C19. Thus, a regular 2×2 bioequivalence study between two formulations of clopidogrel was performed in volunteers selected and unselected for relevant CYP2C19 haplotypes for the Mexican population. It was found that selection of volunteers homozygous for the CYP2C19*1 haplotype, increased the stringency of bioequivalence statistics and resulted in bioinequivalence of a generic clopidogrel compound that otherwise proved equivalent when tested in an open unselected population. They have claimed that augmentation of bioequivalence strictness is expected to result from pharmacogenetic selection of volunteers.

Also, Ortega-Vázquez et al. (2015) explored the possible influence of CYP2C9 (*2, *3 and IVS8-109 A>T), CYP2C19 (*2, *3 and *17) and ABCB1 (1236C>T, 2677G>A/T and 3435C>T) on phenytoin (PHT) plasma concentrations in 64 Mexican Mestizo (MM) patients with epilepsy currently treated with PHT in mono- (n=25) and polytherapy (n=39). Genotype and allele frequencies of these variants were also estimated in 300 MM healthy volunteers. In multivariate models, CYP2C9 IVS8-109 T was significantly associated to higher PHT plasma concentrations (t(64)=2.27; P=0.03). Moreover, this allele was more frequent in the supratherapeutic group as compared with the subtherapeutic group (0.13 *versus* 0.03, respectively; P=0.05, Fisher's exact test). Their results suggested that CYP2C9 IVS8-109 T allele might decrease CYP2C9 enzymatic activity on PHT. Nonetheless, according to the authors, more research is necessary to confirm those findings.

CYP3A4 and CYP3A5 in Mexico and Central America

From the past until 2015, a total of 15 research studies have been completed; from which 12 present clinical application, 3 are related to toxicology and just 1 presents a population approach.

In this regard, the research guided by Alvarez-González et al. (2001) focused on the flavonove Naringin (Nar) which is found in high amount in grapefruit. Since it has been suggested that antimutagenicity may be related to the inhibition of the human enzyme Cytochrome P450 (CYP) 3A4 by Nar they planned and designed a strategy to fulfill three main purposes: (1) to determine whether Nar has a genotoxic effect in mouse in vivo. This was evaluated by measuring the rate of micronucleated polychromatic erythrocytes (MNPE); (2) to determine its antigenotoxic and its anticytotoxic potential on the damage produced by ifosfamide (Ifos). The first study was done by scoring the rate of MNPE, and the second one by establishing the index polychromatic erythrocytes/normochromatic erythrocytes (PE/NE); and (3) to explore whether its antigenotoxic mechanism of action is related to an inhibitory effect of Nar on the expression of the Cyp3a enzyme, an effect which could avoid the biotransformation of Ifos. A single oral administration was used for all groups in the experiment: three groups were given different doses of Nar (50, 250, and 500 mg/kg), other groups received the same doses of Nar plus an administration of Ifos (60 mg/kg), another group treated with distilled water and another with Ifos (60 mg/kg) were used as negative and positive controls, respectively. The micronuclei and the cell scoring were made in blood samples taken from the tail of the animals at 0, 24, 48, 72, and 96 h. The results showed that Nar was neither genotoxic nor cytotoxic with the doses tested, but Ifos produced an increase in the rate of MNPE at 24 and 48 h. The highest value was 24+/-1.57 MNPE per thousand cells at 48 h. The index PE/NE was significantly reduced by Ifos at 24 and 48 h. Concerning to the antigenotoxic capacity of Nar, a significant decrease was observed in the MNPE produced by Ifos at the three tested doses. This effect was dose-dependent, showing the highest reduction in MNPE frequency (54.2%) at 48 h with 500 mg/kg of Nar. However, no protection on the cytotoxicity produced by Ifos was observed. Immunoblot analysis was used to assess the Cyp3a expression in liver and intestinal microsomes from mouse orally exposed to Nar. An induction in the Cyp3a protein was observed in both intestinal and hepatic microsomes from treated mice. This induction correlated with an increase in erythromycin N-demethylase activity. In conclusion, their data suggested that other mechanism(s) are involved in the antigenotoxic action of naringin.

In general, human-derived cell lines fail to express CYPs. And, since CYP3A4 is the predominant cytochrome P450 (CYP) expressed in human liver which contributes to the metabolism of approximately half the drugs in use today. And, since it was previously shown that CYP3A4 mRNA and CYP3A immunoreactive protein are induced by 1alpha,25-dyhydroxyvitamin D(3) (1alpha,25-(OH)(2)D(3)) in the human colon carcinoma cell line Caco-2. Therefore, the aim of Elizondo and Medina-Díaz (2003) was to examine whether

1alpha,25-(OH)(2)D(3) regulates CYP3A4 gene expression in HepG2 cells, a human hepatocarcinoma cell line. Treatment with 1alpha,25-(OH)(2)D(3) resulted in an induction of CYP3A4 mRNA and CYP3A4 immunoreactive protein, 1.5-fold and 4.0-fold respectively, when compared to control cultures, in a time-dependent fashion. Their observations were in agreement with previous reports suggesting a role of 1alpha, 25-(OH)(2)D(3) on CYP3A4 transcription regulation, and demonstrated that this hormone, as in Caco-2 cells, increase CYP3A4 levels in HepG2 cells. Then they concluded that, HepG2 cell cultures treated with 1-alpha,25-(OH)(2)D(3), provides a useful model to study the function of CYP3A4 and its role in drug liver metabolism.

Since calcitriol antiproliferative effects include inhibition of the oncogenic ether-à-go-go-1 potassium channel (Eag1) expression, which is necessary for cell cycle progression and tumorigenesis; research developed by García-Quiroz et al. (2012) made clear that the interaction between calcitriol and astemizole as well as their conjoint antiproliferative action in SUM-229PE, T-47D affect the primary tumor-derived breast cancer cells. Moreover, their results suggested that astemizole synergized calcitriol antiproliferative effects by downregulating CYP24A1, upregulating VDR and targeting Eag1. Thus, their study provided an insight into the molecular mechanisms involved in astemizole-calcitriol combined antineoplastic effect, offering scientific support to the combination of both compounds in further preclinical and clinical studies of neoplasms expressing VDR and Eag1. VDR-negative tumors might also be sensitized to calcitriol antineoplastic effects by the use of astemizole. In conclusion, they suggested a novel combined adjuvant therapy for the management of VDR/Eag1-expressing breast cancer tumors. Since astemizole improves calcitriol bioavailability and activity, decreased calcitriol dosing is advised for conjoint administration.

According to cancer research, involvement of cytochrome P450 genes (CYPs) in breast cancer (BCa) may differ between populations, with expression patterns affected by tumorigenesis. Thus, Bandala et al. (2012) determined the mRNA expression patterns of four cytochrome P450 genes (CYP2W1, 3A5, 4F11 and 8A1) in Mexican women with breast cancer. Expression levels were tested for association with clinical and pathological data of patients. Thereby, they found higher gene expression of CYP2W1, CYP3A5, CYP4F11 in BCa than in adjacent tissues and only low in normal mammary glands in the Mexican population studied by them, while CYP8A1 was only expressed in BCa and adjacent tissues. Interestingly, they found that Ki67 protein expression was associated with clinicopathological features as well as with CYP2W1, CYP4F11 and CYP8A1 but not with CYP3A5. Finally, their results indicated that breast cancer tissues might have a greater capability to metabolize carcinogens and other xenobiotics to active species than normal or adjacent non-tumor tissues.

Due to the increasing research in transplants, it has been documented the variability in CYP3A5 expression associated with differences in tacrolimus bioavailability. Therefore, the research realized by García-Roca et al. (2012) aimed to determine the frequency of CYP3A5*1 and CYP3A5*3 in 291 (124 adults, 167 pediatric) Mexican renal transplant recipients, in order to evaluate the tacrolimus dose requirements by genotype and compared their found genotype frequency data with other population´s data as well. They found out that the CYP3A5 phenotype had a significant impact in tacrolimus bioavailability, as wild-type carriers required higher dosing compared to mutated carriers to achieve similar drug trough levels. Finally, from the Mexican transplant recipients, they reported that 52.2% were

CYP3A5*3*3 and required significantly lower tacrolimus dose than those with CYP3A5*1 allele.

On one hand, clopidogrel is recommended in addition to aspirin to prevent atherothrombotic events in patients with acute coronary syndromes (ACS) and in those undergoing percutaneous coronary intervention (PCI), but in the other hand, recurrent cardiovascular events have ocurred and multiple mechanisms have been associated with no response including genetics factors. Therefore, Isordia-Salas et al. (2012) enrolled 60 patients with ACS undergoing emergent PCI in their research study. Platelet aggregation to adenosine diphosphate and arachidonic acid was assessed by turbidimetric method at 24 hours after dual administration of 300 mg of clopidogrel and 300 mg of acetylsalicylic acid loading dose. They identified a high percent of clopidogrel resistance in Mexican patients with ACS undergoing PCI. However, a normal platelet response to acetylsalicylic acid was observed in most of them. There was no association between CYP3A5*1/*3, PIA1/A2, and T744C polymorphisms with clopidogrel resistance. Consequently, they concluded that more studies are needed to determine the possible interaction between genetics factors, platelet response to clopidogrel and cardiovascular adverse events.

Since pharmacogenetic studies in breast cancer (BC) may predict the efficacy of tamoxifen and paclitaxel and capecitabine toxicity, Alcazar-González et al. (2013) determined the frequency of polymorphisms in the CYP2D6 gene associated with activation of tamoxifen, and those of the genes CYP2C8, CYP3A5 and DPYD associated with toxicity of paclitaxel and capecitabine. They also included a IL-10 gene polymorphism associated with advanced tumor stage at diagnosis. To achieve that, they analyzed 241 BC patients from northeast Mexico. Finding that, for tamoxifen processing, CYP2D6 genotyping predicted that 90.8% of patients were normal metabolizers, 4.2% ultrarapid, 2.1% intermediate and 2.9% poor metabolizers. For paclitaxel and the CYP2C8 gene, 75.3% were normal, 23.4% intermediate and 1.3% poor metabolizers. Regarding the DPYD gene, only one patient was a poor metabolizer. For the IL-10 gene, 47.1% were poor metabolizers. It is important to state that their results made a valuable contribution with information towards personalizing BC chemotherapy in Mexican women.

Concerning to renal transplants, Jacobo-Cabral CO, et al. (Jacobo-Cabral et al., 2014) evaluated the bioavailability of two oral tacrolimus formulations, the innovator Prograf(®) and a formulation commercialized in Mexico with the brand name Limustin(®), in children. Stable Mexican pediatric renal transplant recipients received the product authorized by their social security provider, being either Prograf(®) or Limustin(®). At steady state, blood samples were drawn and tacrolimus blood concentration against time curves was constructed. CYP3A5 genotype was also determined. There was no significant difference in dose or in trough concentrations between formulations. However, AUC and Cmax were significantly higher with Prograf(®). The lower tacrolimus bioavailability with Limustin(®) was observed in both expressers and non-expressers of the functional CYP3A5 protein. Therefore, Limustin(®) exhibited dissimilar pharmaceutical characteristics to the innovator that likely explained the reduced tacrolimus exposure in children. It was quite significant their finding, Limustin(®) resulted inadequate for pediatric use.

It has been documented that levels of enzymes that determine testosterone catabolism such as CYP3A4 have been associated with prostate cancer (PCa) risk. Thus, a study conducted by Reyes-Hernández et al. (2014) evaluated whether PXR-HNF3β/T (rs2472677), PXR-HNF4/G (rs7643645), and CYP3A4*1B (rs2740574) polymorphisms were associated to

PCa, and to test that, a case control-study was performed. The multiple testing analysis showed that the PXR-HNF4/G polymorphism was associated with higher levels of prostate-specific antigen (PSA) in patients with PCa (OR=3.99, p=0.03). This association was stronger in patients diagnosed at the age of 65 years or older (OR=10.8, p=0.006). Although the CYP3A4*1B/*1B genotype was overrepresented in PCa patients, no differences were observed in the frequency of this and PXR-HNF3β/T alleles between controls and cases. Moreover, no significant association was found between these polymorphisms and PSA, Gleason grade, or tumor lymph node metastasis.

In regard to tumor development, tumor response to therapy and protein expression, Floriano-Sanchez et al. (2014), analyzed protein expression in patients with breast cancer (BCa) and in healthy women. Links with some clinic-pathological characteristic were also assessed. Immunohistochemical analyses were conducted on 48 sets of human breast tumors and normal breast tissues enrolled in Hospital Militar de Especialidades de la Mujer y Neonatologia and Hospital Central Militar, respectively, during the time period from 2010 to 2011. They found a significant CYP3A4 overexpression in BCa stroma and gland regions in comparison to healthy tissue. A significant association between protein expression and smoking, alcoholism and hormonal contraceptives use was also observed. Additionally, they observed a positive association between estrogen receptor (ER) and progesterone receptor (PR) in BCa. Thus, they suggested that CYP3A4 expression promotes BCa development and can be used in the prediction of tumor response to different treatments. Finally, they claimed that one therapeutic approach may thus be to block CYP3A4 function.

According to pediatric renal transplants, a review conducted by Medeiros et al. (2015) focused on the fact that transplant recipients receive potent immunosuppressive drugs in order to prevent graft rejection. Therapeutic drug monitoring is the current approach to guide the dosing of calcineurin inhibitors, mammalian target of rapamycin inhibitors (mTORi) and mofetil mycophenolate. Target concentrations used in pediatric patients are extrapolated from adult studies. Gene polymorphisms in metabolizing enzymes and drug transporters such as cytochromes CYP3A4 and CYP3A5, UDP-glucuronosyl transferase, and P-glycoprotein are known to influence the pharmacokinetics and dose requirements of immunosuppressants. Therefore, they highlighted the pharmacogenomics implications in that patient population. They also emphasized that genetic information can help to achieve target concentrations in the early post-transplant period, avoiding adverse drug reactions and drug-drug interactions. Consequently, they revised evidence about genetic studies and transplant outcomes. In addition, a study realized in Cuba by Rodeiro et al. (2013) demonstrated the cytotoxic effects and changes in the P450 system after exposing rat hepatocytes to four polyphenol-rich products widely used in Cuban traditional medicine (Mangifera indica L. (MSBE), Thalassia testudinum (Tt), Erythroxylum minutifolium and confusum extracts). The effects of the main polyphenol in MSBE, mangiferin, were also evaluated. Seven specific P450 activities (CYP1A2, 2A6, 2C9, 2D6 y 3A4) and UDP-glucuronosyltransferases (UGT) were evaluated after 48 h exposure of cells to the products. Their results showed in vitro effects of these natural products on P450 systems, possibly leading to potential metabolic-based interactions.

Toxicological Studies

Concerning to insecticides, technical grade DDT, a commonly used organochloride pesticide, contains 20% of the (o,p'-1,1,1,-trichloro-2,2-bis (p-chlorophenyl)ethane (DDT)), o,p'-DDT isomer. Therefore, Medina-Díaz and Elizondo (2005) analyzed the effects of o,p'-DDT on CYP3A4 gene expression in HepG2 cells. Since DDT alters the activity of hepatic mixed function oxidase and induces expression of cytochrome P450 such as 3A subfamilies, treatment with o,p'-DDT dose-dependently increased levels of CYP3A4 mRNA and the immunoreactive protein, by 13- and 3.8-fold, respectively, relative to untreated cultures. Thus, their findings demonstrated that this insecticide is able to induce CYP3A4 transcription and may play an important role in the modulation of endogenous hormones and xenobiotic metabolism. To complement these results, Medina-Díaz et al. (2007) realized another study to determine the mechanism by which o,p'-DDT induces CYP3A4 expression. Therefore, transactivation and electrophoretic mobility shift assays were carried out, revealing that o,p'-DDT activates the CYP3A4 gene promoter through the pregnane X receptor (PXR). CYP3A4 gene promoter activation resulted in both an increase in CYP3A4 mRNA levels and an increase in the total CYP3A4 activity in HepG2 cells. They also observed induction of CYP3A4 and mouse Cyp3a11 mRNA in the intestine of CYP3A4-transgenic mice after exposure to 1 mg/kg o,p'-DDT. At higher doses, a decrease of CYP3A4 inducibility was observed together with an increase in levels of interleukin 6 mRNA, a proinflammatory cytokine that strongly represses CYP3A4 transcription. Thus, their study indicated that regulation of other genes under PXR control may be altered by o,p'-DDT exposure. Continuing in the same research line, Medina-Díaz et al. (2009) investigated the effect of sodium arsenite and its metabolites monomethylarsonous acid (MMA(III)) and dimethylarsinous acid (DMA(III)) on CYP3A4, PXR, and RXR alpha expression in the small intestine of CYP3A4 transgenic mice. Sodium arsenite treatment increases mRNA, protein and CYP3A4 activity in a dose-dependent manner. However, the increase in protein expression was not as marked as compared to the increase in mRNA levels. Arsenite treatment induces the accumulation of Ub-protein conjugates, indicating that the activation of this mechanism may explain the differences observed between the mRNA and protein expression of CYP3A4 induction. Overall, their results suggested that sodium arsenite and its metabolites induce CYP3A4 expression by increasing PXR expression in the small intestine of CYP3A4 transgenic mice.

Later, Sinues et al. (2007) detected genotypic differences between three populations of healthy volunteers from Northern Spain (204 subjects), Nicaragua (120 subjects), and El Salvador (112 subjects) regarding CYP3A4*1B and CYP3A5*3 polymorphisms. No significant differences were found by comparing allelic frequencies between the two Central American populations. The CYP3A5*3 allele frequency was significantly different ($P < 0.01$) between Central Americans (76%) and Spaniards (91%). By contrast, CYP3A4*1B allele was more prevalent among Central Americans (12.5%) than among North Spaniards (4%) ($P < 0.01$). Analysis of CYP3A4-3A5 genotype combinations revealed that individuals carrying CYP3A4*1B/CYP3A5*1 were more represented in Central Americans (16.9%) than in Spaniards (5.4%), suggesting a marked linkage disequilibrium. Their acquired data was compatible with a higher CYP3A enzyme activity in Central Americans as opposed to Spaniards and other white groups, which could imply serious differences in dose requirements for drugs metabolized by CYP3A and they claim that, the latter exposed should be considered in allele-disease association studies.

CYP2E1 Studies in Mexico

Due to its many substrates, the CYP2E1 enzyme may be involved in such varied processes as gluconeogenesis, hepatic cirrhosis, diabetes, and cancer. Therefore, a total of 28 research studies have been conducted in Mexico. These include 19 toxicology studies, 7 present clinical application and 2 are focused on Amerindian populations.

Applications in Toxicology

The effects of the anthelmintic drug albendazole (ABZ) treatment (i.p. and p.o. administration) on the expression of several cytochrome P450 (CYP) enzymes was evaluated in rat liver in a study conducted by Asteinza et al. (2000). They characterized the spectrum of altered CYP enzymes involved in the metabolism of environmental mutagens and carcinogens, after drug intake. Intraperitoneal administration of ABZ (50 mg/kg body weight/day/three days in corn oil) to rats, caused an induction of hepatic activities of CYP1A1-associated ethoxyresorufin O-deethylase (EROD) 65 fold, CYP1A2-associated methoxyresorufin O-demethylase (MROD) 6 fold, CYP2B1-associated penthoxyresorufin O-dealkylase (PROD) 4 fold, CYP2B2-associated benzyloxyresorufin O-dealkylase (BROD) 14 fold, as well as a partial reduction of CYP2E1-associated 4-nitrophenol hydroxylase (4-NPH) activity. Their findings suggested that oral administration of ABZ at the human therapeutic dose of 20 mg/kg body weight/day/three days produced an increase in CYP1A1/2 protein content 24 h after the first intake. The protein level remained high during the treatment, and up to 72 h after the last administration; basal protein levels were almost recovered 48 h later.

According to the study developed by Montero et al. (2003), [i]Infection of rat liver by Taenia taeniformis metacestodes produced an increase in the total CYP450 content and induced activity of the CYP1A1, CYP2B1 and COH isoforms. Variations in activity and p450 total content were found with increasing time of infection. During increased activity of p450 isoforms, rats were challenged with carcinogens metabolized by the mentioned isozymes and an increased amount of genotoxic damage was found when benzo[a] pyrene, cyclophosphamide and aflatoxin B(1) were used. No change was seen in CYP2E1 activity. Therefore, their results support previous findings regarding an increased susceptibility to genotoxic damage of infected organisms.

Concerning to CYP2E1 regulation by benzene, González-Jasso et al. (2003) investigated CYP2E1 inducibility in liver and peripheral lymphocytes of rats treated with benzene (0-10 mmol/kg body weight (bw), daily for 3 days, i.p., or 0 and 5 mmol/kg bw, daily for 14 days, i.p.) or toluene (0 and 5 mmol/kg bw, daily for 3 days, i.p.) and compared with that of pyridine (5 mmol/kg bw, i.p.) or acetone (5% in drinking water) both daily for 3 days. Acute benzene treatment (5 mmol/kg bw) increased both CYP2E1 apo-protein (2-fold) and p-nitrophenol hydroxylase (p-NPH) activity (1.4-fold) in liver, and CYP2E1 mRNA in both liver (2.2-fold) and peripheral lymphocytes (2.9-fold). The response to toluene was qualitatively similar, although smaller than that to benzene. As expected, acetone and pyridine treatments resulted in a 2- to 3-fold increase of p-NPH activity and CYP2E1 apo-protein content in liver, but not the mRNA levels. In addition, acute benzene and acetone treatments increased the 6-hydroxychlorzoxazone/chlorzoxazone metabolic ratio 1.6- and 3.1-fold, respectively. The subchronic treatment with benzene increased CYP2E1 mRNA and apo-protein from days 2 and 3 to day 14, respectively, whereas the enzyme activity increased transiently on days 3 and 5 only. So, their results showed that acute/subacute benzene and acute toluene treatments induce CYP2E1 expression probably through a similar mechanism which might be different from that of pyridine or acetone. Which means that the former increase mRNA levels, both in liver and in peripheral lymphocytes, whereas the latter stabilized the apo-protein.

In addition to hepatic CYP1A regulation by exogenous compounds, Oropeza-Hernández et al. (2003) researched the effect on liver cytochrome P450 (CYP) by i.p. injections of methoxychlor (MXC) in corn oil at 0, 100, 150, 200 or 250 mg/kg twice daily for 3 days in adult male and female Wistar rats. The MXC injection (100 mg/kg b.w.) caused a similar increase of total CYP content in males and females as compared with controls who received the vehicle only. In males, this increase continued up to 250 mg/kg. As to the induction of specific CYP activities, the effect of MXC was found to be sex dependent with three different patterns. Males showed the greatest increases of ethoxy- and methoxyresorufin-O-dealkylase (EROD and MROD, respectively), two CYP1A1/1A2-related activities. On the contrary, females were more responsive than males for pentoxyresorufin-O-dealkylase (PROD) and benzyloxyresorufin-O-dearylase (BROD), two CYP2B-related activities. Finally, p-nitrophenol hydroxylase (PNPH), a CYP2E1-related activity, showed a similar small, although statistically significant, increase for both sexes. As to CYP apoprotein levels, CYP1A1 and CYP2B1/2B2 showed greater increases in females than in males; whereas, interestingly, CYP2E1 induction was higher in males than in females. Their results overall indicated that gender modulates CYP expression after MXC injection both, qualitatively and quantitatively, and, therefore, this pesticide is not a pure PB inducer. Moreover, the statistically significant increase of CYP3A2 apoprotein expression observed in females and also, to a lower extent, in males, and the decrease of CYP2C11 apoprotein found in males, two sex-related enzymes, may explain the reported endocrine disrupting effect of MXC. They finally stated that, the relevance of the different patterns of rat liver CYP induction observed after MXC treatment, in relationship to the speculated endocrine disrupting potential of MXC in humans potentially exposed to this pesticide, needed further investigation.

In another study developed by Oropeza-Hernández et al. (2003), they studied the induction of cytochrome P450 (CYP) 2E1 in testes and liver and the presence of trifluoroacetylated (TFA) adducts in spermatozoa, testes, liver and plasma of rats subchronically exposed by inhalation to halothane (15 ppm/4 h/day/5 days/week/9 weeks). After halothane exposure, p-nitrophenol hydroxylase (p-NPH) activity increased 3.2-fold and CYP2E1 apo-protein content 7-fold in testes. Whereas in liver, p-NPH increased 2.3-fold and CYP2E1 apoprotein content 1.4-fold. Their results suggested a differential inductive effect of halothane on CYP2E1 in these tissues. Moreover, TFA adducts were present in microsomes of testis and liver and in plasma of halothane-treated rats. The increase in CYP2E1 apoprotein and p-NPH activity observed in testis and liver microsomes suggests that halothane induces its own biotransformation both hepatically and extrahepatically. In addition, the nature of the TFA adducts will depend on the proteins present in each tissue. Also, the presence of TFA adducts in spermatozoa may result from the activation of halothane in the reproductive tract.

Finally, they added that the detailed mechanism of TFA adducts formation and its consequences on the spermatozoa function remain to be fully clarified.

Focusing on the fact that CYP1A2 and CYP2E1 are two of the main cytochrome P450 isoforms involved in the metabolism of commonly used drugs and xenobiotic compounds considered to be responsible for the development of several human diseases, they also could be possible participants. Thus, individual susceptibility to developing these pathologies relies, among other factors, on genetic polymorphisms, which depend on ethnic differences, as the frequency of mutant genotypes varies in different human populations. Accordingly, a study realized by Mendoza-Cantú et al. (2004) investigated the frequency of CYP1A2 5'-flanking region and CYP2E1 *Rsa I/Pst I* polymorphisms in Mexicans by PCR-RFLP methods. They recruited 159 subjects for analyses and mutant allele frequencies of 30% for CYP2E1 *Rsa I/Pst I* sites and 43% for CYP1A2 5'-flanking region were found. They strongly concluded that these frequencies are higher than those previously reported for other human populations.

Continuing with occupational exposure and genetic polymorphisms, Mendoza-Cantú et al. (2006) studied the association between toluene exposure and the CYP2E1 response, as assessed by mRNA content in peripheral lymphocytes or the 6-hydroxychlorzoxazone (6OH-CHZ)/chlorzoxazone (CHZ) quotient (known as CHZ metabolic ratio) in plasma, and the role of genotype (5 -flanking region RsaI/PstI polymorphic sites) in 97 male print workers. Besides, 54% of the study participants were exposed to toluene concentrations that exceeded the maximum permissible exposure level (MPEL). In summary, with further validation, the researchers claimed that CYP2E1 mRNA content in peripheral lymphocytes could be a sensitive and noninvasive biomarker for the continuous monitoring of toluene effects in exposed persons.

Concerning to carcinogenic compounds, cyclohexanol is a basic industrial chemical widely used because of its versatility as an industrial solvent. No studies have been conducted to evaluate the carcinogenic/co-carcinogenic hazards associated to cyclohexanol exposure. Based on this, Márquez-Rosado et al. (2007) researched liver preneoplastic lesions in 344 male Fisher rats which were induced by N-nitrosodiethylamine (150 mg/Kg) i.p., followed by the tumor promoter 2-acetylaminofluorene (2-AAF: 20 mg/kg) orally administered on three consecutive days before partial hepatectomy. The cyclohexanol administration in this hepatocarcinogenesis assay revealed that it has a strong tumor co-promoter potential. There is clear evidence that oxidative stress and the CYP2E1 are components of carcinogenesis. Although no changes in the lipid peroxidation levels were observed between treated and untreated animals, a significant increase in CYP2E1 expression was observed when cyclohexanol was administered 24 h after the last 2-AAF dose. On the other hand, levels of the proliferation markers PCNA and Ki-67 were not increased after treatment with cyclohexanol, but a marked downregulation of the Bax proapoptotic protein was found exclusively in mitochondrial extracts of animals treated with cyclohexanol. Astonishingly, their study represented the first report of the ability of cyclohexanol-induced lesions, when administered simultaneously with 2-AAF, to potentiate the development of preneoplastic liver.

Due to the knowledge that histamine (HA) may bind to cytochrome P450 (CYP450) in rat liver microsomes, the CYP450-HA complex seems to regulate some cellular processes such as proliferation. Therefore, a study leaded by Dávila-Borja et al. (2007) demonstrated that HA increases the activity and protein level of CYP1A1 and CYP2E1, *in vivo*. Since CYP1A1 is associated with polycyclic aromatic hydrocarbon-mediated carcinogenesis and

CYP2E1 with liver damage by oxidative stress. Studies of enzyme kinetics and binding with rat liver microsomes and supersomes were carried out to determine whether HA is a substrate of CYP1A1 and/or a CYP2E1 substrate. The lack of NADPH oxidation in the presence of HA showed that it is not a substrate for CYP1A1. Activity measurements using the O-dealkylation of ethoxyresorufin indicated that HA is a mixed-type inhibitor of CYP1A1 in both microsomes and supersomes. On the other hand, HA induced a significant NADPH oxidation catalyzed by CYP2E1 supersomes, strongly suggesting that HA is a substrate for this isoform. Furthermore, HA is consumed in the presence of CYP2E1-induced microsomes and supersomes, as determined by o-phtalaldehyde complexes with HA by HPLC. Their accurate findings may contribute to a better understanding of the physiological function of CYP450 in relation with inflammation and other physiological processes in which HA may have a relevant role.

Concerning to halomethanes (HMs) and oxidative stress, toxic effects induced by HMs are diverse and include oxidative stress, which is also induced by divalent and polyvalent metals, in mammals. Therefore, a study by Vega-López et al. (2012) found out that high CYP 2E1 and GST theta-like activities were found in viscera of the Toluca silverside Chirostoma riojai from Lake Zumpango (LZ; central Mexico). Formaldehyde, one of the HM metabolites, was correlated with CYP 2E1 activity and also induced lipid peroxidation in viscera. Hepatic CYP 2E1 activity was correlated with GST theta-like activity, suggesting the coupling of both pathways of HM bioactivation and its consequent oxidative damage. Sediment metals, among others, were also responsible for oxidative stress, particularly iron, lead, arsenic and manganese. However, under normal environmental conditions, the antioxidant enzymes of this species sustain catalysis adapted to oxidative stress. Thus, their findings suggested that this fish species apparently has mechanisms of adaptation and recovery that enable it to confront toxic agents of natural origin, such as metals and other substances formed through natural processes, e.g., HMs. This has allowed *C. riojai* to colonize LZ despite the high sensitivity of this species to xenobiotics of anthropogenic origin.

Regarding mosquito mats, Vences-Mejía et al. (2012) assesed the effect of transfluthrin (TF) or D-allethrin (DA) pyrethroid (PYR) vapors, often contained as main ingredients in two commercially available mosquito repellent mats, on cytochrome P450 (CYP) enzymes of rat brain and liver. Immunodetection of CYP2E1 and CYP3A2 proteins revealed their induction in cerebrum and cerebellum, but not in liver microsomes of rats exposed by inhalation to TF or DA. This overexpression of proteins correlated with an increase of their catalytic activities. Therefore, they stated that the specifically increased expression of CYP isoenzymes, due to PYR exposure in the rat brain, could perturb the normal metabolism of endogenous and xenobiotic compounds and leads to increased risks of neurotoxicity by bioactivation, lipid peroxidation and DNA damage.

It is well known that the inducible enzyme CYP2E1 metabolizes several potentially toxic substances including many volatile organic compounds (VOCs). One indirect way to monitor exposure to VOCs may be, therefore, the assessment of CYP2E1 activity in vivo using the chlorzoxazone (CHZ) test, which was employed in the study undertaken by Jiménez-Garza et al. (2012). In their study they compared CYP2E1 activity in two groups of workers: one with a known occupational exposure to VOCs (exposed group) and the other employed in administrative tasks at two universities (control group) from the city of León, Guanajuato, México. To complete the study, (1) passive diffusion monitors were used to evaluate individual levels of exposure to toluene, benzene and ethylbenzene in 48 persons (24 tannery workers and 24 administrative controls) during a 8h work shift; (2) after 12h fasting 500mg CHZ, a selective probe for assessing CYP2E1 activity, was orally administered and, after 2h, a venous blood sample was collected for HPLC plasmatic quantitative determination of CHZ and its mean metabolite 6-hydroxychlorzoxazone. Afterwards, their results were in line with previous findings obtained from shoemakers exposed to various solvents but, interestingly, they were partly in contrast with those of another study in printers. Finally, they concluded that, in spite of the relatively low levels of toluene exposure found for tannery workers, an effect on CYP2E1 activity was evident. Although the mechanism of this interaction is still unknown, the decrease in CYP2E1 activity per se might represent a health risk, considering that these workers may be less protected against other CYP2E1 substrates present in the labor setting or derived from an intentional exposure.

In addition to hepatotoxicity induced by exogenous compounds, induction of CYP2E1 is exerted mainly at posttranscriptional levels through mRNA and protein stabilization, and there is little evidence of xenobiotic induction at the transcriptional level. Therefore, the objective of the study realized by Mejia-Garcia et al. (2013) was to determine whether 2,3,7,8-tetrachlorodibenzo-p-dioxin (TCDD) increased mouse CYP2E1 levels in an AhR-dependent manner and the impact on CCl_4-induced hepatotoxicity. TCDD treatment induced CYP2E1 mRNA and protein levels in mouse liver, and this effect was aryl hydrocarbon receptor (AhR)-dependent. Moreover, TCDD pre-treatment increased the CCl_4-induced alanine aminotransferase (ALT) activity, the extent of CCl_4-induced necrosis, and the number of sinusoidal cells in wild-type animals, while this potentiating effect was not observed in Ahr-null mice. In conclusion, their study accurately revealed that TCDD, probably in an AhR-dependent manner, exacerbated CCl_4-induced hepatotoxicity through induction of CYP2E1.

The development of non-invasive methods aimed to evaluate the effects of many toxicants is required. Although there are some studies conducted in successful ways, a lack of information prevails especially for those substances that could be formed autochthonously in the water bodies, such as halomethanes (HMs). Thus, Dzul-Caamal et al. (2013) studied the induction of pro-oxidant forces (CH_2O, O_2, H_2O_2), oxidative stress (TBARS, RCO) and antioxidant defenses (superoxide dismutase (SOD), catalase (CAT) and glutathione peroxidase (GPx) in the skin mucus layer regarding to the liver of Goodea gracilis exposed to CH_2Cl_2, $CHCl_3$ and $BrCHCl_2$ were also evaluated, in addition to the hepatic cytochrome P450 (CYP 2E1) and glutathione S-transferase theta (GSTT) activities. Regardless of the implicit toxicity involved in the bioactivation of the HMs, carried out by the CYP 2E1 and GST, it was noticeable that this process induces oxidative stress. The usefulness of the mucus layer for the evaluation of the oxidative stress response was demonstrated, despite some peculiar characteristics concerning induction of oxidative stress in liver and skin mucous layer. However, for the understanding of the induction of reactive oxygen species in both targets it is essential to evaluate the activity of antioxidant defenses; otherwise the interpretation of toxic effects elicited by HMs would be erroneous. In the skin mucus layer, lower activities of the enzymes involved in antioxidant defense than in liver were observed. Remarkably, they concluded that the evaluation of the biomarkers in the skin mucus layer involved in the oxidative stress is useful due the consistent response regarding to concentration of the HMs.

It is known that genotoxicity in cells may occur in different ways, direct interaction, production of electrophilic metabolites, and secondary genotoxicity via oxidative stress. Chloroform, dichloromethane, and toluene are primarily metabolized in liver by CYP2E1, producing reactive electrophilic metabolites, and may also produce oxidative stress via the uncoupled CYP2E1 catalytic cycle. Additionally, GSTT1 also participates in dichloromethane activation. Despite the oxidative metabolism of these compounds and the production of oxidative adducts, their genotoxicity in the bone marrow micronucleus test is unclear. Therefore the objective of the work conducted by Belmont-Díaz et al. (2014) was to analyze whether the oxidative metabolism induced by the coexposure to these compounds would account for increased micronucleus frequency. They used an approach including the analysis of phase I, phase II, and antioxidant enzymes, oxidative stress biomarkers, and micronuclei in bone marrow (MNPCE) and hepatocytes (MNHEP). Rats were administered different doses of an artificial mixture of CLF/DCM/TOL, under two regimes. After one administration MNPCE frequency increased in correlation with induced GSTT1 activity and no oxidative stress occurred. Conversely, after three-day treatments oxidative stress was observed, without genotoxicity. In conclusion, the effects they observed indicate that MNPCE by the coexposure to these VOCs could be increased via inducing the activity of metabolism enzymes.

Concerning to aspartame administration in diabetics, a study undertaken by Nosti-Palacios et al. (2014) demonstrated that aspartame consumption and insulin treatment in a juvenile diabetic rat model leads to increase in cytochrome P450 (CYP) 2E1 and CYP3A2 isozymes in brain. Diabetes mellitus was induced in postweaned 21-day-old Wistar male rat by streptozotocin. Animals were randomly assigned to one of the following groups: untreated control, diabetic (D), D-insulin, D-aspartame, or the D-insulin + aspartame-treated group. Brain and liver tissue samples were used to analyze the activity of CYP2E1 and CYP3A2 and protein levels. Their results indicated that combined treatment with insulin and aspartame in juvenile diabetic rats significantly induced CYP2E1 in the cerebrum and cerebellum without modifying it in the liver, while CYP3A2 protein activity increased both in the brain and in the liver. The induction of CYP2E1 in the brain could have important in situ toxicological effects, given that this CYP isoform is capable of bioactivating various toxic substances. Additionally, they concluded that CYP3A2 induction in the liver and brain could be considered a decisive factor in the variation of drug response and toxicity.

In reference to occupational exposure to organic compounds, 1-Bromopropane (1-BP) was introduced into the workplace as an alternative to ozone-depleting solvents and increasingly used in manufacturing industry. The potential exposure to 1-BP and the current reports of adverse effects associated with occupational exposure to high levels of 1-BP have increased the need to understand the mechanism of 1-BP toxicity in animal models as a mean of understanding risk in workers. To reinforce that, the study leaded by Garner et al. (2015) developed a physiologically based pharmacokinetic (PBPK) model for 1-BP in order to examine 2 metabolic pathway assumptions for gas-uptake inhalation study. Based on previous gas-uptake experiments in the Fischer 344 rat, the PBPK model was developed by simulating the 1-BP concentration in a closed chamber. In the model, they tested the hypothesis that metabolism responsibilities were shared by the p450 CYP2E1 and glutathione (GSH) conjugation. Their results showed that 2 metabolic pathways adequately simulated 1-BP closed chamber concentration. Furthermore, the above model was tested by simulating the gas-uptake data of the female rats pretreated with 1-aminobenzotrizole, a general P450 suicide inhibitor, or d,l-buthionine (S,R)-sulfoximine, an inhibitor of GSH synthesis, prior to exposure to 800 ppm 1-BP. Accordingly, they concluded that the comparative investigation on the metabolic pathway of 1-BP through the PBPK modeling in both sexes provides critical information for understanding the role of p450 and GSH in the metabolism of 1-BP and eventually helps to quantitatively extrapolate current animal studies to human.

In relation to CYP2E1 epigenetic regulation, human toluene exposure increases CYP2E1 mRNA and modifies its activity in leucocytes; however, epigenetic implications of this interaction have not been fully investigated. For that reason, a research leaded by Jiménez-Garza et al. (2015) determined promoter methylation of CYP2E1 and other genes known to be affected by toluene exposure. They recruited 48 volunteers, 24 tannery workers exposed to toluene and 24 administrative workers, all of them from the city of León, Guanajuato, México. Afterwards, in the exposed group they found significant correlations between toluene airborne levels and CYP2E1 promoter methylation ($r=-.36$, $p<0.05$), as well as for IL6 promoter methylation levels ($r=.44$, $p<0.05$). Moreover, CYP2E1 promoter methylation levels where higher in toluene-exposed smokers compared to nonsmokers ($p=0.009$). Thus, their results highlighted the importance of considering CYP2E1 epigenetic modifications, as well as its interactions with other genes, as key factors for unraveling the sub cellular mechanisms of toxicity exerted by oxidative stress, which can initiate disease process in chronic, low-level toluene exposure. Therefore, people co-exposed to toluene and tobacco smoke are at higher risk due to a possible CYP2E1 repression.

According to cholesterol and toxicity, obesity and alcohol consumption are risk factors for hepatic steatosis, and both commonly coexist. Due to this, a study conducted by López-Islas et al. (2015) evaluated the effect of ethanol and acetaldehyde on primary hepatocytes obtained from mice fed for two days with a high cholesterol (HC) diet. HC hepatocytes increased lipid and cholesterol content. HC diet sensitized hepatocytes to the toxic effect of ethanol and acetaldehyde. CYP2E1 content increased with HC diet, as well as in those treated with ethanol or acetaldehyde, while the activity of this enzyme determined in microsomes increased in the HC and in all ethanol treated hepatocytes, HC and CW. Oxidized proteins were increased in the HC cultures treated or not with the toxins. Transmission electron microscopy showed stress of the endoplasmic reticulum (ER) and megamitochondria in hepatocytes treated with ethanol as in HC and the ethanol HC treated hepatocytes. ER stress determined by PERK content was increased in ethanol treated hepatocytes from HC mice and CW. Nuclear translocation of ATF6 was observed in HC hepatocytes treated with ethanol, results that indicate that lipids overload and ethanol treatment favor ER stress. Therefore, they concluded that oxidative stress, ER stress, and mitochondrial damage underlie potential mechanisms for increased damage in steatotic hepatocyte treated with ethanol.

Studies with Clinical Applications

It is well known that association studies provide a powerful approach to link DNA variants and genetic predisposition to complex diseases. According to this, a study developed by Montano Loza et al. (2006) determined the genotype and allelic frequencies of genes encoding enzymes involved in alcohol metabolism in alcoholic and nonalcoholic subjects of related ethnicity. A total of 118 individuals of Otomi Mexican Indian ancestry were included. Fifty-nine were chronic alcoholics according to WHO criteria and alcohol dependents according to the Diagnostic and Statistical Manual of Mental Disorders, Fourth Edition (DSM IV) criteria. They were compared to 59 teetotalers or alcohol consumers of <10 g per day. From the studied polymorphisms, a significant difference between alcoholic and nonalcoholic

Otomies was observed only in the CYP2E1/*TaqI*. The common genotype in alcoholics was A1/A2 (54%), and in nonalcoholics the homozygous A2/A2 (63%) (odds ratio [OR]: 0.28; 95% confidence interval [CI]: 0.13-0.60; P=.002). The frequency of the mutant allele A1 was significantly higher in alcoholics than in nonalcoholics (41 vs. 21%; OR: 2.4; 95% CI: 1.3-4.3; P=.003). Their research documented the presence of a polymorphism of CYP2E1 that is overexpressed in alcoholic Otomies, in which the variant allele (A1 of CYP2E1/TaqI) is associated with increased susceptibility to alcoholism. The authors´ appreciation stated that this finding may be an additional factor contributing to the high frequency of liver cirrhosis in Otomies and therefore, would require further investigation.

It is highlighted that a study from Castillejos-López et al. (2008) described an increase of the frequency of Directly Observed Therapy Short-course (DOTS) failure in countries with high rates of mycobacterial drug resistance. This increase could be due to the standardized doses of DOTS results in low or insufficient dosage of drugs in plasma. Several members of cytochrome P450 enzymes superfamily could explain the variations on acetylation velocity and in drug disposition. A population with slow acetylation has a higher risk of toxicity, as that potent inhibition of cytochrome P450 (CYP450) isoforms by isoniazid (CYP2C19 y CYP3A) are dependent of INH plasmatic concentration. This inhibitory effect has been described also for CYP12, CYP2C9 and CYP2E1. INH is metabolized by N-acetyltransferase 2 (NAT2). The wide interethnic and intraethnic variability in acetylation velocity is associated with the polymorphisms of NAT2. Patients with rapid acetylation have plasmatic concentration of INH low or insufficient, which induces treatment failure. In conclusion, the study of genotypes of P450 and NAT2 allowed them to predict therapeutic and individualized dosages.

To reinforce the previously exposed, in a study realized by García-Bañuelos et al. (2012) determined the ADH1B*2, ALDH2*2, and CYP2E1*c2 allele frequencies in healthy control individuals (C) and patients with alcoholic cirrhosis (AC) from western Mexico. Ninety C and 41 patients with AC were studied. Afterwards, they concluded that CYP2E1*c2 allele was associated with susceptibility to AC; meanwhile, ADH1B*2 and ALDH2*2 alleles were not. CYP2E1*c2 allele was associated with AC severity, which could probably be attributed to the oxidative stress promoted by this polymorphic form. Further studies to clearly establish CYP2E1*c2 clinical relevance in the development of alcohol-induced liver damage and its usefulness as a probable prognostic marker, should be performed. Also, increasing the number of patients and including a control group conformed by alcoholic patients free of liver damage may render more conclusive results. Their findings contributed to the understanding of the influence of gene variations in AC development among populations, alcohol metabolism, and pharmacogenetics.

In relation to malignant cell proliferation, lung cancer is the leading cause of cancer mortality in Mexico and worldwide. In the past decade, there has been an increase in the number of lung cancer cases in young people, which suggest an important role for genetic background in the etiology of this disease. Therefore, in a study undertaken by Pérez-Morales et al. (2011) were genetically characterized 16 polymorphisms in 12 low penetrance genes (AhR, CYP1A1, CYP2E1, EPHX1, GSTM1, GSTT1, GSTPI, XRCC1, ERCC2, MGMT, CCND1 and TP53) in 382 healthy Mexican Mestizos as the first step in elucidating the genetic structure of this population and identifying high risk individuals. All of the genotypes analyzed were in Hardy-Weinberg equilibrium, but different degrees of linkage were observed for polymorphisms in the CYP1A1 and EPHX1 genes. The genetic variability of this population was distributed in six clusters that were defined based on their genetic characteristics. The use of a polygenic model to assess the additive effect of low penetrance risk alleles identified combinations of risk genotypes that could be useful in predicting a predisposition to lung cancer. They concluded that estimation of the level of genetic susceptibility showed that the individual calculated risk value (iCRV) ranged from 1 to 16, with a higher iCRV indicating a greater genetic susceptibility to lung cancer.

It has been documented that halomethanes (HMs) can be formed during the chlorination process to obtain drinking water. In liver cells, HMs had been shown to be mutagenic and carcinogenic; however, their bioactivation by CYP 2E1 and GSTT1 is required. Although inhalation is the most common pathway of exposure, reports on the toxic effects induced by HMs in human lung are contradictory. Due to this, a study conducted by Nájera-Martínez et al. (2012) focused on the evaluation of the in vitro cytotoxicity and cell proliferation induced by CH(2)Cl(2), CHCl(3) and BrCHCl(2) in human lung NL20-TA epithelial cells and MRC-5 fibroblasts, and their relationship with CYP 2E1 and GSTT1 activity. High concentrations of these HMs induced cytotoxicity, particularly in cells treated with $BrCHCl_2$. Low concentrations of $BrCHCl_2$ stimulated hyperproliferation of fibroblasts, the most probable consequence of which is regenerative proliferation related to collagen induction. Fibroblasts exposed to $BrCHCl_2$ exhibited low levels of CYP 2E1 activity suggesting that released bromine is able to alter this activity by affecting the active site or auto regulating the activity itself. GSTT1 was up to ten times more active than CYP 2E1 in both cell lines, indicating that potential lung damage is due to formation of pro-carcinogens such as formaldehyde.

In reference to tumor tissues, intratumoral expression of genes encoding Cytochrome P450 enzymes (CYP) might play a critical role not only in cancer development but also in the metabolism of anticancer drugs. Then, a study undertaken by Molina-Ortiz et al. (2014) aimed to compare the mRNA expression patterns of seven representative CYPs in paired tumor and normal tissue of child patients with rabdomyosarcoma (RMS). Using real time quantitative RT-PCR, the gene expression pattern of CYP1A1, CYP1A2, CYP1B1, CYP2E1, CYP2W1, CYP3A4, and CYP3A5 were analyzed in tumor and adjacent non-tumor tissues from 13 child RMS patients. Their data showed that the expression levels of CYP1A1 and CYP1A2 were negligible. Elevated expression of CYP1B1 mRNA and protein was detected in most RMS tumors and adjacent normal tissues. Most cancerous samples exhibited higher levels of both CYP3A4 and CYP3A5 compared to normal tissue samples. Expression of CYP2E1 mRNA was found to be significantly higher in tumor tissue, however no relation was found with protein levels. CYP2W1 mRNA and/or protein are mainly expressed in tumors. In conclusion, they defined the CYP gene expression profile in tumor and paired normal tissue of child patients with RMS. The overexpression of CYP2W1, CYP3A4 and CYP3A5 in tumor tissues suggested that they may be involved in RMS chemoresistance; furthermore, they may be exploited for the localized activation of anticancer prodrugs.

In relation to structural and energetic analysis, docking and molecular dynamics (MD) simulation have been two computational techniques used to gain insight about the substrate orientation within protein active sites, allowing to identify potential residues involved in the binding and catalytic mechanisms. For those reasons, in a study realized by Bello et al. (2014) they combined both methods to predict the regioselectivity in the binding mode of valproic acid (VPA) on three cytochrome P-450 (CYP) isoforms CYP2C9, CYP2C11, and CYP2E1, which are involved in the biotransformation of VPA yielding reactive hepatotoxic intermediate 2-n-propyl-4-pentenoic acid (4nVPA). Therefore, the complexes between these

CYP isoforms and VPA or 4nVPA were studied to explore their differences in binding and energetic stabilization. Docking results showed that VPA and 4nVPA are coupled into CYPs binding site in a similar conformation, but it does not explain the VPA hydrogen atom abstraction. On the other hand, MD simulations showed a set of energetic states that reorient VPA at the first ns, then making it susceptible to a dehydrogenation reaction. For 4nVPA, multiple binding modes were observed in which the different states could favor either undergo other reaction mechanism or ligand expulsion from the binding site. Otherwise, the energetic and entropic contribution pointed out a similar behavior for the three CYP complexes, showing as expected a more energetically favorable binding free energy for the complexes between CYPs and VPA than with 4nVPA.

It is well known that alcohol abuse represents the major identified etiological factor of cirrhosis in México. ADH1B, ALDH2, and CYP2E1 have been considered candidate genes in alcohol-related diseases. Controversial results probably due to ethnic differences, among other factors, have been reported. Mexican Mestizos (MES) derive from the combination of indigenous, Spaniard, and African genes. Huichols (HUI) constitute an indigenous group from western Mexico with no racial admixture. According to the latter exposed, a research conducted by Gordillo-Bastidas et al. (2010) evaluated ADH1B*2, ALDH2*2, and CYP2E1*c2 allele frequencies in healthy Huicholes (HUI) and Mestizos (MES) from western Mexico. Lipid and hepatic profile were also carried out. One hundred and one HUI and 331 MES subjects were studied. Hepatic profile was normal in both groups. HUI showed a better lipid profile than MES independently of genotype. Huichols exhibited the highest CYP2E1*c2 allele frequency of the world documented up to that date; meanwhile, ADH1B*2 and ALDH2*2 were practically absent. This feature could be useful in the understanding of Mexican population gene composition, alcohol metabolism, and alcoholic liver disease development. However, this research group claimed that further association studies are necessary. The heterogeneity of Mexican population was evident by the significantly different distribution of CYP2E1*c2 allele observed among different regions of the country. Lipid and hepatic values were not associated to genotype. This report constituted the first study dealing with gene polymorphisms of alcohol metabolizing enzymes conducted in HUI.

A review realized by Sosa-Macías and Llerena (2013) in relation to genetic polymorphisms of the cytochrome P450 (CYP) genes in Mexican indigenous populations, who are part of the wide ethnic diversity of this country. These native groups have a particular historical trajectory, different from the Mexican Mestizos. This variability may be reflected in the frequency distribution of polymorphisms in the CYP genes that encode enzymes involved in the metabolism of drugs and other xenobiotics. Therefore, these polymorphisms may affect drug efficacy and safety in indigenous populations in Mexico. So, their study aimed to analyze the prevalence of CYP polymorphisms in indigenous Mexicans and compare their results with studies in Mexican Mestizos. Because the extrapolation of pharmacogenetic data from Mestizos is not applicable to the majority of indigenous groups, pharmacogenetic studies directed at indigenous populations need to be developed. Amerindians analyzed in this study showed a low phenotypic (CYP2D6) and genotypic (CYP2D6, CYP2C9) diversity, unlike Mexican Mestizos. The frequency of polymorphisms in the CYP1A1, CYP2C19, CYP2E1, and CYP3A4 genes was more similar among the Amerindians and Mexican Mestizos, with the exception of the CYP1A2 gene, which *1F variant frequency in Mexican Amerindians was the highest described until that date.

LATIN AMERICAN STUDIES OF GENETIC POLYMORPHISMS IN PHASE II ENZYMES

Conjugation reactions play a major role in drug metabolism detoxification. Due to their importance, a total of 24 studies have been conducted in Latin America. Focused on the study of Arylamine N-acetyltransferases (NATs) are 11 documents; also, there are 5 studies for Glutathion-S-Transaminase (GST); only 2 studies about UDP-glucuronosyltransferase (UGT); there are 5 studies for Thiopurine methyltransferase (TPMT), and just 1 study focused on P-glycoprotein (ABCB1) and (ABCC5).

N-Acetyl Tranferases (NAT)

Human biodiversity originates partially from human microevolution, which has produced different populations. This biodiversity is responsible for most of the variability in drug response. Therefore, a study conducted by Jorge and Arias (1995) pointed out the presentation of the methodology employed in population pharmacology studies and general information about the CYP2D6 and NAT2 systems was also given. Their report comprised the results obtained in Embera and Ngawbe Amerindians, who are characterized by a low phenotypic and genotypic CYP2D6 diversity. In regard to NAT2, Amerindians are distinguished by a high allelic frequency of S3 and low ones of S1 and S2, situation that is reversed in Caucasians.

According to research conducted in Amerindians from Central America, Jorge-Nebert et al. (2002) evaluated Six NAT2 single-nucleotide polymorphisms (SNPs) in 105 unrelated Ngawbe and 136 unrelated Embera Amerindians (482 chromosomes) by SNP-specific polymerase chain reaction analysis. 282C>T was the most common synonymous mutation, while 857G>A was the most frequent nonsynonymous inactivating exchange. The allelic frequency of the NAT2*5 series (containing the 341T>C exchange) was 2.4% and 9.9% for Ngawbe and Embera, respectively, five- to 20-times lower than that in Caucasians. The NAT2*6 series (590G>A) showed allelic frequencies of 0% and 3.7%, eight- to 30-times lower than in Caucasians. On the other hand, the NAT2*7 series, characterized by mutation 857G>A, had allelic frequencies (23.3% and 22.8%) that were 10-20-times higher in Amerindians than in Caucasians. Amerindians are characterized by decreased genetic diversity because they display a low number of mutated alleles (four and five for Ngawbe and Embera, respectively) that are present at low proportions (27.6% and 39%), reduced genotypic variability (seven out of 15 and 12 out of 21 possible genotypes) and low heterozygosity (40% and 55.1%) at the NAT2 locus. The NAT2 phenotype was evaluated with caffeine in a subset of 72 Embera. There were no disagreements between genotype and phenotype among rapid and slow acetylators (13/72, 18%). They concluded that, in the Embera, the analysis of three inactivating mutations was sufficient to predict the phenotype in more than 99.5% of these subjects. NAT2 would appear to be of a selectively neutral character given that there was no evidence of adaptation to the prevailing ecology in Amerindians.

In relation to damage biomarkers, Montero et al. (2003) evaluated micronuclei and other biomarkers in oral cells from 11- to 16-year-old girls living in a foster home in the central area of México City. Variables analyzed for possible association with these biomarkers included smoking habits, body mass index, metabolic polymorphisms for NAT1 and GSTM1 and whether the cells were obtained from the cheek or pharynx. Their results indicated that individuals having the NAT1*10 homozygous genotype showed a significant increase in chromatin buds and binucleated cells. When the damage in the cheek was compared with damage in the pharynx, a significant increase in micronuclei and binucleated cells was found for the latter tissue in all the individuals analyzed.

In reference to individualized therapy, different patients exhibit wide variability in the way they respond to medications. Individual differences in drug response can result from environmental factors, as well as genetic determinants. In particular, inherited differences in the metabolism and disposition of drugs can have a great influence on the efficacy and toxicity of medications. Therefore, a study conducted in Mexico by López-López et al. (2004) focused on the pharmacogenetics of drug metabolism. High-through-put genomic technologies serve as the foundation of personalized therapies. Finally, the authors concluded that knowledge of an individual's genetic variability in drug response may be clinically and economically important and could provide the basis for a rational approach to drug prescription in neuropsychiatric disorders.

In accordance with therapeutic failure related to conjugation enzymes, a study conducted by Castillejos-López et al. (2008) described an increase of the frequency of Directly Observed Therapy Short-course (DOTS) failure in countries with high rates of mycobacterial drug resistance. This increase could be due to the standardized doses of DOTS results in low or insufficient dosage of drugs in plasma. Several members of cytochrome P450 enzymes superfamily could explain the variations on acetylation velocity and in drug disposition. A population with slow acetylation has a higher risk of toxicity, as that potent inhibition of cytochrome P450 (CYP450) isoforms by isoniazid (CYP2C19 y CYP3A) are dependent of INH plasmatic concentration. This inhibitory effect has been described also for CYP12, CYP2C9 and CYP2E1. INH is metabolized by N-acetyltransferase 2 (NAT2). The wide interethnic and intraethnic variability in acetylation velocity is associated with the polymorphisms of NAT2. Patients with rapid acetylation have plasmatic concentration of INH low or insufficient which induces treatment failure. The study of genotypes of P450 and NAT2 allowed the investigators to predict therapeutic and individualized dosages.

Focusing on adverse reactions, isoniazid (INH) is a drug extensively used as a prophylactic and therapeutic agent for human tuberculosis (TB). INH is metabolized by the enzymatic activity of N-acetyltransferase 2 (NAT2). Numerous studies have established the correlation between the acetylator phenotype and the NAT2 genotype in several populations; however, little is known regarding Latin-American populations and the pharmacogenetics of NAT2. Therefore, a study realized by Díaz-Molina et al. (2008) aimed to report the molecular genotyping of the NAT2 gene, the acetylator phenotype, and the incidence of INH-related adverse reactions in a group of 25 Mexican individuals enrolled in a prophylactic protocol for TB. Using both, the NAT2 genotyping and acetylation phenotyping approach, they found a ratio of 69.2 and 30.8% of slow and fast acetylators, respectively. Concordance with the NAT2 genotype and phenotype classification was 88% in the bimodal model. Regarding INH-related adverse reactions, only 2 individuals (8%) exhibited declared gastric intolerance. In their study group, they found an association between the NAT2 genotype and acetylator phenotype (OR=7.78, 95% CI, 0.87-87.98, Fisher's exact test, $p<0.05$), but did not find any genotype or phenotype association with the incidence of INH-related adverse reactions (Fisher's exact test, $p>0.05$).

Related to pharmacogenetics screening, specific information about the population pharmacogenetics can be the starting point to study the inheritance of these traits, to design individual drug therapy, and to develop new drugs rationally. Thus, a study realized by Ramos et al. (2011) reported the distribution of NAT2, TPMT, and MTHFR gene polymorphisms in Baja California, Mexico. They found that their population sample exhibited allele and genotype frequencies that are highly similar to those observed in Caucasian populations; although it should be noted that there are slight similarities with those determined in other populations. As allelic variants of drug-metabolizing enzymes are prevalent in their studied population, they concluded that it is important to consider pharmacogenetic testing as part of the standard diagnostic protocols before medication.

It is well known that N-acetyltransferase 2 (NAT2) catalyzes the bioactivation and/or detoxification of drugs and carcinogens. Therefore, a study conducted by Taja-Chayeb et al. (2011) aimed to establish the correlation between the NAT2 genotype and the acetylating phenotype in a Mexican population using sulfamethazine as a probe. From a total of 122 individuals, 73 (59.8%) were slow and 49 (40.2%) were fast acetylators. Eleven individuals (9%) had the wild-type genotype (NAT2*4/NAT2*4). The most frequent genotype was NAT2*4/NAT2*5B observed in 20.66% of individuals. In conclusion, their results showed that an accurate prediction of the acetylation phenotype by genotyping can be achieved in around half of the population. Further studies with a larger number of individuals are required to establish correlations between phenotype and genotype in half of patients having a genotype combined with slow/rapid alleles.

In the same matter, another study leaded by Taja-Chayeb et al. (2012) aimed to examine the distribution and frequency of NAT2 genotypes in the Mexican population. Among 250 samples were amplified and sequenced for the NAT2 gene. They found seven different SNPs; the most frequent allele was 803 A>G (35.8%), followed by 282 C>T, 341 T>C, and 481 C>T. There were no differences in the distribution of SNPs between healthy subjects and cancer patients. These eight polymorphisms defined 26 diplotypes; 11.6% were wild type (NAT2*4/NAT2*4), while the most common diplotype was NAT2*4/NAT2*5B, present in 17.2%. They did not identify other common polymorphisms. Their results were compared with the NAT2 SNPs reported from other populations. All but the Turkish population was significantly different from theirs. Finally, they concluded that the mixed-race Mexican population requires special attention because NAT2 genotype frequencies differ from those in other regions of the world.

Additionally, a study conducted by Salazar-González et al. (2014) in a Mexican Mestizo population evaluated NAT2 expression at the protein level in immune cells, as well as the distribution and frequency of six NAT2 SNPs and their association with anti-TB therapy, by measuring the plasma levels of INH and Acetyl-INH (AcINH). They performed genotyping assays of NAT2 SNPs in 40 TB patients and 121 healthy volunteers by real-time PCR. The phenotypes obtained in the healthy volunteers were as follows; 18.87% of subjects had the rapid acetylator phenotype, 45.45% had the intermediate phenotype and 39.66% exhibited the slow acetylator phenotype. In the TB patient group, 35% of patients had the rapid acetylator phenotype, 32.5% were intermediate and 32.5% showed the slow acetylator phenotype. A high correspondence between the rapid and slow acetylator phenotype with MR was demonstrated. In conclusion, the 282C>T, 341T>C, 481C>T, 590G>A, 803A>G, 857G>A

SNPs of NAT2 gene provides accurate prediction of the acetylator phenotype in Mexican mestizo population. A statistical difference was found in frequency of rapid metabolizer phenotype, which was higher in TB patients. In addition, the expression of NAT2 protein in immune cells can lead to further studies related to its functional role in the innate immune response against M. tuberculosis and other xenobiotics metabolized by this enzyme.

It is well documented that NAT2 polymorphisms lead to three phenotypes: rapid, intermediate and slow acetylators. Thus, the study realized by Bisso-Machado et al. (2015) aimed to research NAT2 diversity in Native Americans. NAT2 exon 2 was sequenced for 286 individuals from 21 populations (Native American and American Mestizos). Excluding the basal/rapid haplotype NAT2*4, the most frequent haplotypes are NAT2*5B (35.95%) in hunter-gatherers and NAT2*7B (20.61%) and NAT2*5B (19.08%) in agriculturalists that were related to the slow phenotype. A new haplotype was identified in two Amerindians. Data from the ~44 kb region surrounding NAT2 in 819 individuals from Africa, East-Asia, Europe and America were used in additional analyses. No significant differences in the acetylator NAT2 haplotype and phenotype distributions were found between Native American populations practicing farming and/or herding and those practicing hunting and gathering, probably because of the absence or weakness of selection pressures and presence of demographic and random processes preventing detection of any selection signal.

Glutathione S-Transferases (GSTs)

It has extensively documented that Glutathione S-transferase (GST) is a dimeric detoxifying isoenzyme, involved in the deactivation of carcinogens, several tobacco-derived carcinogens, and xenobiotics. Thus, a research conducted by Gallegos-Arreola et al. (2003-2004) studied the distribution of GSTT1 gene deletion in peripheral blood DNA samples from 178 healthy controls (41 nonsmokers, 63 passive smokers and 74 smokers) and 52 lung cancer patients. Comparisons between groups showed that there was an increased lung cancer risk for individuals with the GSTT1 null genotype. Cancer patients showed significant differences when compared with controls: nonsmokers, passive smokers, and smokers. Twenty-one percent of lung cancer patients carried the deletion versus 2% among nonsmokers not exposed to passive smoking, 6% among passive smokers, and 5% among smokers. Thus, there is a significant association between this genotype and the possibility to risk of developing lung cancer.

Due to the fact that GST-T1 and GST-M1 null genotypes have been responsible for interindividual variations in the metabolism of arsenic, a known human carcinogen, a study leaded by Drobná et al. (2012) aimed to assess the specific GST genotypes in the Mexican population chronically exposed to arsenic. To achieve that, they have developed a multiplex High Resolution Melting PCR (HRM-PCR) analysis using a LightCycler480 instrument. Using this newly developed multiplex HRM-PCR analysis, they evaluated GST-T1 and GST-M1 genotypes in 504 DNA samples isolated from the blood of individuals residing in Zimapan, Lagunera, and Chihuahua regions in Mexico. They found that the Zimapan and Lagunera populations have similar GST-T1 and GST-M1 genotype frequencies which differ from those of the Chihuahua population. In addition, 14 individuals have been identified as carriers of the double null genotype, i.e., null genotypes in both GST-T1 and GST-M1 genes. Although this procedure did not distinguish between biallelic (+/+) and monoallelic (+/-)

genotypes, it can be used in an automated workflow as a simple, sensitive, and time and money saving procedure for rapid identification of the GST-T1 and GST-M1 positive or null genotypes.

In relation to pollutants present in food, breast milk can also be a potential source of pollutants. Mothers can be exposed to different contaminants as a result of their lifestyle and environmental pollution. Mercury (Hg) and arsenic (As) could adversely affect the development of fetal and neonatal nervous system. Some fish and shellfish are rich in selenium (Se), an essential trace element that forms part of several enzymes related to the detoxification process, including glutathione S-transferase (GST). Due to the previously exposed, a study realized by Gaxiola-Robles et al. (2014) determined the interaction between Hg, As and Se and analyzed its effect on the activity of GST in breast milk. Milk samples were collected from women between day 7 and 10 postpartum. The GST activity was determined spectrophotometrically; total Hg, As and Se concentrations were measured by atomic absorption spectrometry. To explain the possible association of Hg, As and Se concentrations with GST activity in breast milk, generalized linear models were constructed. The model explained 44% of the GST activity measured in breast milk. The GLM suggested that GST activity was positively correlated with Hg, As and Se concentrations. They concluded that the activity of the enzyme was also explained by the frequency of consumption of marine fish and shellfish in the diet of the breastfeeding women.

Concerning pregnancy disorders in humans, a study realized by Sandoval-Carrillo et al. (2014) researched the relationship between null alleles of the glutathione S-transferases (GST) M1 and T1 genes and the risk of preeclampsia. This case-control study involved 112 preeclamptic and 233 normoevolutive pregnant women. The null polymorphisms were genotyped by multiplex polymerase chain reaction (PCR). Their results showed an increased risk of preeclampsia in patients with the GSTT1 null genotype [odds ratio (OR) = 2.21; 95% confidence interval (CI) = 1.14-4.27; P = 0.018]. Their data further showed that a combination of deletion genotypes of the GSTM1 and GSTT1 genes conferred an even higher risk of preeclampsia (OR = 4.56, 95%CI = 1.59-13.09; P = 0.005). Their results provided the first evidence suggesting that a GSTT1 null polymorphism might be associated with preeclampsia in the Mexican mestizo population, and that this risk increases with the combination of both GSTT1 and GSTM1 null polymorphisms.

According to carcinogen detoxification, Jaramillo-Rangel et al. (2015) recently determined the frequencies of polymorphisms in the genes GSTM1, GSTT1, GSTP1, and GSTM3 and also investigated whether an association existed between these genes and breast cancer risk in subjects from northeastern Mexico. Genotypes were determined in 243 women with histologically confirmed breast cancer and 118 control subjects. Gene polymorphisms were analyzed using a DNA microarray. They found an increased breast cancer risk associated to GSTM1 gene deletion polymorphism (OR = 2.19; 95%CI = 1.50-3.21; P = 0.001). No associations between GSTT1, GSTP1, and GSTM3 genotypes and neoplasia risk were observed. In conclusion, they determined the genotype distribution of GST polymorphisms in control subjects and in breast cancer patients from northeastern Mexico. The GSTM1 null genotype was associated to breast cancer risk. Their findings may be used to individualize breast cancer screening and therapeutic intervention in Mexican Mestizo population, which displays ethnic characteristics that differentiate it from other populations in Mexico.

UDP-Glucuronyl Transferases 1 (UGT1)

As stated in literature, UDP-glucuronosyltransferase 1A4 (UGT1A4) is a phase II drug-metabolizing enzyme that catalyzes the glucuronidation of many clinically-important drugs. Moreover, interethnic differences in the genetic polymorphism of UGT1A4 have been reported; however, there is no information in Mexican Mestizos (MMs) and Spaniards (SPs). Furthermore, MM is an admixed population with 26% of Caucasian genes mainly from Spain. Therefore, a study conducted by López M, et al. (López et al., 2013) aimed to investigate the potential differences between 318 SPs and 248 MMs healthy individuals regarding UGT1A4*1b, UGT1A4*2 and UGT1A4*3 alleles and to compare the observed frequencies with those previously reported in different populations. The allelic frequencies of the three UGT1A4 polymorphisms showed interethnic differences between MMs and SPs ($p < 0.05$). The analyzed SNPs variants in this genetic region were not in linkage disequilibrium (LD) for the MM population, suggesting that these mutations have arisen independently in the same genetic background. In contrast, UGT1A4*2 and UGT1A4*3 were in LD in the SP population. Comparison of their data with other in different ethnic groups revealed that the frequencies of UGT1A4*2 and UGT1A4*3 in SP were similar to other Caucasians and higher than in Asians, whereas in MMs were lower than in Caucasians and higher than in Asians only for UGT1A4*2. Their results could be helpful to improve the use of UGT1A4 drug substrates in order to adjust them to the ethnic background of a given population, specifically for Hispanics.

Studies of pharmacogenomics-related traits are increasingly being performed to identify loci that affect either drug response or susceptibility to adverse drug reactions. However, the effect of the polymorphisms can differ in magnitude or be absent depending on the population being assessed. Therefore, in a study conducted by Bonifaz-Peña et al. (2014) they used the Affymetrix Drug Metabolizing Enzymes and Transporters (DMET) Plus array to characterize the distribution of polymorphisms of pharmacogenetics and pharmacogenomics (PGx) relevance in two samples from the most populous Latin American countries, Brazil and Mexico. The sample from Brazil included 268 individuals from the southeastern state of Rio de Janeiro, and was stratified into census categories. The sample from Mexico comprised 45 Native American Zapotecas and 224 self-identified Mestizo individuals from 5 states located in geographically distant regions in Mexico. They evaluated the admixture proportions in the Brazilian and Mexican samples using a panel of Ancestry Informative Markers extracted from the DMET array, which was validated with genome-wide data. A substantial variation in ancestral proportions across census categories in Brazil, and geographic regions in Mexico was identified. They evaluated the extent of genetic differentiation (measured as FST values) of the genetic markers of the DMET Plus array between the relevant parental populations. Although the average levels of genetic differentiation are low, there is a long tail of markers showing large frequency differences, including markers located in genes belonging to the Cytochrome P450, Solute Carrier (SLC) and UDP-glucuronyltransferase (UGT) families as well as other genes of PGx relevance such as ABCC8, ADH1A, CHST3, PON1, PPARD, PPARG, and VKORC1. In conclusion their study showed how differences in admixture history may have an important impact in the distribution of allele and genotype frequencies at the population level.

Thiopurine Methyl Transferase (TPMT)

It is well documented that, Thiopurine methyltransferase (TPMT) catalyzes the inactivation of thiopurine drugs (mercaptopurine, thioguanine and azathioprine) used to treat acute lymphoblastic leukemia, autoimmune diseases and recipients of transplanted organs. Therefore, a study conducted by Isaza et al. (2003) aimed to determine the frequency of the four allelic variants of the TPMT gene, TPMT*2 (G238C), TPMT*3A (G460A and A719G), TPMT*3B (G460A) and TPMT*3C (A719G), in 140 Colombian volunteers of Mestizo origin. They found that 92.1% and 7.9% of the Colombian population corresponded to the phenotypes high and intermediate methylators, respectively. Their results showed that the frequency of mutations and the allelic distribution of the TPMT gene in the Colombian population are similar to the genetic profile found among US and European Caucasian populations, where the *3A allele is prevalent and the *2 allele is currently present.

Accordingly, polymorphisms at the thiopurine S-methyltransferase coding gene (TPMT) determine enzyme activity and consequently, the development of toxicity secondary to thiopurines. Thus, the research leaded by Taja-Chayeb et al. (2008) aimed to analyze 108 DNA samples from volunteer donors and 39 from patients with acute lymphoblastic leukemia (ALL). Their results showed a frequency of functional allele polymorphisms was 17.6%, being the most frequent *3A (n = 13; 4.4%), followed by *3B (n = 5; 1.7%), *3C (n = 5; 1.7%), and *2 (n = 3; 1.0%). From 39 ALL patients, 22 were treated with thiopurines, and five from 10 with a functional polymorphism developed hematological toxicity (4 mild, 1 severe in a patient referred to our Hospital after developing pancytopenia while on treatment with thiopurine). Finally, they concluded that this was the first analysis of the polymorphisms at this gene in Mexican population. Since a direct relation has been documented within functional polymorphisms and enzyme activity, and DHPLC is a highly sensitive, rapid and efficient method, feasible to realize in any phase during treatment of ALL patients, the typing routine of TPMT polymorphisms in ALL patients has been set in their Institution.

As stated in literature, thiopurine S-methyltransferase (TPMT) is a cytosolic enzyme that catalyzes the S-methylation of 6-mercaptopurine and azathioprine. Since ethnic differences in the TPMT genetic polymorphisms have been demonstrated worldwide, a study conducted by Alvarez et al. (2009) researched ethnic differences in the TPMT gene in the Chilean population. The frequency of four allelic variants of the TPMT gene, *2 (G238C), *3A (G460A and A719G), *3B (G460A) and *3C (A719G) were analyzed in 210 Chilean blood donors. They found that the TPMT variants associated to low enzymatic activity, were detected in 16 subjects (8%), who had a heterozygous genotype (*3A in 12; *3C in three and *2 in one subject). No TPMT*3B allelic variant was found. The normal allele (wild-type) was found in 92% of the studied individuals. Finally, they concluded that the allele TPMT*3A, was the most prevalent in th group of Chilean blood donors, as in Caucasian populations.

According to literature, Thiopurine S-methyltransferase (TPMT) is involved in the toxicity and therapeutic efficacy of thiopurine drugs, and its gene exhibits genetic polymorphisms that differ across diverse populations. Four TPMT polymorphisms (TPMT*2, *3A, *3B and *3C) account for 80-95% of alleles that cause reduced enzyme activity. To date, only a single study in the Mexican population involving 108 individuals has been performed, but the regional and ethnic origin of this population was not described. Moreover, information about the TPMT polymorphism in the Mexican population is limited. Therefore, a study conducted by González-Del Angel et al. (2009) determined the TPMT allele and genotype frequencies in a sample of newborns from Mexico City. Three hundred and sixty DNA samples from unrelated, anonymous individuals were obtained from dried blood spots collected on filter paper as part of the Newborn Screening National Program. Their findings reported that from 720 TPMT alleles analysed, 49 (6.81%) were deficiency alleles. The most common deficiency allele was TPMT*3A (5.69%), followed by TPMT*3C (0.56%), TPMT*3B (0.28%) and TPMT*2 (0.28%). Forty-five newborns were heterozygous for one mutant allele (12.5%) and two showed a genotype with two deficiency alleles (0.56%). Despite its unique ethnic composition, their Mexican population exhibited variant allele frequencies that were similar to some Caucasian populations. Finally, their data suggested that approximately 1 in 180 persons born in Mexico City might have low or undetectable TPMT enzyme activity, a frequency that, overall, is somewhat higher than that reported for Caucasian populations generally (1 in 300).

Literature reports state that Thiopurine S-Methyltransferase (TPMT) catalyses the S-methylation of thiopurine drugs, such as 6-mercaptopurine, 6-thioguanine and azathioprine, leading to their inactivation. Individuals who carry TPMT allele variants are more likely to experience life-threatening toxicity when these drugs are given at a standard dose. Wildtype phenotype TPMT*1 exhibits high level of catalytic activity, while all variants manifest decreased enzymatic activity. Ethnic-related differences in the distribution of TPMT variant alleles have been found. In Mexico, limited information is available; so far only two studies have been published and clear differences exist between them. Therefore, a study leaded by Moreno-Guerrero et al. (2013) focused on the determination of allelic variants and genotypes of the TPMT gene in 240 Mexican children with leukemia and solid tumors using DNA extracted from peripheral blood. Results showed that Homozygous wild-type genotype TPMT*1/TPMT*1 was found in 173 patients (72.1%); 67 cases (27.9%) were heterozygous: 18 with genotype TPMT*1/TPMT*3B (7.5%), 17 TPMT*1/TPMT*3C (7.1%), 16 TPMT*1/TMPT*2 (6.7%), 14 TPMT*1/TPMT*3A (5.8%), and 2 (0.8%) were homozygous for two variants: TPMT*2/ TPMT*3B in both groups. The allele frequencies were TPMT*1 in 411 (85.62%), TPMT*3B in 20 (4.1%), TPMT*2 in 18 (3.75%), TPMT*3C in 17 (3.55%) and TPMT*3A in 14 (2.9%). They concluded that a high frequency and diversity of variant TPMT genotypes was found in their series with predominance of the TPMT*3B allele.

It has been stated that folate metabolism plays an essential role in the processes of DNA synthesis and methylation. Deviations in the folate flux resulting from single-nucleotide polymorphisms in genes encoding folate-dependent enzymes may affect the susceptibility to leukemia. Therefore, a study conducted by Gutiérrez- Álvarez et al. (2016) aimed to assess associations among MTHFR (C677T, A1298C) and TPMT (*2, *3A) mutations as well as to evaluate the synergistic effects of combined genotypes for both genes. They recruited 70 children with acute lymphoblastic leukemia, ALL, and 152 age-matched controls (range, 1-15 years). They found that the frequency of the MTHFR A1298C CC genotype was statistically significant (odds ratio [OR], 6.48; 95% 95% confidence intervals [CI], 1.26-33.2; p=0.025). In addition, the combined 677CC+1298AC genotype exhibited a statistically significant result (OR, 0.23; 95% CI, 0.06-0.82; p=0.023). No significant results were obtained from the MTHFR (C677T CT, C677T TT) or TPMT (*2, *3A) genotypes. More importantly, no association between the synergistic effects of either gene (MTHFR and/or TPMT) and susceptibility to ALL was found. Finally, they concluded that the MTHFR A1298C CC genotype was associated with an increased risk of developing childhood ALL. However, a decreased risk to ALL with the combination of MTHFR 677CC+1298AC genotypes was found.

Drug Transporters

ABCB1 y ABCC5

The drug of choice for acute lymphoblastic leukemia (ALL) treatment is methotrexate, which has been associated with a high risk of adverse reactions (ADRs). The xanthine oxidase (XO) polymorphisms, 1936A>G and 2107A>G, as well as the polymorphic variants derived from ATP-binding cassette transporter gene subfamilies, ABCB1 and ABCC5, of drug resistant codifying genes, are implicated as precursors of drug-related neurologic, hepatic, and renal toxicities. Thus, a study conducted by Zaruma-Torres et al. (2015) determined whether the mentioned polymorphisms are risk or protective factors for the development of adverse reactions by methotrexate in their ALL pediatric population. They recruited a total of 35 Mexican children from Centro Estatal de Cancerología-Durango, Mexico diagnosed with ALL. At the same time, a 12-month drug monitoring program was conducted in accordance with WHO-PAHO guidelines for pharmacovigilance. Thus, their results highlighted that the ABCB11936A>G and 2107A>G and ABCC5 3414+434A>C polymorphisms were not associated with methotrexate ADRs. Moreover, single nucleotide polymorphisms (SNPs) of ABCB1 1236C>T (OR 0.19, 95% CI: 0.03-0.9, $p<0.05$) and ABCC5 3933+313T>C (OR 0.12, 95% CI: 0.027-0.58, $p<0.05$) were associated with methotrexate ADRs. Finally, they concluded that SNPs 1236C>T of ABCB1 and ABCC5 3933+313T>C are not associated with the development of typical ADRs by methotrexate, rather, they showed a protective factor for myelosuppression in the studied sick population.

References

Aceves Avila FJ, Esquivel Nava GA, Gallegos Arreola MP, Gómez Meda B, Zúñiga González G, Ramos-Remus. Cyclophosphamide boluses induce micronuclei expression in buccal mucosa cells of patients with systemic lupus erythematosus independent of cytochrome P450 2D6 status. *J Rheumatol.* 2004 Jul; 31(7): 1335-9.

Aguilar B, Rojas JC, Collados MT. Prevalence of CYP2C9 variants in the Mexican population. *Arch Med Res.* 2008 May; 39(4): 463.

Agúndez JA, Ramirez R, Hernandez M, Llerena A, Benítez J. Molecular heterogeneity at the CYP2D gene locus in Nicaraguans: impact of gene-flow from Europe. *Pharmacogenetics.* 1997 Aug;7(4): 337-40.

Alcazar-González GA, Calderón-Garcidueñas AL, Garza-Rodríguez ML, Rubio-Hernández G, Escorza-Treviño S, Olano-Martin E, Cerda-Flores RM, Castruita-Avila AL, González-Guerrero JF, le Brun S, Simon-Buela L, Barrera-Saldaña HA.. Comparative study of polymorphism frequencies of the CYP2D6, CYP3A5, CYP2C8 and IL-10 genes in Mexican and Spanish women with breast cancer. *Pharmacogenomics.* 2013; 14(13):1583-92.

Alvarez L L, Venegas S M, Larrondo L M, Becerra B N, Castro L A, Quera P R. [Thiopurine S-methyltransferase gene polymorphism in Chilean blood donors]. *Rev Med Chil.* 2009; 137(2): 185-92.

Alvarez-González I, Madrigal-Bujaidar E, Dorado V, Espinosa-Aguirre JJ.Inhibitory effect of naringin on the micronuclei induced by ifosfamide in mouse, and evaluation of its modulatory effect on the Cyp3A subfamily. *Mutat Res.* 2001 480-481:171-8.

Arias TD, Jorge LF, Inaba T. No evidence for the presence of por metabolizers of spartein in an Amerindian group: the Cuinas of Panama. *Br J Clin Pharmac* 1986; 21: 547-548.

Asteinza J, Camacho-Carranza R, Reyes-Reyes RE, Dorado-González V V, Espinosa-Aguirre JJ. Induction of cytochrome P450 enzymes by albendazole treatment in the rat. *Environ Toxicol Pharmacol.* 2000; 9(1-2): 31-37.

Bandala C, Floriano-Sánchez E, Cárdenas-Rodríguez N, López-Cruz J, Lara-Padilla E. RNA expression of cytochrome P450 in Mexican women with breast cancer. *Asian Pac J Cancer Prev.* 2012; 13(6):2647-53.

Bello M, Mendieta-Wejebe JE, Correa-Basurto J. Structural and energetic analysis to provide insight residues of CYP2C9, 2C11 and 2E1 involved in valproic acid dehydrogenation selectivity. *Biochem Pharmacol.* 2014; 90(2):145-58.

Belmont-Díaz J, López-Gordillo AP, Molina Garduño E, Serrano-García L, Coballase-Urrutia E, Cárdenas-Rodríguez N, Arellano-Aguilar O, Montero-Montoya RD. Micronuclei in bone marrow and liver in relation to hepatic metabolism and antioxidant response due to coexposure to chloroform, dichloromethane, and toluene in the rat model. *Biomed Res Int.* 2014; 2014: 425070.

Bisso-Machado R, Ramallo V, Paixão-Côrtes VR, Acuña-Alonzo V, Demarchi DA4, Sandoval JR, Granara AA, Salzano FM, Hünemeier T, Bortolini MC. NAT2 gene diversity and its evolutionary trajectory in the Americas. *Pharmacogenomics J.* 2015 Oct 27. doi: 10.1038/tpj.2015.72. [Epub ahead of print].

Bonifaz-Peña V, Contreras AV, Struchiner CJ, Roela RA, Furuya-Mazzotti TK4, Chammas R4, Rangel-Escareño C, Uribe-Figueroa L, Gómez-Vázquez MJ, McLeod HL, Hidalgo-Miranda A, Parra EJ, Fernández-López JC, Suarez-Kurtz G. Exploring the distribution of genetic markers of pharmacogenomics relevance in Brazilian and Mexican populations. *PLoS One.* 2014; 9(11):e112640.

Castelán-Martínez OD, Hoyo-Vadillo C, Sandoval-García E, Sandoval-Ramírez L, González-Ibarra M, Solano-Solano G, Gómez-Díaz RA, Parra EJ, Cruz M, Valladares-Salgado A. Allele frequency distribution of CYP2C9*2 and CYP2C9* 3 polymorphisms in six Mexican populations. *Gene.* 2013 Jul 10;523(2):167-72.

Castillejos-López M de J, García-Sancho MC, Quiñones-Falconi F, Pérez-Padilla JR. [Cytochrome P450 and NAT2 polymorphisms and drug metabolism in DOTS]. Rev Invest Clin. 2008 (1):47-57.

Céspedes-Garro C, Fricke-Galindo I, Naranjo ME, Rodrigues-Soares F, Fariñas H, de Andrés F, López-López M, Peñas-Lledó EM, LLerena A. Worldwide interethnic variability and geographical distribution of CYP2C9 genotypes and phenotypes. *Expert Opin Drug Metab Toxicol.* 2015;11(12):1893-905. doi: 10.1517/17425255.2015.1111871. Epub 2015 Nov 23.

Céspedes-Garro C, Jiménez-Arce G, Naranjo ME, Barrantes R, Llerena A; CEIBA.FP Consortium of the Ibero-American Network of Pharmacogenetics & Pharmacogenomics RIBEF. Ethnic background and CYP2D6 genetic polymorphisms in Costa Ricans. *Rev Biol Trop.* 2014;62(4): 1659-7.

Céspedes-Garro C, Naranjo ME, Ramírez R, Serrano V, Fariñas H, Barrantes R, LLerena A; CEIBA Consortium of the Ibero-American Network of Pharmacogenetics and Pharmacogenomics RIBEF. Pharmacogenetics in Central American healthy volunteers: interethnic variability. *Drug Metabol Personal Ther.* 2015; 30(1):19-31.

Contreras AV, Monge-Cazares T, Alfaro-Ruiz L, Hernandez-Morales S, Miranda-Ortiz H, Carrillo-Sanchez K, Jimenez-Sanchez G, Silva-Zolezzi I. Resequencing, haplotype construction and identification of novel variants of CYP2D6 in Mexican Mestizos. *Pharmacogenomics.* 2011; 12(5):745-56.

Cuautle-Rodríguez P, Llerena A, Molina-Guarneros J. Present status and perspective of pharmacogenetics in Mexico. *Drug Metabol Drug Interact.* 2014; 29(1):37-45.

Dávila-Borja VM, Belmont JA, Espinosa JJ, Moreno-Sánchez R, Albores A, Montero RD. Induction of CYP1A1 and CYP2E1 in rat liver by histamine: binding and kinetic studies. *Arch Toxicol.* 2007; 81(10): 697-709.

Díaz-Molina R, Cornejo-Bravo JM, Ramos-Ibarra MA, Estrada-Guzmán JD, Morales-Arango O, Reyes-Báez R, Robinson-Navarro OM, Soria-Rodríguez CG. Genotype and phenotype of NAT2 and the occurrence of adverse drug reactions in Mexican individuals to an isoniazid-based prophylactic chemotherapy for tuberculosis. genotype in half of that patients having a genotype combined with slow/rapid alleles. *Mol Med Rep.* 2008; 1(6): 875-9.

Dorado P, Sosa-Macias MG, Peñas-Lledó EM, Alanis-Bañuelos RE, Wong ML, Licinio J, Lares-Asseff I, Llerena A. CYP2C9 allele frequency differences between populations of Mexican-Mestizo, Mexican-Tepehuano, and Spaniards. *Pharmacogenomics J.* 2011; 1 1(2):108-12.

Drobná Z, Del Razo LM, Garcia-Vargas G, Sánchez-Ramírez B, González-Horta C, Ballinas-Casarrubias L, Loomis D, Stýblo M. Identification of the GST-T1 and GST-M1 null genotypes using high resolution melting analysis. *Chem Res Toxicol.* 2012; 25(1): 216-24.

Dzul-Caamal R, Olivares-Rubio HF, López-Tapia P, Vega-López A. Pro-oxidant and antioxidant response elicited by CH2Cl2, CHCl3 and BrCHCl2 in Goodea gracilis using non-invasive methods. *Comp Biochem Physiol A Mol Integr Physiol.* 2013; 165(4): 515-27.

Elizondo G, Medina-Díaz IM. Induction of CYP3A4 by 1alpha,25-dyhydroxyvitamin D3 in HepG2 cells. *Life Sci.* 2003 May; 73(2):141-9.

Favela-Mendoza AF, Martinez-Cortes G, Hernandez-Zaragoza M, Salazar-Flores J, Muñoz-Valle JF, Martinez-Sevilla VM, Velazquez-Suarez NY, Rangel-Villalobos H. Genetic variability of CYP2C19 in a Mexican population: contribution to the knowledge of the inheritance pattern of CYP2C19*17 to develop the ultrarapid metabolizer phenotype. *J Genet.* 2015; 94(1):3-7.

Floriano-Sanchez E, Rodriguez NC, Bandala C, Coballase-Urrutia E, Lopez-Cruz J.CYP3A4 expression in breast cancer and its association with risk factors in Mexican women. *Asian Pac J Cancer Prev.* 2014; 15(8): 3805-9.

Fricke-Galindo I, Céspedes-Garro C, Rodrigues-Soares F, Naranjo ME, Delgado Á, de Andrés F, López-López M, Peñas-Lledó E, LLerena A. Interethnic variation of CYP2C19 alleles, 'predicted' phenotypes and 'measured' metabolic phenotypes across world populations. *Pharmacogenomics J.* 2015 Oct 27. doi: 10.1038/tpj.2015.70. [Epub ahead of print].

Fricke-Galindo I, Jung-Cook H, LLerena A, López-López M. Pharmacogenetics of adverse reactions to antiepileptic drugs. *Neurologia.* 2015 May 11. pii: S0213-4853(15)00056-0. doi: 10.1016/j.nrl.2015. 03.005. [Epub ahead of print].

Gallegos-Arreola MP, Gómez-Meda BC, Morgan-Villela G, Arechavaleta-Granell MR, Arnaud-López L, Beltrán-Jaramillo TJ, Gaxiola R, Zúñiga-González G. GSTT1 gene deletion is associated with lung cancer in Mexican patients. *Dis Markers.* 2003-2004; 19(6):259-61.

Garcés-Eisele J, Ruiz-Argüelles A, Estrada-Marín L, Reyes-Núñez V, Vázquez-Pérez R, Guzmán-García O, Coutiño-Medina R, Acosta-Sandria L, Cedillo-Carvallo B. Pharmacogenetic selection of volunteers increases stringency of bioequivalence studies; the case of clopidogrel. *Indian J Pharm Sci.* 2014; 76(4):281-6.

Garcia DA. Warfarin and pharmacogenomic testing: the case for restraint. *Clin Pharmacol Ther.* 2008; 84(3): 303-5.

García-Bañuelos J, Panduro A, Gordillo-Bastidas D, Gordillo-Bastidas E, Muñoz-Valle JF, Gurrola-Díaz CM, Sánchez-Enríquez S, Ruiz-Madrigal B, Bastidas-Ramírez BE. Genetic polymorphisms of genes coding to alcohol-metabolizing enzymes in western Mexicans: association of CYP2E1*c2/CYP2E1*5B allele with cirrhosis and liver function. *Alcohol Clin Exp Res.* 2012; 36(3): 425-31.

García-Quiroz J, García-Becerra R, Barrera D, Santos N, Avila E, Ordaz-Rosado D, Rivas-Suárez M, Halhali A, Rodríguez P, Gamboa-Domínguez A, Medina-Franco H, Camacho J, Larrea F, Díaz L Astemizole synergizes calcitriol antiproliferative activity by inhibiting CYP24A1 and upregulating VDR: a novel approach for breast cancer therapy. *PLoS One.* 2012;7(9):e45063. doi: 10.1371/journal.pone.0045063.

García-Roca P, Medeiros M, Reyes H, Rodríguez-Espino BA, Alberú J, Ortiz L, Vásquez-Perdomo M, Elizondo G, Morales-Buenrostro LE, Mancilla Urrea E, Castañeda-Hernández G. CYP3A5 polymorphism in Mexican renal transplant recipients and its association with tacrolimus dosing. *Arch Med Res.* 2012; 43(4):283-7.

Garner CE, Liang S, Yin L, Yu X. Physiologically based pharmacokinetic modeling for 1-bromopropane in F344 rats using gas uptake inhalation experiments. *Toxicol Sci.* 2015;145(1):23-36.

Gaxiola-Robles R, Labrada-Martagón V, Celis de la Rosa Ade J, Acosta-Vargas B, Méndez-Rodríguez LC, Zenteno-Savín T. Interaction between mercury (Hg), arsenic (As) and selenium (Se) affects the activity of glutathione S-transferase in breast milk; possible relationship with fish and sellfish intake. *Nutr Hosp.* 2014; 30(2): 436-46.

González HM, Romero EM, Chavez T de J, Peregrina AA, Quezada V, Hoyo-Vadillo C. Phenotype of CYP2C19 and CYP3A4 by determination of omeprazole and its two main metabolites in plasma using liquid chromatography with liquid-liquid extraction. *J Chromatogr B Analyt Technol Biomed Life Sci.* 2002; 780(2):459-65.

Gonzalez HM, Romero EM, Peregrina AA, de J Chávez T, Escobar-Islas E, Lozano F, Hoyo-Vadillo C. CYP2C19- and CYP3A4-dependent omeprazole metabolism in West Mexicans. *J Clin Pharmacol.* 2003; 43(11):1211-5.

González I, Peñas-Lledó EM, Pérez B, Dorado P, Alvarez M, LLerena A. Relation between CYP2D6 phenotype and genotype and personality in healthy volunteers. *Pharmacogenomics*. 2008; 9(7):833-40.

González I, Pérez B, Alvarez M, Dorado P, Llerena A. Study of debrisoquine hydroxylation polymorphism (CYP2D6) in the Cuban population compared to Spaniards]. *Med Clin (Barc)*. 2007;128(20):772-4.

González-Del Angel A, Bermúdez-López C, Alcántara-Ortigoza MA, Vela-Amieva M, Castillo-Cruz RA, Martínez V, Torres-Espíndola L. Thiopurine S-methyltransferase (TPMT) genetic polymorphisms in Mexican newborns. *J Clin Pharm Ther*. 2009; 34(6): 703-8.

González-Jasso E, López T, Lucas D, Berthou F, Manno M, Ortega A, Albores A. CYP2E1 regulation by benzene and other small organic chemicals in rat liver and peripheral lymphocytes. *Toxicol Lett*. 2003; 144(1): 55-67.

Gordillo-Bastidas E, Panduro A, Gordillo-Bastidas D, Zepeda-Carrillo EA, García-Bañuelos JJ, Muñoz-Valle JF, Bastidas-Ramírez BE. Polymorphisms of alcohol metabolizing enzymes in indigenous Mexican population: unusual high frequency of CYP2E1*c2 allele. *Alcohol Clin Exp Res*. 2010; 34(1): 142-9.

Gutiérrez-Álvarez O, Lares-Asseff I, Galaviz-Hernández C, Reyes-Espinoza EA, Almanza-Reyes H, Sosa-Macías M, Chairez Hernández I, Salas-Pacheco JM, Bailón-Soto CE. Involvement of MTHFR and TPMT genes in susceptibility to childhood acute lymphoblastic leukemia (ALL) in Mexicans. *Drug Metabol Personal Ther*. 2016 Mar 1;31(1):41-6.

Hernández I, Domínguez-Pérez M, Bucio L, Souza V, Miranda RU, Clemens DL, Gomez-Quiroz LE, Gutiérrez-Ruiz MC. Free fatty acids enhance the oxidative damage induced by ethanol metabolism in an in vitro model. *Food Chem Toxicol*. 2015; 76: 109-15.

Hoyo-Vadillo C, Venturelli CR, González H, Romero E, Cervantes R, Mata N, Ortiz AC, Rincón V, Zarate F, Sosa C, Ramírez-Mayans J. Metabolism of omeprazole after two oral doses in children 1 to 9 months old. *Proc West Pharmacol Soc*. 2005;48:108-9.

Isaza C, Henao J, López AM, Cacabelos R. Allelic variants of the thiopurine methyltransferase (TPMT) gene in the Colombian population. *Methods Find Exp Clin Pharmacol*. 2003; 25(6): 423-9.

Isordia-Salas I, Olalde-Román MJ, Santiago-Germán D, de la Peña NC, Valencia-Sánchez JS. The impact of CYP3A5*1/*3, PIA1/A2 and T744C polymorphisms on clopidogrel and acetylsalicylic acid response variability in Mexican population. *Thromb Res*. 2012; 130(3): e67-72.

Jacobo-Cabral CO, García-Roca P, Reyes H, Lozada-Rojas L, Cruz-Antonio L, Medeiros M, Castañeda-Hernandez G. Limustin®, a non-innovator tacrolimus formulation, yields reduced drug exposure in pediatric renal transplant recipients. *Pediatr Transplant*. 2014; 18(7): 706-13.

Jaramillo-Rangel G, Ortega-Martínez M, Cerda-Flores RM, Barrera-Saldaña HA. Polymorphisms in GSTM1, GSTT1, GSTP1, and GSTM3 genes and breast cancer risk in northeastern Mexico. *Genet Mol Res*. 2015; 14(2):6465-71.

Jiménez-Garza O, Baccarelli AA, Byun HM, Márquez-Gamiño S, Barrón-Vivanco BS, Albores A. CYP2E1 epigenetic regulation in chronic, low-level toluene exposure: Relationship with oxidative stress and smoking habit. *Toxicol Appl Pharmacol*. 2015; 286(3): 207-15.

Jiménez-Garza O, Márquez-Gamiño S, Albores A, Caudillo-Cisneros C, Carrieri M, Bartolucci GB, Manno M. CYP2E1 phenotype in Mexican workers occupationally exposed to low levels of toluene. *Toxicol Lett.* 2012; 210(2): 254-63.

Jorge LF, Arias TD, Griese U, Nebert DW, Eichelbaum M. Evolutionary pharmacogenetics of CYP2D6 in Ngawbe Guaymi of Panama: allele-specific PCR detection of the CYP2D6B allele and RFLP analysis. *Pharmacogenetics.* 1993;3(5):231-8.

Jorge LF, Arias TD. [Human biodiversity and its effects on the pharmacological variability: CYP2D6 and NAT2 enzymes in Amerind populations of Panama, Colombia and Costa Rica]. *Rev Med Panama.* 1995; 20(3):98-107.

Jorge LF, Eichelbaum M, Griese EU, Inaba T, Arias TD. Comparative evolutionary pharmacogenetics of CYP2D6 in Ngawbe and Embera Amerindians of Panama and Colombia: role of selection versus drift in world populations. *Pharmacogenetics.* 1999; 9(2):217-28.

Jorge-Nebert LF, Eichelbaum M, Griese EU, Inaba T, Arias TD. Analysis of six SNPs of NAT2 in Ngawbe and Embera Amerindians of Panama and determination of the Embera acetylation phenotype using caffeine. *Pharmacogenetics.* 2002; 12(1): 39-48.

Lares-Asseff I, Sosa-Macías M, Elizondo-Azuela G, Flores-Pérez C, Flores-Pérez J, Bradley-Alvarez F. Phenotypical expression of CYP2D6 in amerindians of tepehuano origin from Durango, Mexico. *Proc West Pharmacol Soc.* 2005;48:102-107.

Lares-Asseff I, Trujillo-Jiménez F. [Pharmacogenetics and its importance in the clinical]. *Gac Med Mex.* 2001; 137(3):227-36.

Lazalde-Ramos BP, Martínez-Fierro M de L, Galaviz-Hernández C, Garza-Veloz I, Naranjo ME, Sosa-Macías M, Llerena A. CYP2D6 gene polymorphisms and predicted phenotypes in eight indigenous groups from northwestern Mexico. *Pharmacogenomics.* 2014;15(3):339-48.

Llerena A, Alvarez M, Dorado P, González I, Peñas-LLedó E, Pérez B2, Cobaleda J, Calzadilla LR. Interethnic differences in the relevance of CYP2C9 genotype and environmental factors for diclofenac metabolism in Hispanics from Cuba and Spain. *Pharmacogenomics J.* 2014; 14(3):229-34.

Llerena A, Dorado P, Ramírez R, González I, Alvarez M, Peñas-Lledó EM, Pérez B, Calzadilla LR. CYP2D6 genotype and debrisoquine hydroxylation phenotype in Cubans and Nicaraguans. *Pharmacogenomics J.* 2012; 12(2):176-83.

López M, Guerrero J, Jung-Cook H, Alonso ME. CYP2D6 genotype and phenotype determination in a Mexican Mestizo population. *Eur J Clin Pharmacol.* 2005; 61(10):749-54.

López M, Dorado P, Monroy N, Alonso ME, Jung-Cook H, Machín E, Peñas-Lledó E, Llerena A. Pharmacogenetics of the antiepileptic drugs phenytoin and lamotrigine. *Drug Metabol Drug Interact.* 2011; 26(1):5-12.

López M, Dorado P, Ortega A, Peñas-Lledó E, Monroy N, Silva-Zolezzi I, Cobaleda J, Gallego-Aguilera A, Alonso ME, Llerena A. Interethnic differences in UGT1A4 genetic polymorphisms between Mexican Mestizo and Spanish populations. *Mol Biol Rep.* 2013; 40(4): 3187-92.

Lopez-Garcia MA, Feria-Romero IA, Fernando-Serrano H, Escalante-Santiago D, Grijalva I, Orozco-Suarez S. Genetic polymorphisms associated with antiepileptic metabolism. *Front Biosci* (Elite Ed). 2014; 6: 377-86.

López-Islas A, Chagoya-Hazas V, Pérez-Aguilar B, Palestino-Domínguez M, Souza V, Miranda RU, Bucio L, Gómez-Quiroz LE, Gutiérrez-Ruiz MC.. Cholesterol Enhances the Toxic Effect of Ethanol and Acetaldehyde in Primary Mouse Hepatocytes. *Oxid Med Cell Longev*. 2016; 2016:9209825. doi: 10.1155/2016/9209825. Epub 2015 Dec 14.

López-López M, Guerrero-Camacho JL, Familiar-López IM, Jung-Cook H, Corona-Vázquez T, Alonso-Vilatela ME. [Pharmacogenomics: the quest for individualized therapy]. *Rev Neurol.* 2004; 39(11): 1063-71.

López-López M, Peñas-Lledó E, Dorado P, Ortega A, Corona T, Ochoa A, Yescas P, Alonso E, LLerena A. CYP2D6 genetic polymorphisms in Southern Mexican Mayan Lacandones and Mestizos from Chiapas. *Pharmacogenomics.* 2014; 15(15):1859-65.

Márquez-Rosado L, Trejo-Solís C, Cabrales-Romero Mdel P, Arce-Popoca E, Sierra-Santoyo A, Alemán-Lazarini L, Fatel-Fazenda S, Carrasco-Legleu CE, Villa-Treviño S. Co-carcinogenic effect of cyclohexanol on the development of preneoplastic lesions in a rat hepatocarcinogenesis model. *Mol Carcinog*. 2007; 46(7): 524-33.

Marsh S, King CR, Van Booven DJ, Revollo JY, Gilman RH, McLeod HL. Pharmacogenomic assessment of Mexican and Peruvian populations. *Pharmacogenomics*. 2015; 16(5): 441-8.

Medeiros M, Castañeda-Hernández G, Ross CJ, Carleton BC. Use of pharmacogenomics in pediatric renal transplant recipients. *Front Genet.* 2015 Feb 18;6:41. doi: 10.3389/fgene.2015.00041. eCollection 2015.

Medina-Díaz IM, Arteaga-Illán G, de León MB, Cisneros B, Sierra-Santoyo A, Vega L, Gonzalez FJ, Elizondo G. Pregnane X receptor-dependent induction of the CYP3A4 gene by o,p'-1,1,1,-trichloro-2,2-bis (p-chlorophenyl)ethane. *Drug Metab Dispos*. 2007; 35(1): 95-102.

Medina-Díaz IM, Elizondo G. Transcriptional induction of CYP3A4 by o,p'-DDT in HepG2 cells. *Toxicol Lett*. 2005; 157(1): 41-7.

Medina-Díaz IM, Estrada-Muñiz E, Reyes-Hernández OD, Ramírez P, Vega L, Elizondo G. Arsenite and its metabolites, MMA(III) and DMA(III), modify CYP3A4, PXR and RXR alpha expression in the small intestine of CYP3A4 transgenic mice. *Toxicol Appl Pharmacol*. 2009; 239(2): 162-8.

Mejia-Garcia A, Sanchez-Ocampo EM, Galindo-Gomez S, Shibayama M, Reyes-Hernandez O, Guzman-Leon S, Gonzalez FJ, Elizondo G. 2,3,7,8-Tetrachlorodibenzo-p-dioxin enhances CCl4-induced hepatotoxicity in an aryl hydrocarbon receptor-dependent manner. *Xenobiotica*. 2013; 43(2): 161-8.

Mendieta-Wejebe JE, Correa-Basurto J, García-Segovia EM, Ceballos-Cancino G, Rosales-Hernández MC. Molecular modeling used to evaluate CYP2C9-dependent metabolism: homology modeling, molecular dynamics and docking simulations. *Curr Drug Metab.* 2011; 12(6):533-48.

Mendoza-Cantú A, Castorena-Torres F, Bermúdez de León M, Cisneros B, López-Carrillo L, Rojas-García AE, Aguilar-Salinas A, Manno M, Albores A. Occupational toluene exposure induces cytochrome P450 2E1 mRNA expression in peripheral lymphocytes. *Environ Health Perspect*. 2006; 114(4): 494-9.

Mendoza-Cantú A, Castorena-Torres F, Bermudez M, Martínez-Hernández R, Ortega A, Salinas JE, Albores A. Genotype and allele frequencies of polymorphic cytochromes P450 CYP1A2 and CYP2E1 in Mexicans. *Cell Biochem Funct.* 2004; 22(1): 29-34.

Molina-Ortiz D, Camacho-Carranza R, González-Zamora JF, Shalkow-Kalincovstein J, Cárdenas-Cardós R, Nosti-Palacios R, Vences-Mejía A. Differential expression of cytochrome P450 enzymes in normal and tumor tissues from childhood rhabdomyosarcoma. *PLoS One.* 2014; 9(4): e93261.

Montano Loza AJ, Ramirez Iglesias MT, Perez Diaz I, Cruz Castellanos S, Garcia Andrade C, Medina Mora ME, Robles Díaz G, Kershenobich D, Gutierrez Reyes G. Association of alcohol-metabolizing genes with alcoholism in a Mexican Indian (Otomi) population. *Alcohol.* 2006; 39(2): 73-9.

Montero R, Serrano L, Dávila V, Segura Y, Arrieta A, Fuentes R, Abad I, Valencia L, Sierra P, Camacho R. Metabolic polymorphisms and the micronucleus frequency in buccal epithelium of adolescents living in an urban environment. *Environ Mol Mutagen.* 2003; 42(3):216-22.

Montero R, Serrano L, Dávila VM, Ito A, Plancarte A Infection of rats with Taenia taeniformis metacestodes increases hepatic CYP450, induces the activity of CYP1A1, CYP2B1 and COH isoforms and increases the genotoxicity of the procarcinogens benzo[a]pyrene, cyclophosphamide and aflatoxin B(1). *Mutagenesis.* 2003; 18(2): 211-6.

Moreno-Guerrero SS, Ramírez-Pacheco A, Dorantes-Acosta EM, Medina-Sanson A. [Analysis of genetic polymorphisms of thiopurine S-methyltransferase (TPMT) in Mexican pediatric patients with cancer]. *Rev Invest Clin.* 2013; 65(2): 156-64.

Nájera-Martínez M, García-Latorre EA, Reyes-Maldonado E, Domínguez-López ML, Vega-López A. Halomethane-induced cytotoxicity and cell proliferation in human lung MRC-5 fibroblasts and NL20-TA epithelial cells. *Inhal Toxicol.* 2012; 24(11): 762-73.

Nastasi-Catanese JA, Padilla-Gutiérrez JR, Valle Y, Ortega-Gutiérrez F, Gallegos-Arreola MP, Figuera LE. Genetic contribution of CYP2C9, CYP2C19, and APOE variants in acenocoumarol response. *Genet Mol Res.* 2013;12(4):4413-21.

Nosti-Palacios R, Gómez-Garduño J, Molina-Ortiz D, Calzada-León R, Dorado-González VM, Vences-Mejía A. Aspartame Administration and Insulin Treatment Altered Brain Levels of CYP2E1 and CYP3A2 in Streptozotocin-Induced Diabetic Rats. *Int J Toxicol.* 2014; 33(4): 325-331.

Oropeza-Hernández LF, López-Romero R, Albores A. Hepatic CYP1A, 2B, 2C, 2E and 3A regulation by methoxychlor in male and female rats. *Toxicol Lett.* 2003; 144(1): 93-103.

Oropeza-Hernández LF, Quintanilla-Vega B, Reyes-Mejía RA, Serrano CJ, García-Latorre EA, Dekant W, Manno M, Albores A. Trifluoroacetylated adducts in spermatozoa, testes, liver and plasma and CYP2E1 induction in rats after subchronic inhalatory exposure to halothane. *Toxicol Lett.* 2003; 144(1):105-16.

Ortega-Vázquez A, Dorado P, Fricke-Galindo I, Jung-Cook H, Monroy-Jaramillo N, Martínez-Juárez IE, Familiar-López I, Peñas-Lledó E, LLerena A, López-López M. CYP2C9, CYP2C19, ABCB1 genetic polymorphisms and phenytoin plasma concentrations in Mexican-Mestizo patients with epilepsy. *Pharmacogenomics J.* 2015 Jun 30. doi: 10.1038/tpj.2015.45. [Epub ahead of print].

Peñas-Lledó EM, Trejo HD, Dorado P, Ortega A, Jung H, Alonso E, Naranjo ME, López-López M, Llerena A. CYP2D6 ultrarapid metabolism and early dropout from fluoxetine or amitriptyline monotherapy treatment in major depressive patients. *Mol Psychiatry.* 2013;18(1): 8-9.

Pérez-Morales R, Méndez-Ramírez I, Castro-Hernández C, Martínez-Ramírez OC, Gonsebatt ME, Rubio J. Polymorphisms associated with the risk of lung cancer in a healthy

Mexican Mestizo population: Application of the additive model for cancer. *Genet Mol Biol.* 2011; 34(4): 546-52.

Perez-Paramo YX, Hernandez-Cabrera F, Dorado P, Llerena A, Muñoz-Jimenez S, Ortiz-Lopez R, Rojas-Martinez A. Interethnic relationships of CYP2D6 variants in native and Mestizo populations sharing the same ecosystem. *Pharmacogenomics.* 2015;16 (7):703-12.

Perez-Paramo YX, Hernandez-Cabrera F, Rojas-Martinez A, Ortiz-Lopez R. CYP2D6 in Amerindians from Southern Mexico: low variability and higher frequency of functional alleles. *Drug Metabol Personal Ther.* 2015 Oct 17. pii: /j/dmdi.ahead-of-print/dmpt-2015-0017/dmpt-2015-0017.xml.

Petersen DD, Kong AN, Jorge LF, Nebert DW, Arias TD. Debrisoquine polymorphism: novel CYP2D6 gene Bam HI restriction fragment length polymorphism in the Ngawbé Guaymí Indian of Panama. *Pharmacogenetics.* 1991; 1(3):136-42.

Ramos MA, Mares RE, Avalos ED, Hernández A, Hernández R, Lameda R, Malváez AE, Rodríguez CA, Rodríguez R. Pharmacogenetic screening of N-acetyltransferase 2, thiopurine s-methyltransferase, and 5,10-methylene-tetrahydrofolate reductase polymorphisms in Northwestern. Mexicans. *Genet Test Mol Biomarkers.* 2011; 15(5): 351-5.

Reyes-Hernández OD, Vega L, Jiménez-Ríos MA, Martínez-Cervera PF, Lugo-García JA, Hernández-Cadena L, Ostrosky-Wegman P, Orozco L, Elizondo G.The PXR rs7643645 polymorphism is associated with the risk of higher prostate-specific antigen levels in prostate cancer patients. *PLoS One.* 2014; 9(6): e99974.

Rodeiro I, Donato MT, Jimenez N, Garrido G, Molina-Torres J, Menendez R, Castell JV, Gómez-Lechón MJ. Inhibition of human P450 enzymes by natural extracts used in traditional medicine. *Phytother Res.* 2009; 23(2):279-82.12.- Sosa-Macías M, Dorado P, Alanis-Bañuelos RE, Llerena A, Lares-Asseff I. Influence of CYP2D6 deletion, multiplication, -1584C-->G, 31G-->A and 2988G-->a gene polymorphisms on dextromethorphan metabolism among Mexican tepehuanos and mestizos.. *Pharmacology.* 2010; 86(1):30-6.

Rodeiro I, José Gómez-Lechón M, Perez G, Hernandez I, Herrera JA, Delgado R, Castell JV, Teresa Donato M. Mangifera indica L. extract and mangiferin modulate cytochrome P450 and UDP-glucuronosyltransferase enzymes in primary cultures of human hepatocytes. *Phytother Res.* 2013; 27(5): 745-52.

Rojas JC, Aguilar B, Rodríguez-Maldonado E, Collados MT. Pharmacogenetics of oral anticoagulants. *Blood Coagul Fibrinolysis.* 2005; 16(6):389-98.

Salazar-Flores J, Torres-Reyes LA, Martínez-Cortés G, Rubi-Castellanos R, Sosa-Macías M, Muñoz-Valle JF, González-González C, Ramírez A, Román R, Méndez JL, Barrera A, Torres A, Medina R, Rangel-Villalobos H. Distribution of CYP2D6 and CYP2C19 polymorphisms associated with poor metabolizer phenotype in five Amerindian groups and western Mestizos from Mexico. *Genet Test Mol Biomarkers.* 2012;16(9):1098-104.

Salazar-González R, Gómez R, Romano-Moreno S, Medellín-Garibay S, Núñez-Ruíz A, Magaña-Aquino M, Milán-Segovia RC, Portales-Pérez DP. Expression of NAT2 in immune system cells and the relation of NAT2 gene polymorphisms in the anti-tuberculosis therapy in Mexican mestizo population. *Mol Biol Rep.* 2014; 41(12): 7833-43.

Saldaña-Cruz AM, Sánchez-Corona J, Márquez de Santiago DA, García-Zapién AG, Flores-Martínez SE. [Pharmacogenetics and antiepileptic drug metabolism: implication of genetic variants in cytochromes P450]. *Rev Neurol.* 2013; 56(9):471-9.

Sandoval-Carrillo A, Aguilar-Duran M, Vázquez-Alaniz F, Castellanos-Juárez FX, Barraza-Salas M, Sierra-Campos E, Téllez-Valencia A, La Llave-León O, Salas-Pacheco JM. Polymorphisms in the GSTT1 and GSTM1 genes are associated with increased risk of preeclampsia in the Mexican mestizo population. *Genet Mol Res.* 2014; 13(1): 2160-5.

Sinues B, Vicente J, Fanlo A, Vasquez P, Medina JC, Mayayo E, Conde B, Arenaz I, Martinez-Jarreta B. CYP3A5*3 and CYP3A4*1B allele distribution and genotype combinations: differences between Spaniards and Central Americans. *Ther Drug Monit.* 2007;29(4):412-6.

Sosa-Macías M, Dorado P, Alanis-Bañuelos RE, Llerena A, Lares-Asseff I. Influence of CYP2D6 deletion, multiplication, -1584C-->G, 31G-->A and 2988G-->a gene polymorphisms on dextromethorphan metabolism among Mexican tepehuanos and mestizos. *Pharmacology.* 2010; 86(1):30-6.

Sosa-Macías M, Elizondo G, Flores-Pérez C, Flores-Pérez J, Bradley-Alvarez F, Alanis-Bañuelos RE, Lares-Asseff. CYP2D6 genotype and phenotype in Amerindians of Tepehuano origin and Mestizos of Durango, Mexico. *J Clin Pharmacol.* 2006; 46(5):527-36.

Sosa-Macías M, Lazalde-Ramos BP, Galaviz-Hernández C, Rangel-Villalobos H, Salazar-Flores J, Martínez-Sevilla VM, Martínez-Fierro ML, Dorado P, Wong ML, Licinio J, LLerena A. Influence of admixture components on CYP2C9*2 allele frequency in eight indigenous populations from Northwest Mexico. *Pharmacogenomics J.* 2013;13 (6):567-72.

Sosa-Macías M, Llerena A. Cytochrome P450 genetic polymorphisms of Mexican indigenous populations. *Drug Metabol Drug Interact.* 2013; 28(4):193-208.

Taja-Chayeb L, Agúndez JA, Miguez-Muñoz C, Chavez-Blanco A, Dueñas-Gonzalez A. Arylamine N-acetyltransferase 2 genotypes in a Mexican population. *Genet Mol Res.* 2012; 11(2): 1082-92.

Taja-Chayeb L, González-Fierro A, Miguez-Muñoz C, Trejo-Becerril C, Cruz-Hernandez Ede L, Cantu D, Agundez JA, Vidal-Millan S, Gutierrez O, Dueñas-González A. Acetylator status and N-acetyltransferase 2 gene polymorphisms; phenotype-genotype correlation with the sulfamethazine test. *Pharmacogenet Genomics.* 2011;21(12): 894-901.

Taja-Chayeb L, Vidal-Millán S, Gutiérrez O, Ostrosky-Wegman P, Dueñas-González A, Candelaria M. Thiopurine S-methyltransferase gene (TMPT) polymorphisms in a Mexican population of healthy individuals and leukemic patients *Med Oncol.* 2008; 25(1): 56-62.

Vargas-Alarcón G, Ramírez-Bello J, de la Peña A, Calderón-Cruz B, Peña-Duque MA, Martínez-Ríos MA, Ramírez-Fuentes S, Pérez-Méndez O, Fragoso JM. Distribution of ABCB1, CYP3A5, CYP2C19, and P2RY12 gene polymorphisms in a Mexican Mestizos population. *Mol Biol Rep.* 2014; 41(10):7023-9.

Vega-López A, Carrillo-Morales CI, Olivares-Rubio HF, Lilia Domínguez-López M, García-Latorre EA. Evidence of bioactivation of halomethanes and its relation to oxidative stress response in Chirostoma riojai, an endangered fish from a polluted lake in Mexico. *Arch Environ Contam Toxicol.* 2012; 62(3): 479-93.

Vences-Mejía A, Gómez-Garduño J, Caballero-Ortega H, Dorado-González V, Nosti-Palacios R, Labra-Ruíz N, Espinosa-Aguirre JJ. Effect of mosquito mats (pyrethroid-based) vapor inhalation on rat brain cytochrome P450s. *Toxicol Mech Methods.* 2012; 22(1): 41-6.

Villegas-Torres B, Sánchez-Girón F, Jaramillo-Villafuerte K, Soberón X, Gonzalez-Covarrubias V. Genotype frequencies of VKORC1 and CYP2C9 in native and Mestizo populations from Mexico, potential impact for coumarin dosing. *Gene.* 2015; 558(2):235-40.

Zaruma-Torres F, Lares-Asseff I, Reyes-Espinoza A, Loera-Castañeda V, Chairez-Hernández I, Sosa-Macías M, Galaviz-Hernández C, Almanza-Reyes H. Association of ABCB1, ABCC5 and xanthine oxidase genetic polymorphisms with methotrexate adverse reactions in Mexican pediatric patients with ALL. *Drug Metabol Personal Ther.* 2015; 30(3): 195-201.

In: Pharmacogenomics in Latin America
Editor: Luis A. Quiñones
ISBN: 978-1-53611-031-9

Chapter 4

CLINICAL PHARMACOGENOMICS IN SOUTH AMERICA

Juan P. Cayún[1,*], Carla E. Miranda, PhD[1], María A. Lavanderos[1], Matías F. Martínez[1], Paula I. Escalante[1], Marcelo I. Suárez[1], Roberto A. Cerro[1], Christopher A. Sandoval[1], Leslie C. Cerpa[1] and Paulina A. Moreno[1]

Laboratory of Chemical Carcinogenesis and Pharmacogenetics (CQF), Department of Basic-Clinic Oncology, Faculty of Medicine, University of Chile, Santiago, Chile

ABSTRACT

In South America, in recent years, some studies have established allelic frequencies of the most relevant pharmacogenes. Several studies in South America have revealed the genetic diversity and miscegenation process generated after colonization during recent centuries. Additionally, relevant clinical studies have been carried out in areas, such as oncology, cardiology and psychiatry. In this chapter we will briefly describe the development of pharmacogenetics in South America with a pharmacotherapeutic approach.

Keywords: pharmacogenomics, pharmacogenetics, South America, clinical pharmacology

* Corresponding Author E-mail: jpcayun@farmacogenetica.cl.

INTRODUCTION

In recent years, several pharmacogenetic studies have been carried out in South America. We searched pharmacogenetic studies in the PubMed database filtering by studies related to clinical outcome (efficacy, toxicity or pharmacokinetic analysis) in South America. Brazil is the first country in relation to number of studies in the region with one hundred fourteen studies. This is followed by Chile and Argentina with nineteen and twelve studies, respectively, Colombia and Venezuela with five studies, followed by Ecuador with one clinical study related to pharmacogenetics. The most relevant clinical areas regarding number of publications are cardiovascular and system nervous, followed by hematology, infectology and oncology. Next in the list, we observed transplants, gastroenterology, endocrinology and lung diseases, finally, pediatrics, immunology, ophthalmology and gynecology-obstetrics. In relation to the number of publications by year, after 2002 numbers have been increasing constantly in South America with peaks of publications in 2005, 2008 and 2010. In this chapter, we will describe and analyze the studies found in Pubmed database with a pharmacotherapeutic approach. In addition, we will discuss briefly other topics, for example, ethnic differences and endophenotypic characterization.

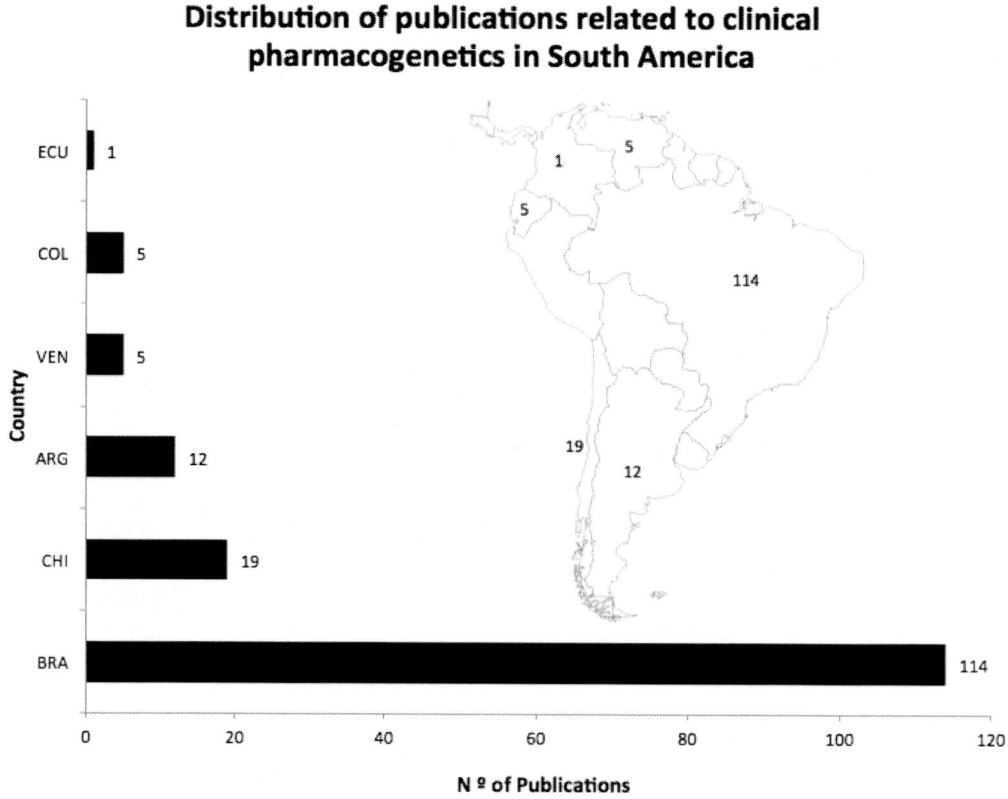

Figure 1. Distribution of publications related to clinical pharmacogenetics in South America (for see data and details of search criteria to visit the next open file: https://drive.google.com/open?id=0BxOdjaxnEWEeMWx5QWFJSWJRTDg).

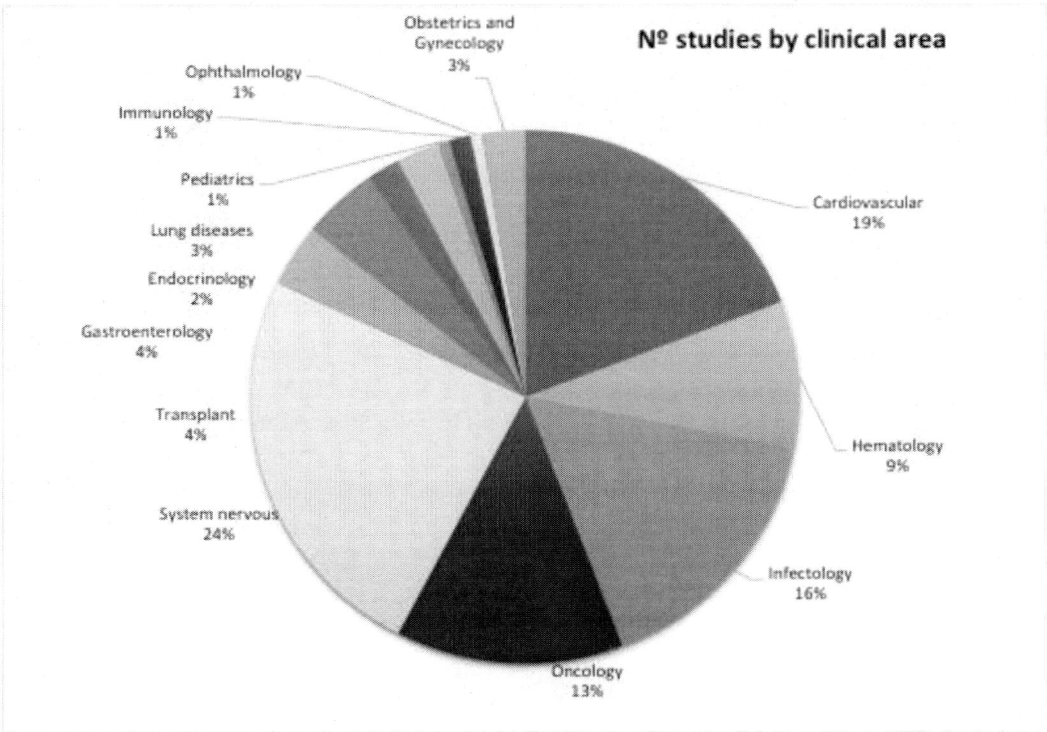

Figure 2. Clinical area frequencies of studies related to clinical pharmacogenetics in South America.

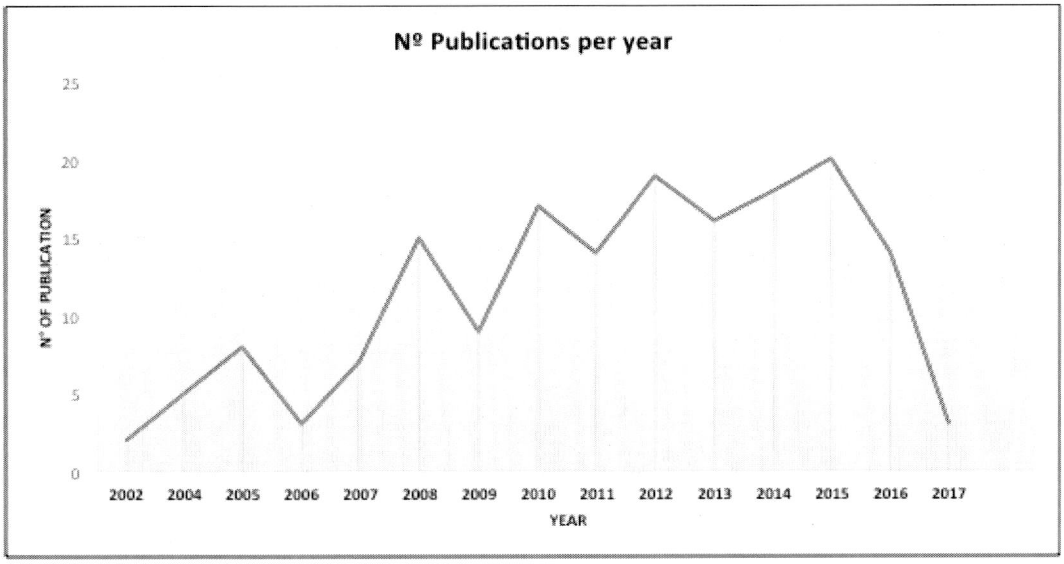

Figure 3. Number of publications per year of clinical studies related to pharmacogenetics in South America.

CYTOCHROME P450 ENZYMES (CYPS)

Dr. Guilherme Suarez-Kurtz's group in Brazil carried out the first report related with polymorphisms in cytochrome P450 enzymes and clinical effect in 2004. They showed the variability of pharmacogenetics regarding *CYP2C9* and the response to anti-inflammatory drugs. The studies were performed in healthy volunteers comparing their pharmacokinetic profiles. This group showed that subjects with the alleles *CYP2C9*2* and *CYP2C9*3* have higher exposure to tenoxicam during single and multiple doses (Vianna-Jorge et al. 2004). Moreover, they showed that areas under the curve (AUC) of subjects with alleles *CYP2C9*2* and *CYP2C9*3* were higher than subjects with only *CYP2C9*1* alleles (Perini et al. 2005), indicating that the influence of polymorphisms in *CYP2C9* have a clear effect on the metabolism of anti-inflammatory drugs in Brazilian subjects. After these studies, several groups have been working on the description of the genotype-phenotype relationship through plasmatic levels in South Americans. For example, one group reported the effect of *CYP2B6* polymorphisms on the high plasma concentration of efavirenz-associated toxicity in Chilean patients (Carr et al. 2010). In addition, Moreno et al., 2012, reported the effect of *CYP3A4/CYP3A5* polymorphisms on the pharmacokinetics of levonorgestrel. Importantly, a connection between the hydroxylation phenotype of dextromethorfan and the *CYP2D6* genotype in Uruguayan (Estevez et al. 1996) and Ecuatorian (Dorado et al. 2012) populations was reported. In addition, a clear effect was shown between the *CYP2D6* genotype and metabolizer phenotype in Chilean subjects through debrisoquine 4-hydroxylase activity as a metabolic ratio (MR) (Varela et al. 2015). Furthermore, they found a percentage of poor metabolizer (PM), similar to that reported in other Hispanic populations (Llerena, Dorado, and Penas-Lledo 2009).

Clinical studies in *CYP2D6* pharmacogenetics have mainly been performed in psychiatry. An association between the *CYP2D6* genotype and neuroleptic treatment in Brazil was observed, but without significant results (Kohlrausch et al. 2008). Recently, the relationship between the *CYP2D6* genotype and refractoriness to antipsychotic treatment was reported, but the group did not find any association (van de Bilt et al. 2015). However, Dos Santos-Júnior et al. reported the association between the *CYP2D6* genotype and body mass index (BMI) and blood pressure in risperidone-treated patients (Dos Santos-Junior et al. 2016) in Brazil.

Additionally, several studies on CYPs were reported in different therapeutic areas using different approaches. In recent years, several clinical studies were carried out in South America in relation to *CYP450* polymorphisms, for example, one of the main genetic polymorphisms reported in CYPs, *CYP3A5*3*, and its influence in the response to calcineurin inhibitors, such as tacrolimus and cyclosporine in organ transplant patients. The effect of *CYP3A5*3* has been reported in Brazilian patients in required doses and blood concentrations of tacrolimus (Genvigir et al. 2016) for immunosuppression after kidney transplantation, similar to the results obtained in other studies in Brazilian kidney transplant (Cusinato et al. 2014) and Colombian liver transplant patients (Buendia et al. 2015). The frequency obtained for this polymorphism is similar in different patient populations in South America, for example, an allelic frequency of 0.28 in Brazil (Genvigir et al. 2016); and a genotypic frequency of 11% to *CYP3A5*1/*1*, 31% to *CYP3A5*1/*3* and 58% to *CYP3A5*3/*3* (Cusinato et al. 2014). Afterward, an allelic frequency of 0.017 in receptors and 0.025 in donors in a Colombia population for liver transplantation was found (Buendia et al. 2015).

In addition, the impact of *CYP3A5*3* has been studied in the response to 3-hydroxy-methylglutaryl CoA reductase (HMG-CoA-R) inhibitors, for example, more effects were reported in response to atorvastatin in Brazilian patients with *CYP3A5*3C* and *CYP3A5*1D* alleles (Estrela et al. 2008). Moreover, others studies have been carried out in hypercholesterolemia with the *CYP3A5*3* genotype but without an effect in the response, for example the report of Rosales et al. in 2012 in Chilean patients treated with atorvastatin (Rosales et al. 2012). In addition, no influence was shown in Brazilian patients treated with simvastatin (Fiegenbaum et al. 2005; Willrich et al. 2013).

Another important gene studied in South Americans is *CYP2C9*. In 2008, Brazilian researchers reported that patients with *CYP2C9*2* and *CYP2C9*3* alleles have a high risk of over-coagulation in treatment with warfarin (Lima et al. 2008). Furthermore, the presence of polymorphisms at *CYP2C9* and the effect of a weekly dose of warfarin in Brazilian patients was reported, in addition to an ethnic component in the outcome (Perini et al. 2008). Later, the impact of *CYP2C9*1*, **2* and **3* was reported in other countries, for example, in Colombia (Palacio et al. 2010). However, no effect was found in this outcome, possibly due to a reduced sample size (Benavides et al. 2015).

UDP-GLUCURONOSYLTRANSFERASES (UGTS)

In relation to UGTs in South America, D'Andrea et al. in Argentina in 2005 evaluated the effect of silymarin and their glucuronidation through rat hepatic microsomes. They found that conjugation of these compounds is related with UGT1A isoenzyme (D'Andrea, Perez, and Sanchez Pozzi 2005). Moreover, Valsecchi et al. in 2007 reported that analysis of thymine-adenine (TA) dinucleotics in the promoter region of the UDP-glucuronosyl-transferase 1A1 enzyme was associated with severe neutropenia in an Argentine patient in treatment with irinotecan for lung cancer (Valsecchi et al. 2007). In addition, Mallea-Gil et al. reported a case report of pegvisomant-Induced cholestatic hepatitis in an acromegalic patient with *UGT1A1*28* polymorphism in Argentina (Mallea-Gil et al. 2016). Afterward, Betonico et al. reported the effects of *UGT1A8, UGT1A9* and *UGT2B7* polymorphisms and the side effects of mycofenolate mofetil (MMF) in Brazil. The authors reported that *UGT1A8 277A* patients have more infection episodes than *UGT1A8 277G* patients when they are treated with a dose of 2 g/day. In addition, they reported that hematological alterations and dose reductions were more frequent in *UGT1A9H4* (-2152T/-275A/-118T9/33T) patients (Betonico et al. 2008). In the endocrinological area, Vargens et al. reported a dosage decrease of thyroxine (T_4) in Brazilian patients with $(TA)_7$ and $(TA)_8$ alleles in treatment of thyroid cancer (Vargens et al. 2011). They also reported additional results in 2014 (Santoro et al. 2014). On the other hand, de Oliveira Almeida et al. in 2014 performed the first study to evaluate *UGT1A1 (TA) n* and warfarin treatment in a Brazilian population. Interestingly, they found that *UGT1A1* $(TA)_n$ variations are related with higher doses of warfarin (de Oliveira Almeida et al. 2014).

GLUTATHIONE-S-TRANSFERASES

The first report related to genetic variations in genes of glutathione-S-transferases (GSTs) was published by Arruda et al. in 1998. These researchers analyzed the frequencies of GSTM1 and GSTP1 deletion in Amazonian Indians. They reported allele frequencies minor than Caucasians population, 0.43 for GSTT1-null and 0.45 for GSTM1-null (Arruda et al. 1998). After that, Quiñones et al. in 1999 published an allele frequency of GSTM1-null of 0.21 in Chilean population (Quiñones et al. 1999) Later, Gaspar et al. in 2002 analyzed the deletion frequencies of *GSTM1* and *GSTT1* genes in seven Amerindian populations of the Amazon region in Brazil (Gaspar et al. 2002), reporting frequencies from 0.19 to 0.38 for Guaraní and Surui populations, respectively. In 2007, a similar study was carried out in Argentina and Paraguay, where they studied eight Amerindian populations. They found frequencies from 0.2 to 0.66 for the deletion of *GSTM1*, while *GSTT1* deletion was present in four populations in less than 0.5 (Bailliet et al. 2007). Over the years, the most important therapeutic area related with genetic variations in GSTs is oncology. The first study in this area was unable to demonstrate any association between GST genotypes and the risk of ovarian cancer (Morari et al. 2006). In 2010, Salinas-Souza et al. published a clinical study in osteosarcoma. They mentioned that *GSTM1-null* patients have a poor clinical response to chemotherapy (carboplatin, cisplatin, ifosfamide, and doxorubicin) in pediatric patients whereas the presence of *GSTM1* and *GSTM3*B* alleles was associated with a better response (Salinas-Souza et al., 2010). That same year, Oliveira et al. reported that the genotype GSTT1/GSTP1105Ile wild-type had a higher response rate to chemotherapy in locally advanced breast cancer (Oliveira et al. 2010). In 2015, a report studied polymorphisms in *GSTT1, GSTM1* and *GSTP1* in 268 pediatric patients with lymphoblastic leukemia in Argentina, however, they did not find a direct association between GST genetic variants and therapeutic response (Araoz et al. 2015). Nevertheless, Weich et al. reported that combined analysis showed that *GSTM1-null/GSTP1-GG* as well as *GSTT1-null/GSTP1-GG* were associated with the development of Chronic myeloid leukemia (CML). In addition, they reported that the *GSTM1* gene was linked with an inferior rate of molecular response and poor survival and *GSTP1-GG* genotype was associated with treatment failure in Argentine patients with CML (Weich et al. 2016). Previously, Oliveira et al. reported an association between *GSTM1-null, GSTT1 non-null, GSTP1-105Ile* and a higher response to chemotherapy in Brazilian breast cancer patients in 2010. Additionally, Acevedo et al. in 2014 reported *GSTM1 non-null, GSTT1 null,* and *CYP1A1*2A* genotypes are associated with survival up to 9-years of follow-up in prostate cancer patients (Acevedo et al. 2014).

THIOPURINE METHYLTRANSFERASE (TMPT)

Reis et al. determined the allelic frequencies for thiopurine-S-methyltransferase (TMPT) in 2003 in a Brazilian population. They estimated the allelic frequency of *TPMT*2* (238G > C rs1800462) as 0.082, *TPMT*3A* as 0.0163 (460G > A/719A> G, rs1800460/rs1142345) and *TPMT*3C* (719A > G rs1142345) as 0.0212. In addition, they didn't find the presence of the *TPMT*3B* allele (460G > A, rs1800460) in this population (Reis, Santoro, and Suarez-Kurtz 2003). In another Brazilian population, the results were similar for *TPMT*3 A*, however,

*TPMT*2, TPMT*3C* were less than the previous study (Boson et al. 2003). The same year, Laróvere et al. reported a 8.2% of variant TPMT alleles in Argentina population (Larovere et al. 2003) and Isaza et al. published a 7,9% of intermediate methylators in Colombian population (Isaza et al. 2003). Silva et al. in 2008 reported the first study of the *TPMT* gene and associated with outcomes in South America. They reported no association between polymorphisms *TPMT*3 A, 3C, 2* and *3B* and adverse events to treatment in Brazilian children with acute lymphoblastic leukemia (Silva et al. 2008). Araoz et al. in 2015 reported similar results in the same type of patients treated with methotrexate and 6-mercaptopurine in Argentina (Araoz et al. 2015). Conversely, Zabala-Fernandez et al. in 2011 found that the presence of *TPMT*2, *3A* and **3C* increases the risk of mielosupression in Venezuelan patients with inflammatory bowel disease and treated with azathioprine (Zabala-Fernandez et al. 2011). In addition, children treated with 6-mercaptopurine that have a variant allele (*TPMT*3A* and *3C*) required lower median cumulative in comparison with wild-type patients (*TPMT*1*) (Farfan et al. 2014). The latter correlates with the phenotype observed when the enzymatic activity in Chilean healthy subjects with a different *TMPT* genotype was measured (Jorquera et al. 2012).

N-Acetyltransferase 2 (NAT-2)

N-acetyltransferase 2 (NAT-2) is an enzyme involved in liver metabolism of anti-tuberculosis drugs (ATD), such as isoniazid. The first study in South America to determine the allelic frequencies of polymorphisms in NAT2 was published in 1993 by Arias et al in Amerindians of Panama and Colombia. They reported allele frequencies of 481T, 590A and 857A in Ngawbé and Emberá Amerindian populations (Arias et al. 1993). Marques et al. published a case-control study of association between genetic polymorphisms and oral cancer susceptibility in Brazil. These researchers reported allele frequencies of 0.35 and 0.43 for NAT*11 in cases and controls, respectively (Marques et al. 2006). In 2007, Texeira et al. reported that *NAT2 * 5B* (341T > C/481C > T/803A > G haplotype) (33%), *NAT2*6A* (282C > T/590G > A haplotype) (26%) *NAT2 * 4* (reference haplotype) (20%), and *NAT2 * 5/* 5* were the most frequent genotypes (31,7%) (Teixeira et al. 2007). In 2008, it was reported that of 254 patients analyzed, 64.3% of patients with hepatotoxicity were slow acetylators (Possuelo et al. 2008). Moreover, in 2011 Texeira et al. reported that slow acetylators presented more incidences of adverse events (hepatotoxicity) associated with anti-tuberculosis drug treatments, compared to intermediate and rapid acetylators in Brazilian patients (Teixeira et al. 2011). Interestingly, smoking seems to be a risk factor for the interaction of the NAT2 phenotype and an increase in the risk of hepatotoxicity (Zaverucha-do-Valle et al. 2014). In Argentina, genotype-phenotype studies have been reported in pediatric patients (Keller et al. 2014) and studies in adults that showed an increased risk of anti-TB drug-induced hepatotoxicity (Chamorro et al. 2013). In another area, slow acetylators have been reported to have significant blood pressure reductions after hydralazine use, with mean 24-h systolic and diastolic blood pressure reductions of 9.2 and 5.5 mmHg in Brazilian patients (Spinasse et al. 2014).

DRUG TRANSPORTERS

In 2011, Rodriguez AC's group in the University of Sao Paulo reported the association between genetic polymorphisms related with organic anion-transporting polypeptide (OATP) transporters and the therapeutic response to atorvastatin in Brazilians with hypercholesterolemia. The authors determined the allelic frequency of three polymorphisms in *SLCO1B1*: 0.32 to c.388G (rs 2306283); 0.16 to c.463A (rs11045819) and 0.12 to c. 521C (rs4149056). Rodriguez et al. found that patients with allele G for the polymorphism c.388A > G presented higher percentage of LDL reduction in comparison to patients with A allele under a dominant model (Rodrigues et al. 2011). In addition, an association between polymorphism rs2306283 in the *SLCO1B1* gene was reported, where they reported greater HDL-C concentrations under treatment with atorvastatin associated with the presence of allele G for 388A > G SNP in Chilean patients (rs2306283) (Prado et al. 2015).

In neurology, Contini et al. reported the presence of genetic polymorphisms and the response to methylphenidate treatment in attention-deficit hyperactivity disorder (ADHD), but without any association (Contini et al. 2012). Then in another area, Coelho et al. in 2013 reported no association between *SLC22A1, SLCO3A1* polymorphisms and virological failure in anti-HIV-1 therapy (Coelho et al. 2013). Recently, Alfirevic et al. in Ecuador reported a study with the relationship between misoprostol and fever (Alfirevic et al. 2015) and Altmann et al reported the prediction of levodopa doses in Parkinson disease (Altmann et al. 2016).

In relation to ATP-binding cassette transporter (ABCs) pharmacogenetics, Sortica et al. in 2012 reported on the influence of ethnicity, geographic origin and genomic ancestry in polymorphisms and haplotype frequencies of drug transporters in Brazilian subjects. The researchers determined in relation to the c.1236C > T (rs1128503) polymorphism in the *ABCB1* gene, allele T has a frequency of 0.43, 0.35 and 0.31 in white, mixed and black populations, respectively. In relation to the variant c.463C > A (rs11045819), the allele A has a frequency of 0.11 in White and mixed populations, and 0.08 for black populations. Whereas, for variant c.521T > C (rs4149056), the C allele has a frequency of 0.13, 0.14 and 0.10 for white, mixed and black populations (Sortica et al. 2012). In 2005 the first association study on ABC pharmacogenetics in South America was reported, Fiegenbaum et al. reported the role of the *ABCB1, CYP3A4,* and *CYP3A5* genes in efficacy and safety of simvastatin treatment. They mentioned that the ABCB1 1236T variant allele had a greater reduction in total cholesterol and LDL (Fiegenbaum et al. 2005). This year, Rodrigues et al. reported an association between T/T carriers (C3435T and G2677T polymorphisms) and higher basal total serum (TC) and LDL cholesterol levels compared with non-T/T carriers (Rodrigues et al. 2005).

In Infectology, Coelho et al. in 2013 reported an association between rs1045642 (3435C > T, *ABCB1*) and rs212091 (198217T > C; 3'-UTR, *ABCC1*) polymorphism and virological failure in anti-HIV-1 therapy (Coelho et al. 2013). In transplantation, Cusinato et al. in 2014 reported that *ABCB1 TTT/TTT* individuals have a higher Co/dose ratio compared with *non-TTT/TTT* individuals in Brazilian kidney transplant patients (Cusinato et al. 2014). Also in Brazil, de Oliveira et al. in 2014 reported that individuals with the *MDR1 3435TT* genotype required a 21% higher dose than that required by *3435CT* and *3435CC* patients (de Oliveira Almeida et al. 2014). Recently, Gengivir et al. reported that patients at 30 days post-kidney transplant with *ABCB1* c.1236TT+c.3435TT+(c.2677TT+TA) genotypes had higher TAC Co/D than those with common or heterozygous genotypes (Genvigir et al. 2016).

VITAMIN K 2,3-EPOXIDE REDUCTASE (VKORC)

Vitamin K antagonist-based anti-coagulant therapy (acenocoumarol, warfarin and phenprocoumon) is currently very important for cardiology, for example, to prevent myocardial infarction and venous thrombosis. However, these drugs duplicate the risk to hemorrhage during the first week of treatment with a high variability between patients (Gage 2006), which can be explained in part through the variability in the gene that codes for the Vitamin K 2,3-epoxide reductase complex subunit 1 (VKORC1). Perini et al. performed the first study of allelic frequency of VKORC1 polymorphisms in South America in Brazil in 2008. In this study researches developed a specific algorithm for Brazilian patients including four polymorphisms in 390 subjects (-1639G > A, 9041G > A, 5808T > G y 6853G > C) (Perini et al. 2008). In 2010 in Colombia, Palacio et al. reported the first study of the genotype-phenotype
association and classified the patient in groups in accordance with the required daily dose (doses 2.28 ± 0. 5 mg/d, 4. 2 ± 0. 76 mg/d and 7. 4 ± 1. 5 mg/d) (Palacio et al. 2010). Palacio et al. found that GG and GA genotype for -1693G > A (rs9923231) polymorphism required a higher daily dose of warfarin (5.17 ± 0.33 mg/d y 4.57 ± 0.28 mg/d, respectively) in comparison to AA genotype (3.38 ± 0.40 mg/d). Also, de Oliveira et al. in 2014 found similar results in Brazilian patients (de Oliveira et al. 2014). Another analyzed variant is the rs397508599 (3730G > A). Botton et al. in 2014 reported that Brazilian patients treated with phenprocoumon required lower doses when these patients had GG genotype in comparison to higher doses in GA and AA patients (Botton et al. 2014). Recently, Benavides et al. in Chilean patients reported that the GG genotype for -1639G > A requires 19.4 mg/week of acenocoumarol, while the GA and AA genotypes require 12.5 mg/week and 8.2 mg/week, respectively (Benavides et al. 2015).

HUMAN LEUKOCYTE ANTIGEN (HLA) SYSTEM

A relevant genetic variability is observed in hypersensitivity reactions to drugs. During hypersensitivity, the human leucocyte antigen (HLA) system plays a central role, because it forms a response against external agents. Severals studies have been carry out in South America in relation to HLA system beacause with a special clinical relevance. In South America some studies have been carried out in native populations in several countries. In 2002 Benitez et al. studied genetic polymorphisms of HLA in the Guaraní population from Paraguay (Benitez et al. 2002), in 2011 Silvera et al. studied these genes in the Wayu population of Colombia (Silvera et al. 2011). Moreover, in 2014, Lorio et al. studied the Tsachilas Indians from Ecuador (Lorio et al. 2014). Infectology is the therapeutic area that is more applicable to HLA polymorphisms. For example, in relation to adverse events related with Abacavir, Moragas et al. reported that the presence of *HLA-B*57:01* is associated with a risk high to have abacavir hypersensitivity syndrome (AHS) in HIV patients in Argentina

(Moragas et al. 2015). The found an allelic frequency of 0.049 for *HLA-B*57:01* in patients with HIV treatment.

Adrenergic Receptors

In relation to adrenergic receptors in South America, Polanczyk et al. published in 2007 a study in Brazilian adolescents with attention-deficit/hyperactivity disorder (Polanczyk et al. 2007). They reported that patients with a G allele at the *ADRA2A* -1291 C > G have an improvement of inattentive symptoms in treatment with methylphenidate. Moreover, Giubergia et al., 2008, found that asthma patients (Giubergia et al. 2008) with Gln27 in beta2-AR genotypes and treated with albuterol in Argentina were associated with a desensitization of the receptor with a decline in the bronchodilator response. Recently, Isaza C in Colombian children didn't find an association between the presence of *Arg16Gly* polymorphisms at *ADRB2* gene and response treatment (Isaza et al. 2012). In addition, Larocca et al in Venezuela reported that Arg/Gly (codon 16) and Gln/Glu (codon 17) genotypes for *ADRB2* were associated with better responses to salbutamol (albuterol) (Larocca et al. 2013). In other therapeutic areas, in 2005 Sookoian et al. analyzed the effect produced by losartan (Sookoian et al. 2005). The most important polymorphism in Alfa-2 adrenergic receptors was *ADRA2A* -1291C > G (rs 1800544).

Dopamine Receptors (DRD)

In 2006, Cordeiro et al. published a study between polymorphisms in dopamine receptors (DPD) and therapeutic failure in patients treated for typical antipsychotics in Brazil, reporting without association in *DRD3 Ser9Gly* rs6280 (Cordeiro et al. 2006). Similar studies have been published in South America, for example, Kohlrausch et al. in 2008 presented a pharmacogenetics study in treatment resistance to typical neuroleptics in Brazilians with European origins. They reported that patients with at least one copy of the T/A/G/A/C haplotype at the *DRD3* gene have more risk to typical neuroleptics (Kohlrausch et al. 2008). Afterward, Ota et al. in 2012 reported an association between a G allele at *DRD1* rs4532 polymorphism and treatment failure in schizophrenia, also in Brazilian patients (Ota et al., 2012). In relation to methylphenidate for attention-deficit/hyperactivity disorder (ADHD), Roman et al. in 2002 reported an association between 19-repeat allele at the dopamine transporter *DAT1* (*SLC6A3*) and poor response to methylphenidate (Roman et al. 2002). In addition, Contini et al. in 2012 reported no association among genetic variants of candidate genes (*SLC6A4, HTR1B, TPH2, DBH, DRD4, COMT,* and *SNAP25*) and outcome and response to methylfenidate treatment in Brazilian patients (Contini et al. 2012).

References

Acevedo, Cristian. A., Luis, A. Quinones., Johanna, Catalan., Dante, D. Caceres., Juan, A. Fulla. & Angela, M. Roco. (2014). "Impact of CYP1A1, GSTM1, and GSTT1

Polymorphisms in Overall and Specific Prostate Cancer Survival." *Urologic Oncology, 32* (3), 280-90. doi:10.1016/j.urolonc.2013.05.010.

Alfirevic, Ana., Jill, Durocher., Anisa, Elati., Wilfrido, Leon., David, Dickens., Steffen, Radisch., Helen, Box., et al. (2015). "Misoprostol-Induced Fever and Genetic Polymorphisms in Drug Transporters SLCO1B1 and ABCC4 in Women of Latin American and European Ancestry." *Pharmacogenomics, 16* (9), 919-28. doi:10.2217/pgs.15.53.

Altmann, Vivian., Artur, F. Schumacher-Schuh., Mariana, Rieck., Sidia, M. Callegari-Jacques., Carlos, R. M. Rieder. & Mara, H. Hutz. (2016). "Influence of Genetic, Biological and Pharmacological Factors on Levodopa Dose in Parkinson's Disease." *Pharmacogenomics, 17* (5), 481-88. doi:10.2217/pgs.15.183.

Araoz, Hilda. Veronica., Karina, D'Aloi., Maria, Eugenia. Foncuberta., Christian, German Sanchez La Rosa., Cristina, Noemi. Alonso., Lilien, Chertkoff. & Marisa, Felice. (2015). "Pharmacogenetic Studies in Children with Acute Lymphoblastic Leukemia in Argentina." *Leukemia & Lymphoma, 56* (5), 1370-78. doi:10.3109/10428194.2014.951844.

Bailliet, G., Santos, M. R., Alfaro, E. L., Dipierri, J. E., Demarchi, D. A., Carnese, F. R. & Bianchi, N. O. (2007). "Allele and Genotype Frequencies of Metabolic Genes in Native Americans from Argentina and Paraguay." *Mutation Research, 627* (2), 171-77. doi:10.1016/j.mrgentox.2006. 11.005.

Benavides, Felipe., Nicole, Grossman., Helena, Poggi., Elena, Nieto., Antonio, Bertran., Daniel, Araos., Marcos, Vasquez., et al. (2015). "[Effect of VKORC1 and CYP2C9 variants on dosage of oral anticoagulants in Chilean individuals]." *Revista medica de Chile, 143* (11), 1369-76. doi:10.4067/S0034-98872015001100001.

Benitez, O., Loiseau, P., Busson, M., Dehay, C., Hors, J., Calvo, F., Durand Mura, M. & Charron, D. (2002). "Hispano-Indian Admixture in Paraguay Studied by Analysis of HLA-DRB1 Polymorphism." *Pathologie-Biologie, 50* (1), 25-29.

Betonico, G. N., Abbud-Filho, M., Goloni-Bertollo, E. M., Alvarenga, M. P. S., Guillemette, C., Villeneuve, L., Benoit-Biancamano, M. O. & Pavarino-Bertelli, E. C. (2008). "Influence of UDP-Glucuronosyltransferase Polymorphisms on Mycophenolate Mofetil-Induced Side Effects in Kidney Transplant Patients." *Transplantation Proceedings, 40* (3), 708-10. doi:10.1016/j.transproceed.2008.03.007.

Boson, W. L., Romano-Silva, M. A., Correa, H., Falcao, R. P., Teixeira-Vidigal, P. V. & De Marco, L. (2003). "Thiopurine Methyltransferase Polymorphisms in a Brazilian Population." *The Pharmacogenomics Journal, 3* (3). 178-82. doi:10.1038/sj.tpj.6500175.

Botton, Mariana. R., Patricia, P. Viola., Eliane, Bandinelli., Tiago, L. L. Leiria., Luis, E. P. Rohde. & Mara, H. Hutz. (2014). "A New Algorithm for Weekly Phenprocoumon Dose Variation in a Southern Brazilian Population: Role for CYP2C9, CYP3A4/5 and VKORC1 Genes Polymorphisms." *Basic & Clinical Pharmacology & Toxicology, 114* (4), 323-29. doi:10.1111/bcpt.12172.

Buendia, Jefferson. Antonio., Esteban, Otamendi., Maria, Cecilia. Kravetz., Fernando, Cairo., Andres, Ruf., Maria, de Davila., Yanina, Powazniak., et al. (2015). "Combinational Effect of CYP3A5 and MDR-1 Polymorphisms on Tacrolimus Pharmacokinetics in Liver Transplant Patients." *Experimental and Clinical Transplantation: Official Journal of the Middle East Society for Organ Transplantation, 13* (5), 441-48.

Carr, Daniel. F., Charles, J. L. la Porte., Munir, Pirmohamed., Andrew, Owen. & Claudia, P. Cortes. (2010). "Haplotype Structure of CYP2B6 and Association with Plasma Efavirenz Concentrations in a Chilean HIV Cohort." *The Journal of Antimicrobial Chemotherapy*, *65* (9), 1889-93. doi:10.1093/ jac/dkq260.

Chamorro, Julian. G., Jorge, P. Castagnino., Rosa, M. Musella., Mabel, Nogueras., Federico, M. Aranda., Ana, Frias., Mabel, Visca., Omar, Aidar., Silvia, Peres. & Gabriela, F. de Larranaga. (2013). "Sex, Ethnicity, and Slow Acetylator Profile Are the Major Causes of Hepatotoxicity Induced by Antituberculosis Drugs." *Journal of Gastroenterology and Hepatology*, *28* (2), 323-28. doi:10.1111/jgh.12069.

Coelho, Antonio. V. C., Suedja, P. S. Silva., Luiz, C. A. de Alencar., Gabriele. Stocco., Sergio, Crovella., Lucas, A. C. Brandao. & Rafael, L. Guimaraes. (2013). "ABCB1 and ABCC1 Variants Associated with Virological Failure of First-Line Protease Inhibitors Antiretroviral Regimens in Northeast Brazil Patients." *Journal of Clinical Pharmacology*, *53* (12), 1286-93. doi: 10.1002/jcph.165.

Contini, Veronica., Marcelo, M. Victor., Guilherme, P. Bertuzzi., Carlos, A. I. Salgado,, Felipe, A. Picon., Eugenio, H. Grevet., Luis, A. Rohde., Paulo, Belmonte-de-Abreu. & Claiton, H. D. Bau. (2012). "No Significant Association between Genetic Variants in 7 Candidate Genes and Response to Methylphenidate Treatment in Adult Patients with ADHD." *Journal of Clinical Psychopharmacology*, *32* (6), 820-23. doi:10.1097/JCP. 0b013e318270e727.

Cordeiro, Quirino., Karen, Miguita., Elisabete, Miracca., Hélio, Elkis. & Homero, Vallada. (2006). "Investigation of Possible Association between Ser9Gly Polymorphism of the D3 Dopaminergic Receptor Gene and Response to Typical Antipsychotics in Patients with Schizophrenia." *Sao Paulo Medical Journal*, *124* (3), 165-67. doi:10.1590/S1516-318020060 00300013.

Cusinato, Diego. Alberto. C., Riccardo, Lacchini., Elen, A. Romao., Miguel, Moyses-Neto. & Eduardo, B. Coelho. (2014). "Relationship of CYP3A5 Genotype and ABCB1 Diplotype to Tacrolimus Disposition in Brazilian Kidney Transplant Patients." *British Journal of Clinical Pharmacology*, *78* (2), 364-72. doi:10.1111/bcp.12345.

D'Andrea, Vanesa., Leonardo, M. Perez. & Enrique, J. Sanchez. Pozzi. (2005). "Inhibition of Rat Liver UDP-Glucuronosyltransferase by Silymarin and the Metabolite Silibinin-Glucuronide." *Life Sciences*, *77* (6), 683-92. doi:10.1016/j.lfs.2005.01.011.

de Oliveira, Almeida., Vanessa, Cristina., Daniel, Dias. Ribeiro., Karina, Braga. Gomes. & Ana, Lucia Brunialti Godard. (2014). "Polymorphisms of CYP2C9, VKORC1, MDR1, APOE and UGT1A1 Genes and the Therapeutic Warfarin Dose in Brazilian Patients with Thrombosis: A Prospective Cohort Study." *Molecular Diagnosis & Therapy*, *18* (6), 675-83. doi:10.1007/s40291-014-0121-4.

Dorado, Pedro., Natalia, Heras., Esther, Machin., Francisco, Hernandez., Enrique, Teran. & Adrian, Llerena. (2012). "CYP2D6 Genotype and Dextromethorphan Hydroxylation Phenotype in an Ecuadorian Population." *European Journal of Clinical Pharmacology*, *68* (5), 637-44. doi:10.1007/s00228-011-1147-8.

Dos Santos-Junior, Amilton., Taciane, Barbosa Henriques., Maricilda, Palandi de Mello., Osmar, Henrique Della Torre., Lucia, Arisaka Paes., Adriana, Perez Ferreira-Neto., Leticia, Esposito Sewaybricker., et al. (2016). "Pharmacogenetics of Risperidone and Cardiovascular Risk in Children and Adolescents." *International Journal of Endocrinology*. 2016:5872423, doi:10.1155/2016/5872423.

Estevez, F. M., Giusti, S. Parrillo. & Oxandabarat, J. (1996). "Enzyme Polymorphism on the Metabolic O-Demethylation of Dextromethorphan in a South American Population." *Medicina*, *56* (4), 378-82.

Estrela, R. C. E., Santoro, A. B., Barroso, P. F., Tuyama, M. & Suarez-Kurtz, G. (2008). "CYP3A5 Genotype Has No Impact on Plasma Trough Concentrations of Lopinavir and Ritonavir in HIV-Infected Subjects." *Clinical Pharmacology and Therapeutics*, *84* (2), 205-7. doi:10. 1038/clpt.2008.12.

Farfan, Mauricio. J., Carolina, Salas., Cristina, Canales., Felipe, Silva., Milena, Villarroel., Katherine, Kopp., Juan, P. Torres., Maria, E. Santolaya. & Jorge, Morales. (2014). "Prevalence of TPMT and ITPA Gene Polymorphisms and Effect on Mercaptopurine Dosage in Chilean Children with Acute Lymphoblastic Leukemia." *BMC Cancer*, *14* (April), 299. doi:10.1186/1471-2407-14-299.

Fiegenbaum, Marilu., Fabiano, R. da Silveira., Cezar, R. Van der Sand., Luiz, Carlos Van der Sand., Maria, E. W. Ferreira., Renan, C Pires. & Mara, H Hutz. (2005). "The Role of Common Variants of ABCB1, CYP3A4, and CYP3A5 Genes in Lipid-Lowering Efficacy and Safety of Simvastatin Treatment." *Clinical Pharmacology and Therapeutics*, *78* (5), 551-58. doi:10. 1016/j.clpt.2005.08.003.

Gage, Brian F. (2006). "Pharmacogenetics-Based Coumarin Therapy." Journal Article, Research Support, N.I.H., Extramural, Review. *Hematology. American Society of Hematology. Education Program*, 467-73. doi:10.1182/asheducation-2006.1.467.

Gaspar, Pedro A., Mara, H. Hutz., Francisco, M. Salzano., Kim, Hill., A, Magdalena. Hurtado., M., Luiza. Petzl-Erler., Luiza, T. Tsuneto. & Tania, A. Weimer. (2002). "Polymorphisms of CYP1a1, CYP2e1, GSTM1, GSTT1, and TP53 Genes in Amerindians." *American Journal of Physical Anthropology*, *119* (3), 249-56. doi:10.1002/ajpa.10128.

Genvigir, Fabiana D. V., Patricia, C. Salgado., Claudia, R. Felipe., Elena, Y. F. Luo., Camila, Alves., Alvaro, Cerda., Helio, Jr Tedesco-Silva., et al. (2016). "Influence of the CYP3A4/5 Genetic Score and ABCB1 Polymorphisms on Tacrolimus Exposure and Renal Function in Brazilian Kidney Transplant Patients." *Pharmacogenetics and Genomics*, *26* (10), 462-72. doi:10.1097/FPC. 0000000000000237.

Giubergia, Veronica., Luis, Pablo Gravina., Claudio, Castanos., Lilien, Chertkoff. & Mario, Grenoville. (2008). "Influence of beta2-Adrenoceptor Polymorphisms on the Response to Chronic Use of Albuterol in Asthmatic Children." *Pediatric Pulmonology*, *43* (5), 421-25. doi:10.1002/ppul.20759.

Iorio, A., De Angelis, F., Garzoli, A., Battistini, A. & De Stefano, G. F. (2014). "HLA-DQA1 and HLA-DQB1 Genes in Tsachilas Indians from Ecuador: New Insights in Population Analysis by Human Leukocyte Antigens." *International Journal of Immunogenetics*, *41* (3), 222-30. doi:10.1111/iji.12116.

Isaza, Carlos., Juan, C. Sepulveda-Arias., Bertha, Ines Agudelo., William, Arciniegas., Julieta, Henao., Gloria, L. Porras. & Leonardo, Beltran. (2012). "beta(2) -Adrenoreceptor Polymorphisms in Asthmatic and Non-Asthmatic Schoolchildren from Colombia and Their Relationship to Treatment Response." *Pediatric Pulmonology*, *47* (9). 848-55. doi:10.1002/ppul.22521.

Jorquera, Andres., Sandra, Solari., Valeska, Vollrath., Irene, Guerra., Jose. Chianale., Colomba, Cofre., Alexis, Kalergis., Patricio, Ibanez., Susan, Bueno. & Manuel, Alvarez-Lobos. (2012). "[Phenotype and genotype of thiopurine methyltransferase in Chilean individuals].” *Revista medica de Chile, 140* (7), 889-95. doi:10.4067/S0034-98872012000700009.

Keller, Guillermo Alberto., Lucas, Fabian., Matias, Gomez., Claudio, Daniel Gonzalez., Roberto, Alejandro Diez. & Guillermo, Di Girolamo. (2014). “Age-Distribution and Genotype-Phenotype Correlation for N-Acetyltransferase in Argentine Children under Isoniazid Treatment.” *International Journal of Clinical Pharmacology and Therapeutics, 52* (4), 292-302. doi:10.5414/CP201957.

Kohlrausch, Fabiana B., Clarissa, S. Gama., Maria, Ines Lobato., Paulo, Belmonte-de-Abreu., Sidia, M. Callegari-Jacques., Alejandro, Gesteira., Francisco, Barros., Angel, Carracedo. & Mara, H. Hutz. (2008). “Naturalistic Pharmacogenetic Study of Treatment Resistance to Typical Neuroleptics in European-Brazilian Schizophrenics.” *Pharmacogenetics and Genomics, 18* (7), 599-609. doi:10.1097/FPC.0b013e328301a763.

Larocca, Nancy., Dolores, Moreno., Jenny, Valentina Garmendia., Olga, Velasquez., Joana, Martin-Rojo., Carlos, Talamo., Alexis, Garcia., & Juan, Bautista De Sanctis. (2013). “Beta 2 Adrenergic Receptor Polymorphisms, at Codons 16 and 27, and Bronchodilator Responses in Adult Venezuelan Asthmatic Patients.” *Biomedical Papers of the Medical Faculty of the University Palacky, Olomouc*, Czechoslovakia, *157* (4). 374-78. doi:10.5507/bp.2012.084.

Lima, M. V., Ribeiro, G. S., Mesquita, E. T., Victer, P. R. & Vianna-Jorge, R. (2008). “CYP2C9 Genotypes and the Quality of Anticoagulation Control with Warfarin Therapy among Brazilian Patients.” *European Journal of Clinical Pharmacology, 64* (1), 9-15. doi:10.1007/ s00228-007-0385-2.

Llerena, Adrian., Pedro, Dorado. & Eva, M. Penas-Lledo. (2009). “Pharmacogenetics of Debrisoquine and Its Use as a Marker for CYP2D6 Hydroxylation Capacity.” *Pharmacogenomics, 10* (1), 17-28. doi:10.2217/ 14622416.10.1.17.

Mallea-Gil, Maria Susana., Ignacio, Bernabeu., Adriana, Spiraquis., Alejandra, Avangina., Lourdes, Loidi. & Carolina, Ballarino. (2016). “Pegvisomant-Induced Cholestatic Hepatitis in an Acromegalic Patient with UGT1A1 (*) 28 Mutation.” *Case Reports in Endocrinology*, 2016:2087102. doi:10.1155/2016/2087102.

Moragas, M., Belloso, W. H., Baquedano, M. S., Gutierrez, M. I., Bissio, E., Larriba, J. M., Fay, F., et al. (2015). “Prevalence of HLA-B*57:01 Allele in Argentinean HIV-1 Infected Patients.” *Tissue Antigens, 86* (1), 28-31. doi:10. 1111/tan.12575.

Morari, Elaine Cristina., Andre, Bacellar Costa Lima., Natassia, Elena Bufalo., Janaina, Luisa Leite., Fabiana, Granja. & Laura, Sterian Ward. (2006). “Role of Glutathione-S-Transferase and Codon 72 of P53 Genotypes in Epithelial Ovarian Cancer Patients.” *Journal of Cancer Research and Clinical Oncology, 132* (8), 521-28. doi:10.1007/s00432-006-0099-3.

Munoz, S., Vollrath, V., Vallejos, M. P., Miquel, J. F., Covarrubias, C., Raddatz, A. & Chianale, J. (1998). “Genetic Polymorphisms of CYP2D6, CYP1A1 and CYP2E1 in the South-Amerindian Population of Chile.” *Pharmacogenetics, 8* (4), 343-51.

Ota, Vanessa Kiyomi., Leticia, Nery Spindola., Ary, Gadelha., Airton, Ferreira dos Santos Filho., Marcos, Leite Santoro., Denise, Maria Christofolini., Fernanda, Teixeira Bellucco., et al. (2012). “DRD1 rs4532 Polymorphism: A Potential Pharmacogenomic Marker for Treatment Response to Antipsychotic Drugs.” *Schizophrenia Research, 142* (1-3), 206-8. doi:10.1016/j.schres.2012.08.003.

Palacio, Lina., Diana, Falla., Ignacio, Tobon., Fernando, Mejia., John, E. Lewis., Ariel, F. Martinez., Mauricio, Arcos-Burgos. & Mauricio, Camargo. (2010). "Pharmacogenetic Impact of VKORC1 and CYP2C9 Allelic Variants on Warfarin Dose Requirements in a Hispanic Population Isolate." *Clinical and Applied Thrombosis/hemostastasis: Official Journal of the International Academy of Clinical and Applied Thrombosis/Hemostasis*, *16* (1), 83-90. doi:10.1177/1076029608330472.

Perini, J. A., Struchiner, C. J., Silva-Assuncao, E., Santana, I. S. C., Rangel, F., Ojopi, E. B., Dias-Neto, E. & Suarez-Kurtz, G. (2008). "Pharmacogenetics of Warfarin: Development of a Dosing Algorithm for Brazilian Patients." *Clinical Pharmacology and Therapeutics*, *84* (6), 722-28. doi:10.1038/clpt.2008.166.

Perini, Jamila A., Rosane, Vianna-Jorge., Ariane, R Brogliato. & Guilherme, Suarez-Kurtz. (2005). "Influence of CYP2C9 Genotypes on the Pharmacokinetics and Pharmacodynamics of Piroxicam." *Clinical Pharmacology and Therapeutics*, *78* (4), 362-69. doi:10.1016/j.clpt.2005.06.014.

Polanczyk, Guilherme., Cristian, Zeni., Julia, P. Genro., Ana, P. Guimaraes., Tatiana, Roman., Mara, H. Hutz. & Luis, A. Rohde. (2007). "Association of the Adrenergic alpha2A Receptor Gene with Methylphenidate Improvement of Inattentive Symptoms in Children and Adolescents with Attention-Deficit/hyperactivity Disorder." *Archives of General Psychiatry*, *64* (2), 218-24. doi:10.1001/ archpsyc.64.2.218.

Possuelo, L. G., Castelan, J. A., de Brito, T. C., Ribeiro, A. W., Cafrune, P. I., Picon, P. D., Santos, A. R., et al. (2008). "Association of Slow N-Acetyltransferase 2 Profile and Anti-TB Drug-Induced Hepatotoxicity in Patients from Southern Brazil." *European Journal of Clinical Pharmacology*, *64* (7), 673-81. doi:10.1007/s00228-008-0484-8.

Prado, Yalena., Nicolas, Saavedra., Tomas, Zambrano., Jenny, Lagos., Alexy, Rosales. & Luis, A Salazar. (2015). "SLCO1B1 c.388A>G Polymorphism Is Associated with HDL-C Levels in Response to Atorvastatin in Chilean Individuals." *International Journal of Molecular Sciences*, *16* (9), 20609-19. doi:10.3390/ijms160920609.

Reis, Marcelo., Ana, Santoro. & Guilherme, Suarez-Kurtz. (2003). "Thiopurine Methyltransferase Phenotypes and Genotypes in Brazilians." *Pharmacogenetics*, *13* (6), 371-73, doi:10.1097/01.fpc.0000054091.48725.eb.

Rodrigues, A. C., Rebecchi, I. M. M., Bertolami, M. C., Faludi, A. A., Hirata, M. H. & Hirata, R. D. C. (2005). "High Baseline Serum Total and LDL Cholesterol Levels Are Associated with MDR1 Haplotypes in Brazilian Hypercholesterolemic Individuals of European Descent." *Revista Brasileira de Pesquisas Medicas E Biologicas [Brazilian Journal of Medical and Biological Research]*, *38* (9), 1389-97. doi:/S0100-879X2005000900014.

Rodrigues, Alice C., Paula, M. S. Perin., Sheila, G. Purim., Vivian, N. Silbiger., Fabiana, D. V. Genvigir., Maria, Alice V. Willrich., Simone, S. Arazi., et al. (2011). "Pharmacogenetics of OATP Transporters Reveals That SLCO1B1 c.388A > G Variant Is Determinant of Increased Atorvastatin Response." *International Journal of Molecular Sciences*, *12* (9), 5815-27. doi:10.3390/ ijms12095815.

Roman, Tatiana., Claudia, Szobot., Silvia, Martins., Joseph, Biederman., Luis, A Rohde. & Mara, H Hutz. (2002). "Dopamine Transporter Gene and Response to Methylphenidate in Attention-Deficit/hyperactivity Disorder." *Pharmacogenetics*, *12* (6), 497-99.

Rosales, Alexy., Marysol, Alvear., Alejandro, Cuevas., Nicolas, Saavedra., Tomas, Zambrano. & Luis, A. Salazar. (2012). "Identification of Pharmacogenetic Predictors of Lipid-Lowering Response to Atorvastatin in Chilean Subjects with Hypercholesterolemia." *Clinica Chimica Acta; International Journal of Clinical Chemistry*, *413* (3-4), 495-501. doi:10. 1016/j.cca.2011.11.003.

Rothhammer, F., Silva, C., Callegari-Jacques, S. M., Llop, E. & Salzano, F. M. (1997). "Gradients of HLA Diversity in South American Indians." *Annals of Human Biology*, *24* (3), 197-208.

Salinas-Souza, Carolina., Antonio, S. Petrilli., & Silvia, R. C. de Toledo. (2010). "Glutathione S-Transferase Polymorphisms in Osteosarcoma Patients." *Pharmacogenetics and Genomics*, *20* (8), 507-15. doi:10.1097/FPC. 0b013e32833caa45.

Santoro, Ana B., Daniela, D. Vargens., Mateus, de Camargo Barros Filho, Daniel, A. Bulzico., Luiz, Paulo Kowalski., Ricardo, M. R. Meirelles., Daniela, P. Paula., et al. (2014). "Effect of UGT1A1, UGT1A3, DIO1 and DIO2 Polymorphisms on L-Thyroxine Doses Required for TSH Suppression in Patients with Differentiated Thyroid Cancer." *British Journal of Clinical Pharmacology*, *78* (5), 1067-75. doi:10.1111/ bcp.12437.

Silva, Marcilene Rezende., Benigna, Maria de Oliveira., Marcos, Borato Viana., Mitiko, Murao. & Alvaro, Jose Romanha. (2008). "Thiopurine S-Methyltransferase (TPMT) Gene Polymorphism in Brazilian Children with Acute Lymphoblastic Leukemia: Association with Clinical and Laboratory Data." *Therapeutic Drug Monitoring*, *30* (6), 700-704. doi:10. 1097/FTD.0b013e31818b0f31.

Silvera, Carlos., Gilberto, Vargas-Alarcon., Cristina, Areces., Diego, Rey., Carlos, Parga-Lozano., Pablo, Gomez-Prieto., Luz, Barbolla., Jorge, Martinez-Laso., & Antonio, Arnaiz-Villena. (2011). "HLA Genes in Wayu Amerindians from Colombia." *Immunological Investigations*, *40* (1), 92-100. doi:10.3109/08820139.2010.517390.

Sookoian, Silvia., Gustavo, Castano., Silvia, I. Garcia., Pedro, Viudez., Claudio, Gonzalez. & Carlos, J. Pirola. (2005). "A1166C Angiotensin II Type 1 Receptor Gene Polymorphism May Predict Hemodynamic Response to Losartan in Patients with Cirrhosis and Portal Hypertension." *The American Journal of Gastroenterology*, *100* (3), 636-42. doi:10.1111/ j.1572-0241.2005.41168.x.

Sortica, Vinicius de A., Elida, B. Ojopi., Julia, P. Genro., Sidia, Callegari-Jacques., Andrea, Ribeiro-Dos-Santos., Manoel, Odorico de Moraes., Marco, A. Romano-Silva., Sergio, D. J. Pena., Guilherme, Suarez-Kurtz. & Mara, H. Hutz. (2012). "Influence of Genomic Ancestry on the Distribution of SLCO1B1, SLCO1B3 and ABCB1 Gene Polymorphisms among Brazilians." *Basic & Clinical Pharmacology & Toxicology*, *110* (5), 460-68. doi:10.1111/j.1742-7843.2011.00838.x.

Spinasse, Lizania Borges., Adalberto, Rezende Santos., Philip, Noel Suffys., Elizabeth, Silaid Muxfeldt. & Gil, Fernando Salles. (2014). "Different Phenotypes of the NAT2 Gene Influences Hydralazine Antihypertensive Response in Patients with Resistant Hypertension." *Pharmacogenomics*, *15* (2), 169-78. doi:10.2217/pgs.13.202.

Teixeira, Raquel L. F., Antonio, B Miranda., Antonio, G. Pacheco., Marcia, Q. P. Lopes., Joseane, Fonseca-Costa., Marcelo, F. Rabahi., Hedi, M. Melo., et al. (2007). "Genetic Profile of the Arylamine N-Acetyltransferase 2 Coding Gene among Individuals from Two Different Regions of Brazil." *Mutation Research*, *624* (1-2), 31-40. doi:10.1016/j.mrfmmm.2007.03.015.

Teixeira, Raquel Lima de Figueiredo., Renata, Gomes Morato., Pedro, Hernan Cabello., Ligia, Mayumi Kitada Muniz., Adriana, da Silva Rezende Moreira., Afranio, Lineu Kritski., Fernanda, Carvalho Queiroz Mello., Philip, Noel Suffys., Antonio, Basilio de Miranda. & Adalberto, Rezende Santos. (2011). "Genetic Polymorphisms of NAT2, CYP2E1 and GST Enzymes and the Occurrence of Antituberculosis Drug-Induced Hepatitis in Brazilian TB Patients." *Memorias Do Instituto Oswaldo Cruz, 106* (6), 716-24.

Valsecchi, Matias., Juan, Garberi., Silvia, Ferrandini., Roxana, Berenguer., Ernesto, Trini. & Pedro, Politi. (2007). "[A prevalent genetic variety of UDP-glycuronosyl transferase predicts high risk of irinotecan toxicity]." *Medicina, 67* (1), 57-60.

van de Bilt, M. T., Prado, C. M., Ojopi, E. P. B., Sousa, R. T., Loch, A. A., Zanetti, M. V., Talib, L. L. & Gattaz, W. F. (2015). "Cytochrome P450 Genotypes Are Not Associated with Refractoriness to Antipsychotic Treatment." *Schizophrenia Research.*, doi:10.1016/j.schres.2015.08.002.

Varela, Nelson., Luis, A. Quiñones., Jana, Stojanova., Joselyn, Garay., Dante, Cáceres., Silvia, Cespedes., Jaime, Sasso. & Carla, Miranda. (2015). "Characterization of the CYP2D6 Drug Metabolizing Phenotypes of the Chilean Mestizo Population through Polymorphism Analyses." *Pharmacological Research, 101* (November), 124-29. doi:10.1016/j.phrs.2015.07.020.

Vargens, Daniela D., Ronaldo, R. S. Neves., Daniel, A. Bulzico., Elida, B. Ojopi., Ricardo, M. R. Meirelles., Cencita, N. Pessoa., Carolina, M. Prado., Pedro, A. Goncalves., Vera, L. G. Leal. & Guilherme, Suarez-Kurtz. (2011). "Association of the UGT1A1-53(TA)n Polymorphism with L-Thyroxine Doses Required for Thyrotropin Suppression in Patients with Differentiated Thyroid Cancer." *Pharmacogenetics and Genomics, 21* (6), 341-43. doi:10.1097/FPC.0b013e3283448d19.

Vianna-Jorge, Rosane., Jamila, A. Perini., Edson, Rondinelli. & Guilherme, Suarez-Kurtz. (2004). "CYP2C9 Genotypes and the Pharmacokinetics of Tenoxicam in Brazilians." *Clinical Pharmacology and Therapeutics, 76* (1), 18-26. doi:10.1016/j.clpt.2004.03.002.

Weich, Natalia., Cristian, Ferri., Beatriz, Moiraghi., Raquel, Bengio., Isabel, Giere., Carolina, Pavlovsky., Irene, B. Larripa. & Ariela, F. Fundia. (2016). "GSTM1 and GSTP1, but Not GSTT1 Genetic Polymorphisms Are Associated with Chronic Myeloid Leukemia Risk and Treatment Response." *Cancer Epidemiology, 44* (October), 16-21. doi:10.1016/j.canep.2016.07.008.

Willrich, Maria Alice V., Alice, C Rodrigues., Alvaro, Cerda., Fabiana, D. V. Genvigir., Simone, S. Arazi., Egidio, L. Dorea., Marcia, M. S. Bernik., et al. (2013). "Effects of Atorvastatin on CYP3A4 and CYP3A5 mRNA Expression in Mononuclear Cells and CYP3A Activity in Hypercholeresterolemic Patients." *Clinica Chimica Acta; International Journal of Clinical Chemistry, 421* (June), 157-63. doi:10.1016/j.cca.2013.03.007.

Zabala-Fernandez, William., Manuel, Barreiro-de Acosta., Ana, Echarri., Daniel, Carpio., Aurelio, Lorenzo., Javier, Castro., David, Martinez-Ares., et al. (2011). "A Pharmacogenetics Study of TPMT and ITPA Genes Detects a Relationship with Side Effects and Clinical Response in Patients with Inflammatory Bowel Disease Receiving Azathioprine." *Journal of Gastrointestinal and Liver Diseases: JGLD, 20* (3), 247-53.

Zaverucha-do-Valle, Camila., Sergio, P. Monteiro., Kenia, B. El-Jaick., Leonardo, A. Rosadas., Marli, J. M. Costa., Marcel, S. B. Quintana., & Liane, de Castro. (2014). "The Role of Cigarette Smoking and Liver Enzymes Polymorphisms in Anti-Tuberculosis Drug-Induced Hepatotoxicity in Brazilian Patients." *Tuberculosis* (Edinburgh, Scotland), *94* (3), 299-305. doi:10.1016/j.tube.2014.03.006.

In: Pharmacogenomics in Latin America
Editor: Luis A. Quiñones
ISBN: 978-1-53611-031-9

Chapter 5

COST-BENEFIT ANALYSIS IN PHARMACOGENOMICS: A DECOMPENSATED RATIO

Fabrício Rios-Santos*[1,*]*, PhD, Cinthia Vila Nova Santana*[2,†]*,
Luiz Alexandre Magno*[2,‡]*, PhD and Antonio Macho*[1,§]*, PhD

[1]Departamento de Ciências Básicas em Saúde, Faculdade de Medicina, Universidade Federal de Mato Grosso, Cuiabá, MT, Brazil
[2]Instituto de Ciências Biológicas, and Instituto Nacional de Ciência e Tecnologia de Medicina Molecular, Faculdade de Medicina, Universidade Federal de Minas Gerais, Belo Horizonte, MG, Brazil

ABSTRACT

Increased evidence of large-scale clinical genetic studies suggests that pharmacogenomics (PGx) is ready for clinical implementation. This assumption rests on the general perception that PGx testing can be used to guide drug therapy selection, improve drug dosing, and prevent side effects. Efforts to control healthcare budgets are essential and a major limitation for PGx implementation has been the lack of prospective studies considering whether PGx health benefits justify its costs as compared with current practice. In this chapter, we focus on a thorough appraisal of the framework in cost–effectiveness analysis as we believe it still is necessary to ensure how the "benefits" have been measured in these studies with respect to the relative costs. Improvements in the quality of care are inevitable, and their costs may offer good value as seen in the best-recognized examples of genotype-guided treatment providing more rapid therapy achievements. Our discussion points out that simple cost–effectiveness models should be expanded to match the research question, thus avoiding inaccurate cost–benefit scenarios and impossible standards of evidence.

* fabriciorios@yahoo.com.
† cinthiavns@gmail.com.
‡ lavmagno@gmail.com.
§ amachoq@gmail.com.

Keywords: pharmacogenomics, pharmacogenetics, pharmacoeconomics, Latin America, cost-benefit

INTRODUCTION

Considerable progress has been made in basic pharmacogenetics research towards the individualization of drug therapy. However, little has been unequivocally shown in favor of the potential benefits of pharmacogenetics testing in clinical practice. Few Cost-Benefit Analysis (CBA) data are extracted from clinical trials, which, in turn, are considered a prerequisite for Pharmacogenetics (PGx) testing implementation. Yet, is this the right way to deal with PGx science? If the principles of PGx therapy preconize individualized medicine, would PGx principles be lost in a population-based approach?

Moreover, much has been discussed about genotyping price, and direct costs. The theory of "price definition" depends of the demand, which is low for PGx testing, and price will go down naturally when PGx testing becomes popular. If genotyping costs seem irrelevant in regard to the benefits, the central problem is that most economic remarks about the PGx implementation are made because many studies have been inadequately designed.

We focused this chapter to highlight such specific points at the interface between costs and benefits. We are convinced that the main issue is not the cost, but how PGx research will be interpreted to obtain full benefits. Furthermore, the high price of some genotyping methods is justified by the elevated number of SNPs (*Single Nucleotide Polymorphism*) used, which does not necessarily increase clinical validity (Cafe Oliveira et al., 2016, Madania et al., 2012). These technologies demonstrate that biotechnology is growing faster than relevant clinical data. In fact, we may ask if it is necessary to genotype a whole marker panel since many reports lack explicit statements on how to translate this information to be used in clinical drug therapy. It is unnecessary to adapt the laboratory or modify personnel training, because molecular biology is currently being used in many clinical applications. This being the case, costs in PGx testing should be viewed from those laboratory facilities already engaged in molecular biology.

For some authors, pharmacogenomics will be cost-effective solely for chronic diseases in which years of inefficient drug therapy could be avoided (Lichter & Kurth, 1997), but acute diseases may also be a good target for pharmacogenomics, provided that the disease did not respond to conventional drug therapy doses or when severe adverse drug reactions exist.

Therefore, we will discuss how clinical evidence is a pre-requisite for any CBA, and, moreover, how economic analysis has an intrinsic perspective deviation over one major PGx principle: "personalized medicine" (PM).

EVIDENCE FOR PHARMACOGENETICS BENEFITS

Benefits of PGx testing have become a reality, and some evidence shows that, when prescribing drugs, PGx improves both the safety and efficacy of therapy. There are a number of examples showing differences in drug response because of genetic variation with commercial available genetic diagnosis kits to predict such responses.

Regarding the benefits that could be introduced by PGx, the use of Evidence Based Medicine (EBM) is highly recommended, because the study design itself brings explicit guarantees or exposes limitations for its consolidation. Taking into account that the most acceptable definition of EBM is "*the conscientious, explicit and judicious use of current best evidence in making decisions about the care of patients,*" PGx is conceptually focused on this clinic perspective.

The fundamental precept of EBM is that there is a hierarchy in the quality of information (Figure 1). However, considering the amount of information on PGx and given a significant number of conflicting results regarding the validity of certain markers as indicative of their phenotypes, analyzing the validity of PGx testing still remains a central problem.

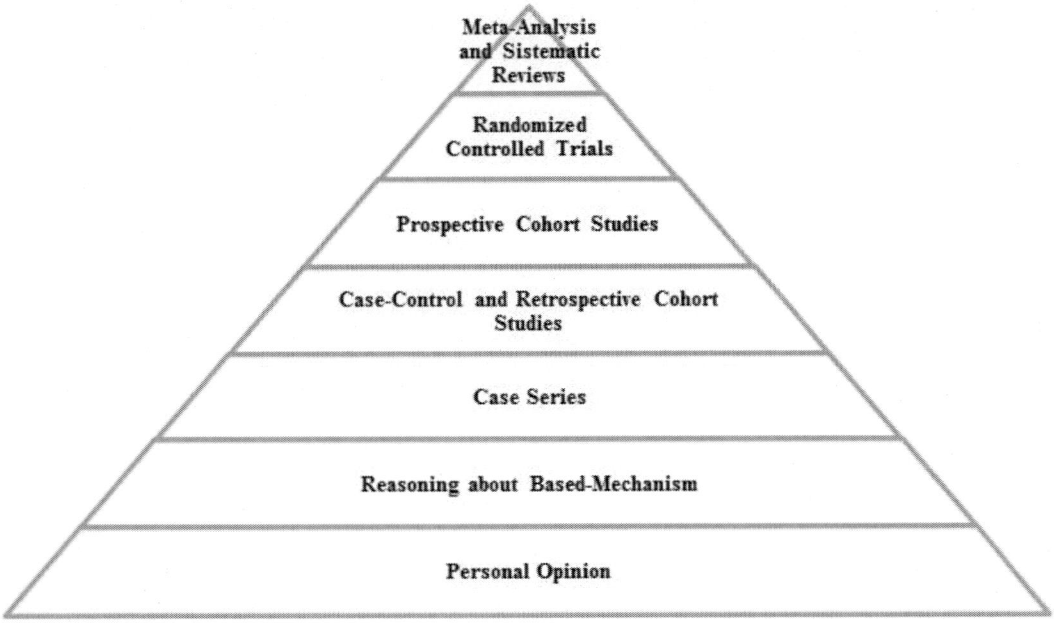

Figure 1. Evidence Based Medicine (EBM). Basic pyramid of the hierarchical Information of Medical Studies.

Unfortunately, compared with the great number of PGx association studies, the amount of evidence supporting pharmacogenetics tests, derived from Randomized Controlled Trials (RCTs), has been rather limited until now. In addition, most studies are poorly characterized regarding patient characteristics, clinical outcome, and phenotype definition, usually investigating a limited number of mutations in only a few genes. Moreover, the majority of predictions are based on case reports or retrospective studies without clearly examining other genetic and non-genetic factors that could also alter the phenotype or outcome. In other words, even in the screening of PGx markers, the most relevant results should be obtained through well-controlled studies, such as RCTs carried out under strongly regulated conditions, and should include as many appropriate candidate genes as possible.

Critical analysis of published clinical studies is a fundamental condition for future investigation of the appropriate cost. Without a proper evaluation of the statistical relevance, sample size, study design, design bias of design, and a suitable determination of qualitatively and quantitatively reliable results, any data about economic analysis would not be true to reality. Moreover, as appointed by the Committee for Medicinal Products for Human Use (CHMP) from the European Medicine Agency, aside from the possible poor quality of the analysis, other important pitfalls are commonly identified in published studies. They include: analyses of non-relevant Single Nucleotide Variations (SNV), analysis of somatic instead of germline DNA (when germline DNA analysis is intended), use of non-PGx design for making claims on PGx markers, non-relevant endpoints selected for the basis of the study, and failure to take into account the pharmacology of the drug in the design of the study (EMA, 2016).

Even when RCT extrapolations have be made with caution, there are a great number of factors to be considered. For instance, in regard to adverse drug reactions (ADR) detection, the selection of patients eligible for RCTs is generally constructed using those who are more vulnerable to ADRs and may not be representative of all patients receiving the treatment. Also, the severity or staging of the disease, as well as comorbidities or multiple drug use in RCTs, may not reflect those found in routine clinical practice and should be considered (Rothwell, 2005). Likewise, the most fragile populations, such as pediatric, geriatric, and pregnant patients, are often underrepresented in RCTs (Bartlett et al., 2005; Cheng, 2013; Sultana et al., 2013). Then, the inclusion criteria for RCT patients should be clearly defined and reported to avoid limitations in drawing conclusions (Sultana et al., 2013, Shapiro et al., 2000).

In addition, traditional RCTs only allow for the estimation of the average treatment effect in the overall study population rather than in a marker-defined sub-population, which would be more appropriate. Therefore, alternative trial designs need to be considered for the evaluation and application of PGx guided therapies (FDA, 2010; Freidlin et al., 2010). However, even with these limitations, RCTs remain the best approach to establishing the clinical utility of PGx testing (Mandrekar & Sargent, 2009a and b).

THE RELEVANCE OF CLINICAL STUDY DELINEATION

That said, we must keep in mind that we first need exhaustive and well-controlled evidence analysis to carry out any valid pharmacoeconomic analyses, because we cannot make any meaningful cost analysis without knowing the benefits.

However, with some systematic reviews aimed at demonstrating an overall conclusion from pooled clinical studies, few of them follow an accurate guideline and with appropriate records of effectiveness. Furthermore, most of them lack standardized methods to conduct an economic analysis. For instance, in a systematic review of 2008, only one study included economic data from a RCT, and no RCT was performed with pharmacoeconomic goals (Vegter et al., 2008). In short, to talk properly of cost-benefits in an evaluation, more consistent and exhaustive RCTs with economic variables should be performed to obtain solid data that could be properly included in appropriate systematic pharmacoeconomic reviews.

Considering the above remarks, a list of important criteria could be proposed for carrying out pharmacoeconomic analysis pertaining to PGx interventions. Vegter et al. (2008) suggest a useful checklist, highlighting critical points of relevance (Table 1). However, other important considerations need to be taken into account, as discussed below.

Table 1. Checklist for performing pharmacoeconomic analysis on pharmacogenetic applications*

Points to be taken in consideration	Observations
Disease under study	The relevance and economic impact of the disease and/or treatment of adverse events under study should be determined
Association between genotype and phenotype	Always: - Use preferably meta-analysis, randomized controlled trials and large cohort studies. - Review and mention studies providing new insights or conflicting results. - Analyze allele frequencies, and test characteristics on sensitivity and specificity.
Compare treatments	Evaluate all current treatments, relevant adverse events and drug efficacy, and determine an alternative treatment based on pharmacogenetics.
Type of economic analysis	Preferably cost-utility or cost-effectiveness analysis
Study perspective	Societal perspectives are preferred.
Time horizon[1] and discount rate[2]	The time horizon should be long enough to include all costs and effects; discounting rates should be guideline-based and be included in the sensitivity analysis.
Sensitivity analysis	Include uncertainty variables, especially in treatment costs and effects, screening costs, genotype distribution, and test parameters on sensitivity and specificity.

* Adapted from: Vegter, S., et al. (2008). "Pharmacoeconomic evaluations of pharmacogenetic and genomic screening programmes: a systematic review on content and adherence to guidelines." *Pharmacoeconomics* 26:569.

[1] Time horizon is the length of time over which an investment is made or held before it is liquidated.

[2] Discount rate is the rate of return used to determine the present value of future cash flows.

Even if a good pharmacoeconomic RCT indicates that a specific PGx test has a good cost-benefit relationship, with relatively high precision, it should be mentioned that it would be completely inaccurate to extend such results to any other population, because the allelic differences or functional polymorphisms would be significantly different. It is perhaps one of the most frequent errors when PGx tests are generalized to be used worldwide. If we assume that a genotype is associated with greater or lesser responsiveness/toxicity to a certain drug, the frequency of these alleles will influence the economic analysis (Veenstra et al., 2009). For instance, *HLA-B* genotyping is normally used for the prevention of some ADR, such as abacavir hypersensitivity syndrome (associated with the *HLA-B*57:01*) or increased risk of Stevens–Johnson syndrome and toxic epidermal necrolysis in response to carbamazepine treatment (associated with the variant allele *HLA-B*15:02*) (Leckband et al., 2013). Specifically, *HLA-B*15:02* is most prevalent in Oceanian and Asian populations, and may even drastically vary within these regions. In Chinese population, it may vary from 1 to 12% or more (the Yunnan province seems reach values as high as 36%). Nevertheless, values decreased in other proximal locations, such as Malaysia and Thailand (6–8%), India (2-6%), Korea (0.5%), and Japan (0.1%), thus demonstrating this variability. Out of this geographical region, the variant allele is quite rare (0-0.02% in European and African populations) (Leckband et al., 2013). In this context, it becomes reasonable to state that the benefit value of such PGx testing will vary among different sub-populations and needs to be validated and adjusted in different countries, especially those with clearly distinct ethnicity (Pena et al., 2011; Talbot et al., 2010). In the same way, if *one drug does not fit all*, a similar pattern of diagnostic markers could not be used indiscriminately for any population.

THE FRONTIER BETWEEN INDIVIDUALIZED AND COLLECTIVE BENEFITS, AND THE COST DILEMMA

It is worthwhile to mention that EMB creates a conceptual dilemma. Both EMB and PM have different scopes: in the case of PM, each patient would have the right to be properly treated in an individualized way, and for EBM and its own directive, the best treatment is focused for a population with a similar clinical profile. In other words, and as stated by José de Leon in his manuscript "*Evidence-Based Medicine versus Personalized Medicine: Are They Enemies?,*" "*while the EBM approach emphases on RCTs to establish the best treatment for the average patient and ignores the outliers, PM focuses on the outliers*" (de Leon, 2012). Furthermore, even the bases of both concepts have a distinct financial origin: while RCTs have a great deal of support from the pharmaceutical industry, most research in the PGx area is rooted in the public and academic fields (Swen et al., 2007). However, nowadays, it seems clear that PM and EBM have a fundamental ethical intersection that puts such approaches side-by-side: the individual, and not society, is the focus of medical care. The fundamental role of PM, as anticipated by Sir William Osler in 1891, remains the same: we still need to look for personal traits in the overall population to make an adjustment in pharmacotherapy (Osler, 1891).

The definition of pharmacoeconomy specified by the International Society for Pharmacoeconomics and Outcomes Research (ISPOR)[1] clearly assumes the social and collective approach of this science (Pashos et al., 1998). However, economic arguments alone cannot be used to refuse the best medical treatment to an individual patient from a pharmacogenetics perspective. Above all, it is an ethical challenge rather than a sanitary or marketing limitation. Thus, in contraposition to "Classical EBM," an emerging "Personalized EBM" should be redefined as "*the conscientious, explicit and judicious use of current best evidence in making decisions about the care of a well clinical defined patient.*" When, for a genetic reason, a group of individuals responds differently from the majority of treated ones, PGx has the mission to individualize care, regardless of the cost. Health is a universal human right.

Fortunately, advances in PGx marker identification showed that patient selections, based on a molecular marker (also known as "enrichment"), is a reasonably strategy to avoid adverse effects and the unnecessary administration of drugs, despite the economic burden of the use of such PGx. For instance, cetuximab is effective only in *KRAS* wild-type colon cancer patients. At least, $600 million could be saved annually by avoiding the inefficient administration in refractory patients (Shankaran et al., 2009). Regardless of the economic evidence that supports or disapproves the introduction of PGx tests in clinical practice, when the main health problem involves survival and/or maintaining human dignity, discussions about money will be irrelevant, as long as there is sufficient evidence of effectiveness and

[1] "Field of study that evaluates individual, enterprise and market behavior in relation to the use of products, services and pharmaceutical programming, and frequently focuses on costs and the consequences of its utilization."

applicability. Consider another case, assuming a high level of PGx evidence, in which only 1% of individuals may die if submitted to a contraindicated treatment, they should have the right to access PGx technology and, therefore, the proper treatment, even they pay for treatment and diagnosis in a direct-to-consumer market service. The cost of such screening should be discussed by government agencies, private insurance companies, and other health providers, since the main purpose of PGx is to gain a better individual medical care system through personalized medicine. It is clear that the analysis of evidence and applicability precedes any pharmacoeconomic analysis, given that the higher the sensibility, specificity, and applicability of a test, the higher its economic utility.

Official PGx Consolidation Efforts for Clinical Practice

Despite the availability of PGx tests, physician use of clinical pharmacogenetics is scarce. It is caused in part by a perceived lack of clinical utility, inadequate or non-existent professional guidelines, and limited reimbursement from private insurance companies or government plans. This behavior is generally due to contradictory or confusing evidence in the literature or lack of appropriate EBM or pharmacoeconomic papers. Using their own criteria, some agencies and organizations have been seeking to identify evidence specifications for the inclusion of PGx evaluations in their clinical routine, as well as provide adequate guidelines for physicians. All of them include evidence-based principles for analyzing applications and assigning a "level of evidence" score. Among these, we highlight the databases of the Pharmacogenomics Knowledge Base (PharmGKB), the Clinical Pharmacogenetics Implementation Consortium (CPIC), and the Office of Public Health Genomics of the Center for Disease Control and Prevention (CDC).

PharmGKB provides six levels of evidence, based on multiples criteria (replications, statistical significances, odds ratio, and others). According to PharmGKB (Whirl-Carrillo et al., 2012), **Level 1A** indicates a variant-drug combination endorsed to a PGx guideline in use at CPIC or other medical societies, implemented at a Pharmacogenomics Research Network (PGRN) site, or in another major healthcare system. **Level 1B** represents a variant-drug combination in which the preponderance of evidence shows an association. This association must be replicated in more than one cohort with significant p-values and preferably will have a strong size effect. **Level 2A** – Defined for a variant-drug combination with moderate evidence of an association. The association must be replicated, but there may be some studies without statistical significance, and/or with a small size effect. In addition, the variant will be within a so-called VIP (Very Important Pharmacogene), as defined by PharmGKB. Variants in Level 2A are between known pharmacogenes and, consequently, functional significance is more likely. **Level 2B** – When the variant-drug combination reaches the same criteria as Level 2A without the necessity of being within a VIP. **Level 3** - Indicates a variant-drug combination based on a single significant (not yet replicated) association or, in multiple studies, lacking clear evidence of an association. **Level 4** - Annotation based on a case report, non-significant study or only on *in vitro*, molecular, or functional assay evidence.

The CDC usually assumes the challenge to guide practicing physicians to stay current in emerging fields, including PGx technologies. In our context, CDC's effort is to bring genomic approaches to physicians and other stakeholders and a degree of evidence supporting implementation in clinical routine by providing a tier classification. Along with EGAPP[2] members from CDC (Dotson et al., 2014), the tier classification involves outside participation by other consolidated groups, such as PharmGKB.

Table 2. Representative list of drugs with Clinical Pharmacogenetics Implementation Consortium guidelines

Drug	Gene of interest	PGx on US FDA label	CDC Tier classification*
Abacavir	*HLA-B*	Genetic testing recommended	Tier 1
Amitriptyline	*CYP2D6*	Actionable PGx	Tier 2
Azathioprine	*TPMT*	Genetic testing recommended	Tier 2
Capecitabine	*DPYD*	Actionable PGx	Tier 2
Carbamazepine	*HLA-B*	Genetic testing required	Tier 1
Clomipramine	*CYP2D6*	Actionable PGx	Tier 2
Clopidogrel	*CYP2C19*	Genetic testing recommended	Tier 2
Codeine	*CYP2D6*	Actionable PGx	Tier 2
Desipramine	*CYP2D6*	Actionable PGx	Tier 2
Doxepin	*CYP2D6*	Actionable PGx	Tier 2
Fluorouracil	*DRYD*	Actionable PGx	Tier 2
Imipramine	*CYP2D6*	Actionable PGx	Tier 2
Ivacaftor	*CFTR*	Genetic testing required	Tier 1
Mercaptopurine	*TPMT*	Genetic testing required	Tier 2
Nortriptyline	*CYP2D6*	Actionable PGx	Tier 2
Peginterferon Alfa-2B	*IFNL3*	Actionable PGx	Tier 2
Phenytoin	*CYP2C9*	Actionable PGx	Tier 2
Rasburicase	*G6PD*	Genetic testing required	Tier 1
Thioguanine	*TPMT*	Actionable PGx	Tier 2
Trimipramine	*CYP2D6*	Actionable PGx	Tier 2
Warfarin	*CYP2C9*	Actionable PGx	Tier 2
	VKORC1	Actionable PGx	Tier 2

* Tier 1 defines genetic tests with strong evidence supporting its routine use in clinical practice. Tier 2 defines genetic tests with some evidence of benefit for a select subset of high-risk patients. All drugs have CPIC (Clinical Pharmacogenetics Implementation Consortium) level A and PharmGKB level of evidence 1A. PGx: Pharmacogenetics.

Adapted from Chang et al. (2015). "Clinical application of pharmacogenetics: focusing on practical issues." *Pharmacogenomics* 16:1733.

The CDC guidelines are stratified into three tiers for a series of health-related genomic tests, based on information from Medicaid coverage decisions, clinical practice guidelines, systematic reviews, FDA labels information, and USA government Centers for Medicare (Dotson et al., 2014). Briefly, **Tier 1** applications are defined by the CDC's Office of Public Health Genomics (OPHG) as "*those having significant potential for positive impact on public health based on available evidence-based guidelines and recommendations.*" Thus, Tier 1 applications incorporate the highest level of evidence/readiness for clinical routine. **Tier 2** applications represent tests of promising utility, but requiring more consolidated studies and, therefore, are not yet recommended for implementation in clinical practice. Tier 2 is especially important for some subsets of high-risk patients and to highlighting future

[2] "Evaluation of Genomic Applications in Practice and Prevention."

strategies for clinical trials. **Tier 3** describes applications not suitable for clinical implementation and with evidence that strongly discourages their use (Chang et al., 2015; Green et al., 2015) or that shows them to be neither harmful nor helpful in clinical practice (Dotson et al., 2014).

Finally, the Clinical Pharmacogenetics Implementation Consortium (CPIC) was founded by both the National Institute of Health's PGRN and the PharmGKB organization. The CPIC has undertaken a substantial effort to promote reliable recommendations for the implementation of PGx tests in routine clinical practice and translating PGx tests into clinical recommendations. CPIC guidelines can be easily accessed in the specialized Clinical Pharmacology and Therapeutics journal, but a representative list of drug guidelines based on PGx is shown in Table 2. Note that not all are classified by CDC as recommended for clinical practice (Tier 2). Contrary to other classifications, CPIC guidelines focus much more on suggesting how to optimize drug therapy based on PGx tests rather than how tests should be ordered or how much they cost.

COMMON PHARMACOECONOMIC CONCEPTS IN PGX RESEARCH

Pharmacoeconomic studies have its own terminology, and although the aim of this chapter is not to delve into these concepts, some definitions become important since studies differ significantly on the methods and concepts used. First, three key concepts need to be clarified -efficacy, effectiveness, and efficiency-, which, although commonly used as synonyms, have distinct applications. *Efficacy* is the response to a treatment obtained in conditions considered optimal, controlled, usually coming from clinical phase III studies. *Effectiveness* is obtained under routine conditions, in the usual way, approaching the behavior of clinical practice, such as that observed in phase IV studies, where multiple variables can modify the outcome. *Efficiency*, in turn, incorporates the ratio of costs in its analysis and is synonymous with cost-effectiveness. Efficiency shows us the extent of the benefit when incorporated into the real world with its real economic costs. From a marketing perspective (usually adopted by financial healthcare agencies), the best decisions should be associated within the best value choice. As shown in the classic diagram of Figure 2, the goal is always to achieve the best ratio between effectiveness and cost. The successful consolidation of any technology is determined by the highest effectiveness achieved at the lowest possible cost or, in other words, at greater efficiency (indicated by the D quadrant in Figure 2). Logically, one may consider a pharmacoeconomic analysis only after evaluating the effectiveness of the intervention (in our case, the PGx impact on the outcome). Without effectiveness, it makes no sense to carry out a pharmacoeconomic analysis.

We have to consider that costs represent the value of all investments (from the equipment to human labor) used in carrying out the service. These overall costs may be classified as direct, indirect, and intangible (Eisenberg, 1989; Rothstein, 2003). Direct costs are those directly related to the services, for example the costs of genotyping tests, staff remuneration, investment in equipment, and even the recovery of invested capital. The direct costs in other areas are those considered the main factor limiting the incorporation of a given technology. However, the costs for implementation of PGX in clinical practice should be viewed with great discretion, as once the real impact of the test results is demonstrated, other cultural and global economic factors could hamper its implementation. Cultural factors include the possible lack of knowledge of medical practitioners in how to use or interpret such examinations and lack of familiarity with the existence of such tests. Among the economic factors, the most common one would be the laboratory's concern of not recovering the costs because of the uncertainty in demands. However, PGx tests are widely used in developed countries to enhance the portfolio of services and the laboratory's reputation, in addition to sharing costs with other molecular exams.

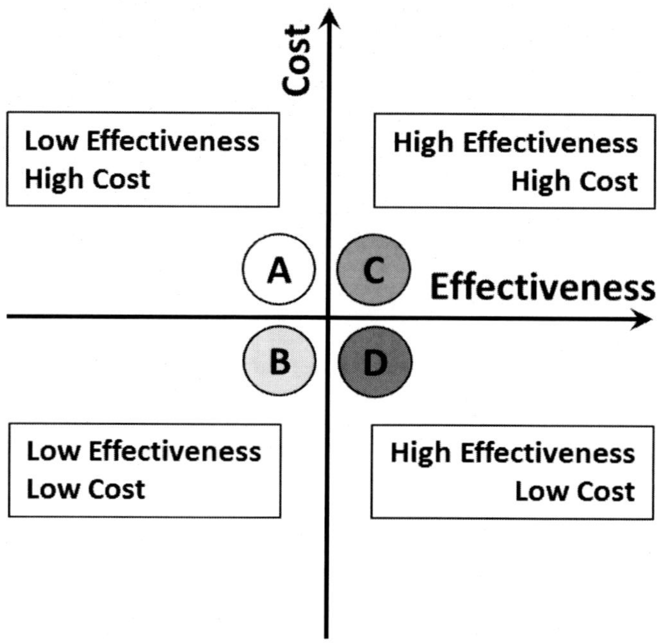

Figure 2. Classic Diagram of Cost/Effectiveness. In a pharmacoeconomic analysis, there is an order of preference of the measures to be taken. In this diagram, we can see that efficiency should always be assessed at the lowest possible cost (D). The quadrants (A) through (D) represent the different options in crescent order of choice.

In our viewpoint, direct costs can be interpreted at least in two different situations, those that involve 1) a high or low impact on public health or 2) a high or low impact on individual health. Public and private insurance funding will primarily invest in those tests that have a significant effect on preventing serious adverse effects, as well as in genotyping for the selection of drugs that would have a lower cost. On a personal level, the discussion would be much broader, involving reimbursement contracts with insurers and the person's financial capacity and interest in carrying out an examination. For example, when a rare genotype is associated with a high risk of death, whether by therapeutic failure or toxicity of a drug, the pharmacoeconomic data would show a high cost for its implementation in routine clinical practice and lead to trouble to be borne by the insurer. However, if the test ensures a high positive predictive value, it would still be carried out by an individual who could afford the cost of a genetic test. This situation would be very similar to others the person had already done in further medical segments, such as PCR for detection of pathogens –such as chlamydial infection-, fetal sexing and paternity.

We also have the possibility to evaluate the indirect and intangible costs in PGx testing. Indirect costs are those related to the consequences (economic or humanitarian) of the introduction of such technology or the absence thereof, and can be measured by the prolongation of the disease or even death. Intangible costs are perhaps the most neglected and the more complex to be evaluated in economic research, because they are related to the quality of life that the intervention brings. Despite the difficulty of this quantification (which is why they are called *intangibles*) and to be measured in a short time, some authors now incorporate Quality of Life assessments in their studies (Plumpton et al., 2016).

Consequently, the costs have a close relationship with the measure of patient outcome that we seek to assess, and rarely are the costs from "not-introducing the PGx testing" and "the quality of life" incorporated. Thus, these indirect and intangible costs include a wide variety of approaches that need to be considered, such as the prevention of severe adverse events, increased quality of life, and adherence and maintenance of the treatment. Pharmacoeconomy should comprise the evaluation of technical yields, clinical efficiency, sadety, economic efficacy, organizational impact, and its social and ethical implications (Mossialos, 1997). A single clinical study could hardly address all possible aspects of the direct, indirect, and intangible costs, but it is clear that the consolidation of clinical evidence and the strength of business market expansion will play key roles in determining the success of the use of PGx markers within the clinical routine.

Pharmacoeconomy was initially organized in accordance with the cost element (which tends to be more constant) and in relation to the evaluated outcome. With this differentiation, various methods have emerged (Areda et al., 2011; Venturini & Johnson, 2002), of which Cost Minimization Analysis (CMA), Cost-Effectiveness Analysis (CEA), Cost-Benefit Analysis (CBA), and Cost-Utility Analysis (CUA) are especially noteworthy. Their advantages and disadvantages are summarized in Table 3. Although several authors have been making efforts to demonstrate the cost-effectiveness of some PGx applications, extrapolation of these results should be made with caution. The implementation of the pharmacoeconomic principles applied to PGx cannot be limited to the development of financial calculations for the simple determination of costs in diagnostic tests and economic benefits in damage reduction. Although it is important to determine the overall costs (direct, indirect, and intangible) for genotyping, such studies will always have limited and temporary applicability; limited because the results cannot be freely extrapolated to any population, not only by the genetic variability between countries, but also by significant differences in local costs and business interests, and temporary because, with the great emergence of genotyping technologies and interested users, the genotyping costs are rapidly falling in the market, resulting in many cost-benefit studies being quickly outdated.

Cost-minimization analysis is the simplest form of economic evaluation, in which only the costs will be subject to comparisons, as efficacy or effectiveness will be considered as technically equal in the compared methods. They have a more limited application and could be used when comparing different genotyping techniques. It assesses the cost differential for a specific unit of effectiveness, i.e., clinical results. The years of life saved, shorter hospitalization or the occurrence of adverse effects fall into this category. Usually, it is a more specific analysis, often disregarding its impact on the quality of life of patients, which should not be disregarded. In response, many authors have been seeking to expand the CEA through cost-utility studies by defining parameters such as gain in quality-adjusted life-years (QALY), difference in clinical effect, incremental cost per QALY or incremental cost for life-year saved, and cost per adverse reaction/event avoided, thus enhancing discussions about the real impact of the use of PGX in clinical practice.

Table 3. Categories of pharmacoeconomic analysis

Method	Description	Comments
Cost Minimization Analysis (CMA)	Finds the program with the lowest cost among those of equal benefit	Although simple, this approach is hard to apply to PGx, since it includes only limited costs. It is justified when alternatives of comparable programs or therapies produce clinically equivalent results.
Cost Effectiveness Analysis (CEA)	The results of CEA are expressed by a cost/effectiveness ratio. Effectiveness is measured as higher survival, lower incidence of adverse reactions.	Although CEA is the most common analysis, it is difficult to establish comparisons between studies of different diseases (for instance, asthma and hypertension), due to differences in the measurement of primary effectiveness.
Cost Utility Analysis (CUA)	Considers the relationship between costs of a treatment and its benefits to the health-related quality of life of the patient, as well as the risks of adverse drug reactions. CUA is applicable in studies aimed at comparing different treatments, mainly focused on chronic patients.	Despite being an improvement over CEA, as it introduces the patient's level of satisfaction with the treatment, it is still difficult to measure some utilities from different sectors, such as health costs in relation to education.
Cost Benefit Analysis (CBA)	CBA is used to compare positive and negative consequences of alternative uses of resources, and it has a monetary unit as a measure of outcome.	Its use is more focused on macroeconomic issues, given that it is very difficult in clinical practice to convert subjective outcomes, such as quality of life, satisfaction. or pain intensity in monetary units. This type of instrument evaluates the economic viability of social projects.

Adapted from Areda et al., 2011. Pharmacoeconomy: An indispensable tool for the rationalization of health costs. *Braz. J. Pharm. Sci.*, 47:231 and Venturini & Johnson, 2002. Introduction to pharmacoeconomic principles and application in pharmacy practice. *Calif. J. Health Syst. Pharm.*, 14:6.

Some authors have also used indirect predictions (or simulations) of the efficiency of a particular diagnostic tool from secondary data obtained from literature, such as the cost of treatment, frequency of adverse reactions, and the financial impact of their prevention (such as reduced hospitalization). For instance, Stallings and cols (Stallings et al., 2006) developed a model for evaluating potential cost savings on healthcare costs in asthma patients, using data from retrospective claims databases, and concluded that the genetic variant prevalence, test cost and the cost of choosing the wrong treatment were key parameters in the economic viability of pharmacogenomics in clinical practice. However, this approach has an economic logic and is often limited to collective interest criteria, whether public by the governments or private in the marketing sphere. The introduction of the analysis of effectiveness to the economic world significantly altered the conclusions on the relevance of introducing a PGx test in clinical practice and should be critically reviewed, because it could vary with the change in the local scene from an economic, formative, and technical point of view, inter alia.

In summary, PGx evaluation prior to pharmacological treatment is economically viable provided the savings gained by avoiding ineffective treatment and adverse effects are greater than the costs of testing, taking into account that the economic viability will depend on specific circumstances of its use. Also, from an ethical and individual viewpoint, the benefits of a well evidenced PGx will always be superior to the costs.

Conclusion

Medical services continue to foment discussions on the costs of covering new technologies in the healthcare system, not only for PGx technologies, and it seems irreversible that advances in pharmacogenetics will gradually be introduced in governments' healthcare strategies, private reimbursement policies, and in other less developed countries. Clearly, there is great potential for pharmacogenetics to improve the risk-benefit profile of treatments as well as reduce healthcare costs by avoiding adverse drug reaction expenses. Nonetheless, many more pharmacoeconomic studies will be needed to satisfactorily measure the economic impact of any PGx testing implementation. Finally, not just the costs to the healthcare system should be considered, but also the user's preference in a direct to consumer payment. Once the real contribution of genotyping for a specific individualized therapy has been confirmed, costs will be the least significant factor that would block the implementation of PGx in clinical practice.

References

Areda CA, Bonizio RC, Freitas Od. Pharmacoeconomy: an indispensable tool for the rationalization of health costs. *Braz J Pharm Sci.* 2011;47:231-40.

Bartlett C, Doyal L, Ebrahim S, Davey P, Bachmann M, Egger M, et al. The causes and effects of socio-demographic exclusions from clinical trials. *Health Technol Assess.* 2005;9(38):iii-iv, ix-x, 1-152.

Cafe Oliveira LN, Muniz-Sobrinho Jda S, Viana-Magno LA, Oliveira Melo SC, Macho A, Rios-Santos F. Detection of multidrug-resistant *Mycobacterium tuberculosis* strains isolated in Brazil using a multimarker genetic assay for *katG* and *rpoB* genes. *Braz J Infect Dis.* 2016;20(2):166-72.

Chang MT, McCarthy JJ, Shin J. Clinical application of pharmacogenetics: focusing on practical issues. *Pharmacogenomics.* 2015;16(15):1733-41.

Cheng H. Randomized, controlled trials: Gold or bronze? *J Am Med Dir Assoc.* 2006;7(9):611-2.

de Leon J. Evidence-based medicine versus personalized medicine: are they enemies? *J Clin Psychopharmacol.* 2012;32(2):153-64.

Dotson WD, Douglas MP, Kolor K, Stewart AC, Bowen MS, Gwinn M, et al. Prioritizing genomic applications for action by level of evidence: a horizon-scanning method. *Clin Pharmacol Ther.* 2014;95(4):394-402.

Eisenberg JM. Clinical economics. A guide to the economic analysis of clinical practices. *JAMA*. 1989;262(20):2879-86.

EMA (European Medicines Agency), Committee for Medicinal Products for Human Use (CHMP). Guideline on good pharmacogenomic practice: European Medicines Agency (EMA); 2016 [updated 28/04/2016]. Available from: http://www.ema.europa.eu/docs/en_GB/document_ library/Scientific_guideline/2016/05/WC500205758.pdf.

FDA (U.S. Food and Drug Administration). Draft Guidance for Industry: adaptive design clinical trials for drugs and biologics, 2010 [updated 02/2010]. Available from: http://www.fda.gov/downloads/Drugs/.../ Guidances/ucm201790.pdf.

Freidlin B, McShane LM, Korn EL. Randomized clinical trials with biomarkers: design issues. *J Natl Cancer Inst*. 2010;102(3):152-60.

Green RF, Dotson WD, Bowen S, Kolor K, Khoury MJ. Genomics in Public Health: Perspective from the Office of Public Health Genomics at the Centers for Disease Control and Prevention (CDC). *Healthcare* (Basel, Switzerland). 2015;3(3):830-7.

Leckband SG, Kelsoe JR, Dunnenberger HM, George AL, Jr., Tran E, Berger R, et al. Clinical Pharmacogenetics Implementation Consortium guidelines for *HLA-B* genotype and carbamazepine dosing. *Clin Pharmacol Ther*. 2013;94(3):324-8.

Lichter JB, Kurth JH. The impact of pharmacogenetics on the future of healthcare. *Curr Opin Biotechnol*. 1997;8(6):692-5.

Madania A, Habous M, Zarzour H, Ghoury I, Hebbo B. Characterization of mutations causing rifampicin and isoniazid resistance of *Mycobacterium tuberculosis* in Syria. *Pol J Microbiol/Polskie Towarzystwo Mikrobiologow*. 2012;61(1):23-32.

Mandrekar SJ, Sargent DJ. (a). Clinical trial designs for predictive biomarker validation: theoretical considerations and practical challenges. *J Clin Oncol*. 2009;27(24):4027-34.

Mandrekar SJ, Sargent DJ. (b). Clinical trial designs for predictive biomarker validation: one size does not fit all. *J Biopharm Stat*. 2009;19(3):530-42.

Mossialos E. Citizens' views on health care systems in the 15 member states of the European Union. *Health Econ*. 1997;6(2):109-16.

Osler W. Recent Advances in Medicine. *Science*. 1891;17(425):170-1.

Pashos C, Klein E, Wanke L. ISPOR Lexicon. NJ, USA1998. 72 p.

Pena SD, Di Pietro G, Fuchshuber-Moraes M, Genro JP, Hutz MH, Kehdy Fde S, et al. The genomic ancestry of individuals from different geographical regions of Brazil is more uniform than expected. *PLoS One*. 2011;6(2):e17063.

Plumpton CO, Roberts D, Pirmohamed M, Hughes DA. A Systematic Review of Economic Evaluations of Pharmacogenetic Testing for Prevention of Adverse Drug Reactions. *Pharmacoeconomics*. 2016;34(8):771-93.

Rothstein MA. Pharmacogenomics: Social, Ethical, and Clinical Dimensions: Wiley; 2003.

Rothwell PM. External validity of randomised controlled trials: "to whom do the results of this trial apply?" *Lancet*. 2005;365(9453):82-93.

Shankaran V, Bentrem DJ, Mulcahy MF, Bennett CL, Benson III AB, editors. Economic implications of Kras testing in metastatic colorectal cancer (mCRC). 2009 Gastrointestinal Cancers Symposium; 2009: ASCO University.

Shapiro SH, Weijer C, Freedman B. Reporting the study populations of clinical trials. Clear transmission or static on the line? *J Clin Epidemiol*. 2000;53(10):973-9.

Stallings SC, Huse D, Finkelstein SN, Crown WH, Witt WP, Maguire J, et al. A framework to evaluate the economic impact of pharmacogenomics. *Pharmacogenomics*. 2006; 7(6):853-62.

Sultana J, Cutroneo P, Trifiro G. Clinical and economic burden of adverse drug reactions. *J Pharmacol Pharmacother*. 2013;4(Suppl 1):S73-7.

Swen JJ, Huizinga TW, Gelderblom H, de Vries EG, Assendelft WJ, Kirchheiner J, et al. Translating pharmacogenomics: challenges on the road to the clinic. *PLoS Med*. 2007;4(8):e209.

Talbot J, Magno LA, Santana CV, Sousa SM, Melo PR, Correa RX, et al. Interethnic diversity of *NAT2* polymorphisms in Brazilian admixed populations. *BMC Genet*. 2010;11:87.

Veenstra DL, Higashi MK, Phillips KA. Assessing the cost-effectiveness of pharmacogenomics. *AAPS PharmSci*. 2000;2(3):E29.

Vegter S, Boersma C, Rozenbaum M, Wilffert B, Navis G, Postma MJ. Pharmacoeconomic evaluations of pharmacogenetic and genomic screening programmes: a systematic review on content and adherence to guidelines. *Pharmacoeconomics*. 2008;26(7):569-87.

Venturini F, Johnson KA. Introduction to pharmacoeconomic principles and application in pharmacy practice. *Calif J Health Syst Pharm*. 2002;14(1):6-14.

Whirl-Carrillo M, McDonagh EM, Hebert JM, Gong L, Sangkuhl K, Thorn CF, et al. Pharmacogenomics knowledge for personalized medicine. *Clin Pharmacol Ther*. 2012;92(4):414-7.

In: Pharmacogenomics in Latin America
Editor: Luis A. Quiñones
ISBN: 978-1-53611-031-9

Chapter 6

PHARMACOGENOMICS, REGULATORY AFFAIRS AND PUBLIC HEALTH

Diadelis Remirez Figueredo*[*]*, PhD
National Centre for Quality Control of Drugs, Cuba

ABSTRACT

The science of pharmacogenomics has advanced significantly in the last five years. The Pharmacogenomics helps identify interindividual variabilities in drug response (both toxicity and effectiveness). This information will make it possible to individualize therapy with the intent of maximizing effectiveness and minimizing risk. The objective of this chapter is to present an overview about the international regulations about this topic and to present briefly the introduction of this science in Cuba. It was done a revision in the international literature about the existing regulations, guidance, concept paper, etc. The chapter illustrates the general requirements for regulation, e.g., reception, codification and sample storage, biomarkers, ethical consideration as well as it is explained the relation of this discipline with pharmacokinetics studies, bioequivalence trials and pharmacovigilance systems. Cuban guidance will be introduced which is focused to pharmacogenetic studies during the clinical phases of drug development. Pharmacogenetic has several advantages in order to get rational use of drugs but still there are many challenges which will be shown in this work. The hope for the future is that through personalized medicine, doctors and patients will be able to make better-informed choices about treatment. This treatment will avoid the adverse drug reaction to the medication and will improve the diagnosis diseases as well as the prevention and treatment of diseases.

Keywords: pharmacogenetics, pharmacogenomics, pharmacovigilance, regulatory, public health

[*] Corresponding Author E-mail: diade.remirez@infomed.sld.cu.

INTRODUCTION

Pharmacogenetics, one of the cornerstones of personalized medicine, has the potential to change the way in which health care is offered by stratifying patients into various pretreatment categories, such as likely responders, likely non-responders or likely to experience adverse drug reactions. In order to advance drug development and regulatory science, regulatory agencies globally have promulgated guidelines on pharmacogenetics for nearly a decade (Evans, 2003).

Pharmacogenomics helps in identifying inter-individual variability in drug response (both toxicity and effectiveness). This information will make it possible to individualize therapy with the intent of maximizing effectiveness and minimizing risk beside that, pharmacogenomics allows optimize pharmacovigilance by identifying risk of adverse reactions and to improve the design of clinical trials by stratifying group population. Thus, it is important to regulate this subject in order to minimize the adverse drug reactions, make decisions based on risk benefit criteria, and allow the rational use of drugs based on other criteria and to avoid the discrimination of people (Gibsburg & Willard, 2009).

The main mission of any regulatory agency is to control the quality, safety and efficacy of drugs. The main regulatory agencies around the world: Food and Drug Administration (FDA) from United States of America, Health Canada (Canada), European Medicines Agency (EMA) from Europe and Pharmaceuticals and Medical Devices Agency (PMDA) from Japan have issued guidance's about pharmacogenomics as well as the International Conference on Harmonization (ICH) which is integrated by FDA, EMA, PMDA and Pharmaceutical companies.

There are different regulatory dispositions related with pharmacogenomic studies; for example: concept paper, reflection paper, drafts, position paper, which explains how to implement the regulations and guidance about pharmacogenomic assays (FDA, 2016).

EMA is the regulatory agency with more regulations about this topic, followed by FDA and International Conference of Harmonization (ICH). These documents explain about the samples reception, the codification, the use of biomarkers. Recently, EMA published a new guide in relation with good practices for pharmacogenomic moreover there are guides which include the importance of Pharmacogenomic in the prescription as well as the drug rescue from the market and pharmacogenetic methodologies in pharmacokinetics studies, etc. On the other side, World Health Organization, in the technical report series, appears as potential risk the declaration of genetic polymorphism for its importance in the drug metabolized by polymorphic enzymes e.g., Cytochrome P-450 (CYP) 3A4 metabolize Indinavir and nelfinavir and promethazine is metabolized by CYP 2D6 (WHO, 2006).

Each regulatory agency has settled their guides according to the rational use of drug for their population, the safety and efficacy of the drugs and taking into account the context of every country for the further implementation.

In general the guidance's published are formed by the following chapters (EMA, 2006):

- Introduction
- Background
- Objectives and Scope

- Terms and Definitions
- Regulatory Requirements

Introduction: In this chapter it is explained a general summary of the regulatory disposition.

Background: Refers about the previous report about the topic of the guidance.

Objectives and Scope: Specify the aims of the regulatory disposition, and its scope should indicate whether the guideline concern a selected area of medicinal product development where limited experience is available and knowledge is fast evolving requiring the need for easy updates and flexibility.

Concerning to the regulatory requirements is mentioned the requirements recommended or demanded related with the codification of samples, the obligation in the use of biomarkers, ethical aspects, etc.

MAIN ITEMS IN THE GUIDELINES

Terms and Definitions

The uses of terms in this subject have been harmonized and these have been accepted by the international scientific community (Regulatory, academics, ethical committee, and health professionals).

Actually the terms pharmacogenomic and pharmacogenetics are frequently used interchangeably. The achievement of widely accepted working definitions of the two would be a useful first approach to applying pharmacogenetics and pharmacogenomics in clinical trials. It is important to single out pharmacogenetics and pharmacogenomics from the wider field of genetic testing as the latter encompasses different level of concerns especially in terms of sensitivity of sample handling, data and trial results management (ICH, 2016).

Pharmacogenetics: is the study of interindividual variations in DNA sequence related to drug response.

Pharmacogenomics: is the study of the variability of the expression of individual genes relevant to disease susceptibility as well as drug response at cellular, tissue, individual or population level. The term is broadly applicable to drug design discovery, and clinical development.

Other terms are also identified like, Mutation, Alleles, Single nucleotide polymorphism, Genomic Biomarker, Gene, Genotype, Phenotype, Locus (EMA, 2016).

MANAGEMENT AND STORAGE SAMPLES

The sample identification is very important for getting traceability of the results. According the guidelines published related with pharmacogenomic studies the samples and data can be identified in 4 general categories (Ricci et al., 2011).

1) Identified data: The samples are identified with personal identifiers such as (name, identification numbers, like social security or national insurance number), the right identification offers privacy protection similar to general healthcare confidentiality in everyday medical practice.
2) Coded Data and Samples. The data and coded samples are labeled at least with a unique code and do not carry any personal identifiers. These samples can have a unique or second label, the second code offers additional confidentiality, and second code is linked to the first code by a key. It is possible to trace the data or samples back to the individual by the use of both coding keys.
3) Anonymised Data and Samples: Anonymous data and samples are initially single or double coded but then the link between the subject's identifiers and the unique code (s) are subsequently deleted. Once the link has been deleted it is no longer possible to trace the data and samples back to the individual through the coding key (s). Anonymisation is intended to prevent subject re-identification.
4) Anonymous Data and Samples. Anonymous data and samples are never labelled with personal identifiers and therefore there is no potential to trace back genomic data and samples to an individual subject.

On the other side, the suitable storage is a key aspect for sample preservation, at the same time to the period of time for protecting the sample is very important, which can take several years. The biological samples could have variable quantities of nucleases in certain conditions, for this reason is important that samples have acceptable integrity in the storage conditions selected which should be checked and validated. All these process, reception codification and storage should fulfillment of good pharmacogenomic and clinical practices (EMA, 2016).

USE OF BIOMARKERS

Significant pharmacogenomic research has focused on understanding the molecular mechanism underlying certain adverse reactions and on recognizing biomarkers (BMs) that identify individuals at risk.

A genomic biomarker is a measurable DNA and/or RNA characteristic that is an indicator of normal biologic process, pathogenic processes, and/or response to therapeutic or other interventions (EMA, 2016).

A genomic biomarker could, for example, be a measurement of:

The expression of a gene
The function of a gene
The regulation of a gene.
There are 2 main types of BMs.

1) Predictive BMs: Are those that provide clues towards response (safety or efficacy or metabolic) to a particular therapeutic intervention, especially drug therapy. Evaluation of clinical utility of such predictive markers is facilitated by pivotal trials

conducted in defined patient populations, selected and grouped based on the marker (s).

2) Prognostic BMs: Those that indicate disease prognosis, that may not have an intrinsic relation to specific intervention, either drug therapy or otherwise. Thus prognostic BM may or may not provide the basis for a clinical decision or influence the decision algorithm for treatment or intervention. However, studies evaluating prognostic GBMs may provide a scientific background of the natural history of the disease, facilitate development of additional other biomarkers (genomic or non-genomic) and contribute to drug development indirectly.

Another important aspect is the critical parameters for the choice Biomarker assay.

The intended use of the BMs should be thought before development and validation of the chosen assay.

Critical Parameters for the Choice Biomarker Assay (EMA, 2016)

1) Assay-specific considerations. These include, known attributes of analytical sensitivity, diagnostic sensitivity, specificity, accuracy, repeatability, reproducibility, linear range of quantitative assays including control of known relevant interference, and limits of detection.
2) Preanalytical factors: General principles of specimen acquisition regarding BMs, sample type, patient or subject selection criteria, conditions and preparation for sampling, sample handling, e.g., storage conditions, extraction procedure.
3) Analytical factors: Assays protocol, assay platform including amplification efficiency, linearity, precision, dynamic range as well as limit of detection, calibrators and software and algorithms used for the interpretation of results, performance variables.
4) Post analytical factors: Data handling and processing, relevant published data, meta data and standards available, comparative performance with relevant standard if available or state of the art test.
5) Validation steps in the development of an assay for a pharmacogenomic biomarkers: Assay performance evaluation: Validation of analytical performance, validation of in vivo clinical performance as relevant for context and intended uses (i.e sensitivity and specificity in detecting clinically relevant response), further plans in post market surveillance to confirm clinical utility.

Therefore, a biomarker should be qualified as early as possible for promoting its use in drug development when reasonable evidence for a particular context of use is available.

Another important point to consider is that a biomarker should be qualified internationally rather than by a single regulatory agency because most drugs are currently developed globally, and conducting a MRCT has become a standard strategy for drug development. For global drug developments, an internationally qualified biomarker is necessary so that the data can be submitted to multiple regulatory agencies for a regulatory review and decision-making (EMA, 2016).

A big challenge is 'biomarker qualification'. A PGx biomarker to be used in drug developments should be qualified and accepted by a regulatory agency because use of an unqualified and unacceptable biomarker may result in misinterpretation of the acquired data due to false signals (false-positive or -negative signal) and, therefore, may not be used in regulatory decision-making. Biomarker qualification by a regulatory agency is an important process to qualify the objective and context of use of the biomarker before it can be widely used in drug development. To confirm the acceptability of the biomarker, each agency – PMDA, the FDA and the EMA – has established a biomarker qualification process. Thus, in many cases the identified biomarkers are used for more than one drug and consequently the same biomarker can be used for different indications, for example, Glivec for several types of leukemia but also for stromal tumours (Otsubo et al., 2013). Figure 1 shows some of the differences in required pharmacogenetics testing between EMA and FDA. The vast majority of drugs/78%) have similar label requirements for diagnostic testing in both geographies.

Biomarkers open a new era for pharmaceutical companies concerning to the Companion diagnostics for drugs mainly for cancer treatment in order to guarantee the safety and efficacy of the drugs and the reduction of the cost (Berryessa et al., 2013).

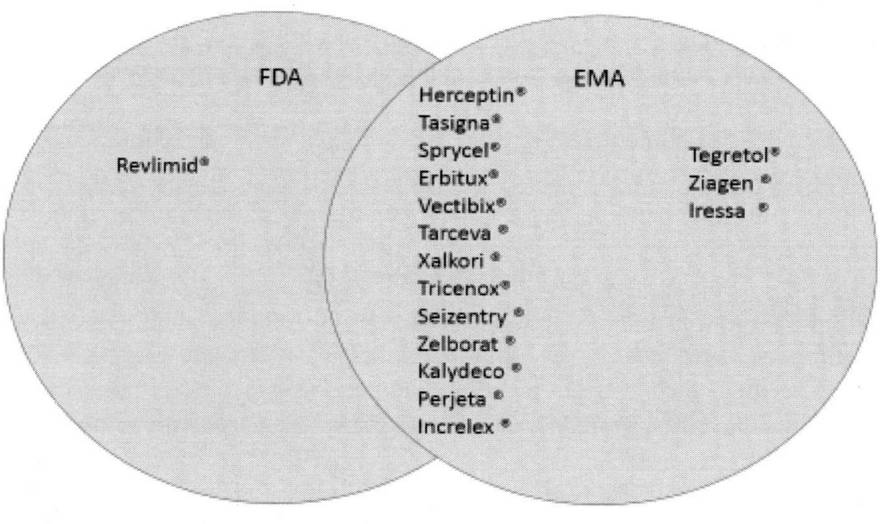

Figure 1. Drug required pharmacogenetic companion diagnostic testing.

Ethical Issues

This is a big challenge in this subject, particularly as science and technology continue to advance very rapidly. Whole genome sequencing, for example, is poised to eliminate the need for individual genetic tests, thus raising ethical concerns about the creation of genetic information which individuals may or may not want to know and which may or may not remain privately secured. Ethical Committee has a great responsibility, should approve the pharmacogenomic studies taking into account, Balancing risk-benefit, Ethical responsibilities of all the participants in the study, The patients need all necessary information to make the own decision. All anticipatable information of expected benefits or expected harms. Concern of individual participants regarding anonymity, privacy and confidentiality should be respected and should be addressed in a research agreement the discrimination should not be allowed and the protocol should always refer the alternative treatment in case the patient according the result cannot take the drug assayed (Issa et al., 2002).

Another important point is the Investigation in biological samples with genetic material because (Berryessa et al., 2013):

1) Genetic material is unique for each person and does not change along the time. It means that patient will be potentially identified.
2) Because DNA is stable. Would be capable of multiple researches. Many of them are not in related to the goals for which they were gotten.
3) The samples that will be taken for pharmacogenomic assays could be useful in order to know the diseases which the subject does not want to know.
4) Because genetic material is common for parents and brothers, the finding could have implications for subject relatives what shows as results individual ethical problems.

Pharmacogenetics allows researchers to conduct gene profiling to answer questions about patient responses to medicines, which results in the design of safer and more effective medicines. The science and its applications are real today and will be increasingly utilized in coming years. While it is extremely unlikely that individuals will be excluded from health insurance because of their response (or lack) to a particular drug, or that they will be subject to employment exclusions (in hiring, promoting or job responsibilities), ethical issues are central to policy debate about the appropriate use of pharmacogenetic testing and its related benefits (Berryessa et al., 2013).

The European regulatory strategy adopted in recent years to raise awareness via informing health-care professionals by adding pharmacogenomic information in drug label is evolving and is now increasingly providing practical guidance on why, when and how to obtain pharmacogenomic individual patient's data to facilitate pharmacogenomics (PGx)-guided drug treatment.

To further promote the scientifically sound integration of PGx in product development and consequently the product label and patient treatment, the EMA sets recommendations and requirements for the investigation and incorporation of PGx in drug development and surveillance/ pharmacovigilance.

In addition, the Agency has elaborated guidance on the importance of identification and validation of genomic biomarkers 10–13 and established a number of activities (Ehrman et al., 2015).

Drug labels form an intrinsic and integral part of the marketing authorization and are intended to guide patient treatment.

The Summary product characteristics (SmPC) is the basis of information for health-care professionals on how to use the medicinal product safely and effectively and the SmPC thus sets out key elements of drug benefits and risks relevant to the clinical use of the product defined during the medicine regulatory assessment process. Regulatory recommendations on how pharmacogenomic information shall be presented in the EU labels have been published (EC, 2016).

The description and place of pharmacogenomic information in the label (SmPC section) has also an important impact on reimbursement not only for the drug but also for the related companion diagnostic test used and potentially liability implications for the treating health-care professionals.

Almost 15% of EMA-evaluated medicines contain pharmacogenomic information in their label that directly impacts patient treatment. These sections include Therapeutic indications, Posology and method of administration and Contraindications etc (EC, 2016).

In Table 1 it is shown, the information in each chapter.

Table 1. Types of PGx information for labeling

Section of Label.	Pharmacogenomic (PG) information.
Therapeutic indications	If the product's indication depends on a particular genotype or the expression of a gene or a particular phenotype, then this should be stated in the indication.
Dosage and administration.	Where necessary, dosage adjustments in patients with a particular genotype should be stated (with cross-reference to other relevant sections for further detail as appropriate).
Contraindications.	Linked to a particular genotype.
Special warning and precautions	Subjects or patients with a specific genotype or phenotype might either not respond to the treatment or be at risk of a pronounced pharmacodynamic effect or adverse reaction. These may arise because of non-functioning enzyme alleles, alternative metabolic pathways (governed by specific alleles) or transporter deficiencies. Such situations should be clearly described if known.
Drug Interactions.	If interactions with other medicinal products depend on polymorphisms of metabolizing enzymes or certain genotypes, then this should be stated.
Undesirable effects.	This section may include information on any clinically relevant differences specifically observed in patients with a specific genotype.
Overdose.	If applicable, counteractive measures based on genetic factors should be described.
Pharmacodynamic properties.	Any relevant pharmacogenetics information from clinical studies may be mentioned here. This should include any data showing a difference in benefit or risk depending on a particular genotype or phenotype.
Pharmacokinetic properties.	Variations with respect to polymorphic metabolism should be described, if clinically relevant, in quantitative terms.

More than 200 drug labels in the US, corresponding to about 10% of drugs approved by the FDA, contain pharmacogenetics information, still a relatively small figure. But it shows that a significant number of relationships between genetic markers and pharmacokinetic or drug response phenotypes are potentially relevant. Both at Food and Drug Administration and at European Medicines Agency (EMA) pharmacogenomic information in drug labels is increasingly present and consequently tailored drug therapy to patients' genetic make-up can lead to improved benefit-risk balance of drug treatment by optimization of the target population and by tailored choice of drug treatment and drug dosages resulting in improved drug efficacy including minimization of adverse drug reactions (ADRs) (Eichelbaum et al., 2006).

There are several differences in how the main agencies deal with critical issues in the application of pharmacogenetics to pharmacokinetics parameters and thee are highlighted in Table 2.

Table 2. Summary of differences between the three regulatory guidelines on pharmacogenetics. (Malliepard et al., 2013)

Issue	Regulatory agency.		
	European Medicinal Agency.	Pharmaceutical and Medical Devices Agency, Japan.	US Food and Drug Administration.
Development phases covered in guideline or guidance.	Preclinical and clinical development (Phase I-IV, focusing on PK).	Clinical development (Phases I-IV).	Early clinical development (Phases I and II).
Banking of DNA samples.	Highly recommended.	Recommended.	Recommended.
Genomic testing	Required	Recommended	Recommended
In vitro cut-off values*	> 50%	None	None
In vitro cut-off values*	> 25%	None	None

*It is firm requirement only when in vitro (> 50%) or in vivo (> 25%) cut-off values are met. For when pharmacogenetics-related testing is requires in pharmacokinetics studies.

Health Canada, the Canada Regulatory Agency, has adopted ICH guidance Definitions for Genomic Biomarkers, Pharmacogenomics, Genomic Data and Sample Coding Categories E-15. In general the regulatory agencies have exchanged through different meeting, working party about Pharmacogenomic. There is consensus among the regulatory authorities concerning this topic.

Current Status of Pharmacogenomics in Latin-American Countries

Several studies have been done with Latin-American population related with the study of the variability of pheno- and genotypes in Hispanics. Most of these studies have been carried out through Ibero American Network of Pharmacogenomic and Pharmacogenetic. Studies related with the polimorphism of CYP isoenzymes (CYP 2C9, 2C19, 2D6) and variability in the drugs response have been done with population from Costa Rica, Peru, Uruguay, Cuba, Argentina, Nicaragua, Ecuador, Chile, Colombia, México. One of the studies describes the frequency of the most relevant pharmacogenetic biomarkers and metabolic phenotypes in Central American healthy volunteers and to determine its interethnic variability. Twenty-six original research articles on allelic, genotypes or metabolic phenotype frequencies were analyzed, in which a total number of 7611 Central American healthy volunteers were included (6118 were analyzed for genotype and 1799 for metabolic phenotype). No reports were available for population from Belize and Honduras. The CYP2D6*4and *5 frequencies in Amerindian populations from Costa Rica have shown to be among the highest frequencies so far reported in the world. Furthermore, NAT2*5and *6 presented high frequencies in admixed populations than in Amerindians, but, inversely, the NAT2*7was more frequent in Amerindians compared to an admixed population. Likewise, different patterns of distribution have been shown in HLA-A*02, *03 and HLA-B*07among Native populations from Latin America. Reports on Central American populations were also found for the CYP2C19, LDLR, CYP2E1, MDR1, G6PD, TP53, CYP1A2, CYP3A4 and CYP3A5 biomarkers, but no data were available for the other 91 pharmacogenetic biomarkers revised in Central American populations. Differences in the frequency of some pharmacogenetic biomarkers and metabolic phenotypes were found, showing interethnic variability within Central American and with other Latin American populations (Céspedes-Garro et al., 2014, Rodeiro et al., 2012).

The main implications for the implementation in Latin-American are: the population are very heterogeneous, so that there is great variability in the drug response, another important aspect is the access to the drugs for every people is not equal is limited, according to the economical support, for this reason, the persons could be discriminated for using specific drugs, it means that people need the medicines and they cannot get them. There is a fragmentation of health care system according the health insurance. Latin-American is a continent which imports drugs and posologies, the drugs are sold in these countries but they have not assayed in them, another barrier is related to the need for clear guidelines for the use of pharmacogenomics in clinical practice due to the cost of trials.

Some of the possible solutions are: to create global development programmes, in several countries rather use bridging studies, the vital need is the education of health professional and the community, particular attention for special populations, like children and geriatrics patients, other relevant aspect is access to the information, and trials for the populations of Latin American countries. Pharmacogenetics should be introduced with the focus on the benefit for the majority of the population (Quiñones et al., 2014; Llerena, 2015).

Considerations about Cuba

Cuba is a country with heterogeneous population, with a growing development of biological product, which are subject to pharmacogenomic studies, these products are mainly for cancer treatment, for this reason is very important the right response to the patients (25). On the other side there are some pharmacogenetic studies with Cuban population through

Pharmacogenetic Iberoamerican Network. Some of them are: It was demonstrated on debrisoquine hydroxylation in a Cuban population, moreover, differences on the frequency of ultrarapid metabolizers. The frequency of poor and ultrarapids metabolizers between Cubans and Spaniards have been determined, these results could explain inter-individual and interethnic differences on drug response such as side effects or the therapeutic failures among Cuban patients receiving treatment with CYP2D6 substrates (Gonzalez et al., 2007).

The role of CYP2D6 activity variation in a sample of Cuban women with regard to their risk of eating disorder symptoms was evaluated and the results showed that that there is a relationship between individual at risk of bulimia symptoms and increased CYP2D6 hydroxylation capacity in healthy Cuban women which supported previous finding about the relationship between eating disorders and CYP2D6 active genes (Lledó et al., 2012).

Taking into account the previous resulted and development of Cuban biotechnology, The Cuban Regulatory Agency, has clinical regulatory framework, which involves 5 main guidance (CECMED, 2016).

1) Requirements for authorization and modification of clinical trials.
2) Good Clinical Practices in Cuba.
3) Requirements for notification and reports of serious and unexpected adverse events in the clinical trials.
4) Requirements for clinical trials phase I and II with local products under investigation destined to the Cancer and AIDS treatment.
5) Requirements for availability and bioequivalence studies.

Recently it has been elaborated a guidance for carrying out pharmacogenetic studies during the clinical phases of drug development, it is oriented to the Industry, and this guide is focused to give some recommendations about this assays for example the use and type of biomarkers, sample codification, ethical aspect, a proposal of consent informed is proposed. This guide is about to be approved.

OTHER IMPORTANT ASPECTS FOR PHARMACOGENOMIC REGULATIONS

Bioequivalence Studies

In bioequivalence studies, intra-individual variability (CVw) is critical in determining sample size. In particular, highly variable drugs may require enrolment of a greater number of subjects. We hypothesize that a strategy to reduce pharmacokinetic CVw and hence sample size and costs would be to include subjects with decreased metabolic enzyme capacity for the drug under study. Regulatory agencies indicate that bioequivalence studies must be conducted in homogeneous but representative samples of the general population, ensuring external validity of the results. The pharmacogenomic assays are very useful for bioequivalence studies so that if the metabolic enzymatic capacity of the subjects is known for the assayed drug, this is clearly essential for the analysis of drug safety and efficacy to ensure that the results can be generalized to the whole population. However, as the main purpose of bioequivalence studies is to assess differences among drug products' bioavailabilities, decreasing intra-individual variability might increase the accuracy of determinations of drug-related factors (González-Vacarezza et al., 2012).

Use of Pharmacogenomic Methodologies in the Pharmacovigilance Evaluation of Medicinal Products

Some genomic biomarkers may predict drug exposure or the risk status of a patient related to adverse drug reactions (ADR). Genomic factors may play a role in the pathogenesis of both predictable and unpredictable ADRs as well as in clinical progression of diseases and rescue drug withdrawn from the market. Currently, there is limited information on the utilization of a genomic biomarker during follow up (post marketing) or on the effect of labeling with genomic information.

It is proposed guidelines to further discuss the following aspects (EMA, 2016).

1. Systematic consideration of pharmacogenomic effects and the implications of genomic biomarker use in the target population in the risk management plan (RMP) for:

a) Suspected/identified lack of efficacy/effectiveness of a relevant medicinal product related to the use of a genomic biomarker.
b) Safety concerns of a relevant medicinal product related to the use of a genomics biomarker.

2. Early consideration of when post authorization genomic data may need to be monitored or collected to confirm appropriate dose and co-medication, as well as to provide information or advice based on identified genomic biomarkers.

3. Collection and storage of genomic material (e.g., DNA or other) during clinical trials and upon the occurrence of serious ADR, l ack effectiveness post authorization or unexpected worsening of the condition.

4. Methodologies for post authorization safety studies and post authorization efficacy/ effectiveness studies regarding pharmacogenomic and biomarkers related issues (for adverse drug reaction and for lack of effectiveness) in the post marketing setting.

5. Consideration of the level and type of evidence for identification of signals, and how to report to the competent authorities (e.g., in RMP updates, periodic safety update reports published studies etc).

6. Consideration of risk minimization measures depending upon the importance of the possible clinical implications.

7. Labelling issues

a) What pharmacogenomic information to include in the product information (PI) and in which sections.
b) Assessing the impact of information in the product information on the use of the medicinal products.

c) Consideration of monitoring the effectiveness of genomic biomarker use in a clinical setting if there are requirements or recommendations in the product information on the use of genomic biomarkers.

The document is expected to provide for both industry and Regulatory Authorities regarding the application of pharmacogenomic methodologies in the pharmacovigilance evaluation of medicinal products and to support the development of methodologies for monitoring of the effectiveness of genetic biomarker use in the clinical setting.

Use of Pharmacogenetic Methodologies in the Pharmacokinetics Evaluation of Medicinal Products

The pharmacokinetics of many medicinal products is prone to interindividual variability, which is caused by several factors such as gender, age, weight, impaired renal and hepatic function and genetics. For drugs where pharmacogenetics is important, for pharmacokinetic variability there are guidelines which recommend that pharmacogenetics should be implemented in the drug development process. Genetic variants can influence a drug pharmacodynamics but also the absorption, distribution, metabolism and excretion of a drug. Furthermore, pharmacogenetics may also influence the formation, distribution and elimination of metabolites and this should be remembered if there are metabolites that may affect the efficacy and/or safety of the administered drug. Genotypes leading to absent decreased or increased enzyme or transport protein activity affecting the pharmacokinetics of the investigated drug and major pharmacologically active metabolites should be considered. Studies of the effect of pharmacogenetics on the pharmacokinetics of an active substance (parent and/or active metabolite) and its implication for efficacy and safety during development are generally required when the magnitude of the interindividual variation in drug exposure is so high as to likely influence the safety and/or efficacy of the drug in genetically variable populations. Factors that identify such a situation are (EMA, 2016):

a) In vitro and/or in vivo studies indicate that known functionally polymorphic enzyme or transporter is likely to represent an important pathway in the metabolism or distribution or the drug or
b) In vitro and/or in vivo studies that known functionally polymorphic enzyme or transporter is likely to represent an important pathway in the formation, elimination or distribution of a pharmacologically active or toxic metabolite, or
c) In vivo studies indicate substantial interindividual differences in the pharmacokinetics of the drug likely to influence the efficacy or safety of the drug in the variable subpopulation, which cannot be explained by other intrinsic or extrinsic factor:

Studies on the effect of pharmacogenetics on the pharmacokinetics of an active substance and its implications for efficacy and safety are generally recommended during development if:

d) Available in vitro data indicate that a human polymorphic enzyme or transporter contributes to the pharmacokinetics of the active substances but the quantitative role may be low based on the in vitro data or,
e) There is high interindividual pharmacokinetic variability or there are pharmacokinetics outliers with higher or lower exposure to the active substance which cannot attributed to other known intrinsic or extrinsic factors, but which possibly can give rise to clinical efficacy and safety concerns based on the existing knowledge, or
f) Major differences in pharmacokinetics are observed in different ethnic groups, which cannot be attributed to other known intrinsic or extrinsic factors.

Other recommendations have been made on how to implement pharmacogenetics during the different phases of clinical development, starting with in vitro studies conducted before investigation of the medicinal product in man. As a general rule, genotyping of the population included in a drug-drug interaction study for a relevant gene is recommended when pharmacogenetics are expected to affect the pharmacokinetics of any of the drugs included in the study. Because interactions might differ in subgroups of different pharmacogenetic genotypes, genotyping for the enzymes and transporters involved in the interaction should be carried out when appropriate (van Schie et al., 2011)).

Conclusion

Consideration of pharmacogenetics is also important in global drug development. Pharmacogenetic analysis in multi-regional clinical trials (MRCTs) will provide useful scientific data for understanding similarities and differences in drug responses (efficacy and/ or safety) among various ethnicities. Specifically, when large differences in pharmacokinetics (PK) parameters among different populations is observed, pharmacogenetic analyses are useful for the examination of the reason or reasons for the differences and to set an appropriate dose for each population in later clinical trials (such as an exploratory dose-finding study) (Warner et al., 2011).

Pharmacogenomics-guided drug development has been implemented in practice in the last decade, resulting in increased labeling of drugs with pharmacogenomic information. However, there are still many challenges remaining in utilizing this process.

Main Challenges

- Education for health professionals and the community.
- Lack of familiarity with pharmacogenomics data.
- Resistance to the routine use of pharmacogenomics in medical care.
- Legal assurance.
- Interaction of the parties involved (patients, health-care professionals, authorities, health insurance companies and scientists.

As it comes to clinical translation, PGx is faced with big hopes and high expectations by everybody involved: patients who demand effective treatment free of adverse effects; physicians in need of guidance for selecting the most appropriate drug and the right dose for the patient; health care providers who have to find ways to improve medical care while reducing cost at the same time; regulatory agencies who need proof of concept to issue guidelines and laws, and also drug developers who are in fear of losing their costly drug candidates due to unforeseen toxicity in late stages of development (34).

In short integration of pharmacogenomics in clinical practice needs training of healthcare professionals and citizens, moreover legal and regulatory guidelines and safeguards will be needed. The answers to the questions of which patient should receive which drug and dose will be not easy, but we believe that the approach offered by pharmacogenomics should be incorporated into the decision-making process. A more rational use of expensive treatment drugs together with actions to minimize patient toxic events and its consequences, would dramatically reduce medical costs as an added benefit.

References

Agarwal A, Ressier D, Snyder G. The current and future state of companion diagnostics. *Pharmacogenomics and Personalized Medicine.* 2015: 8, 99-110.

Berryessa CM, Cho MK. Ethical, legal, Social and policy. Implications of behavioral genetics. *Annu Rev. Genomics Hum. Genet.* 2013; 14: 515-534.

CECMED, http://www.cecmed.cu/reglamentacion/aprobadas (Accessed September 12, 2016).

Céspedes-Garro C, Jiménez-Arce G, Naranjo ME, Barrantes R, Llerena A; CEIBA.FP Consortium of the Ibero-American Network of Pharmacogenetics & Pharmacogenomics RIBEF. Ethnic background and CYP2D6 genetic polymorphisms in Costa Ricans. *Rev Biol Trop.* 2014;62(4): 1659-7.

EC, European Commission "Guideline on summary of product characteristics (SmPC)" http//ec.europa.eu/heatlh/files/eudralex/vol-2/c/smpc_guideline_ rev2_en.pdf.

Ehrman F, Caneva L, Prasad K, Paulmich M, Malliepard M, LLerena A Ingelman-Sundberg M and Papaluca-Amati M. Pharmacogenomics information in drug labels: European Medicines Agency perspective. *The Pharmacogenomics Journal,* 2015, 15, 201-210.

Eichelbaum M, Igelman-Sundberg M and Evans W.E Pharmacogenomics and individualized drug therapy. *Annu. Rev. Med.* 2006. 57, 119-137.

EMA, European Medicines Agency, http://www.ema.europa.eu/ema/index.jsp?curl= pages/regulation/general/general_content_000411.jsp&mid=WC0b01ac05800 Accessed September 12, 2016.

Evan WE. Mc Leod HL Pharmacogenomics. Drug targets and side effects. *N. Engl. J. Med.* 2003; 348: 538-49.

FDA, fwww.fda.org www.ema.eu www.ich.org (accessed on August 1st, 2016).

Ginsburg GS, Willard HF. Genomic and personalized medicine: foundations and applications. *Transl. Res.* 2009; 154 (6): 277-87.

González I, Pérez B, Alvárez M, Dorado P y Llerena A. Estudio farmacogenético del polimorfismo metabólico de la debrisoquina (CYP2D6) en la población cubana en relación con la española. *Med. Clin. (Barc).* 2007. 128 (20): 772-4.

González-Vacarezza N, Abad-Santos F, Carcas Sansuan A, DoradoP, Peñas Lledó E, Estevez-Carrizo F and Llerena A. Use of pharmacogenetics in bioequivalence studies to reduce sample size: an example with mirtazapine and CYP2D6. *The Pharmacogenomics Journal,* 2012 1-4.

ICH, international conference for Armonization. http://www.ich.org/home. html (Accessed on October 30, 2016).

Issa AM, Ethical perspectives on pharmacogenomic profiling in the drug development process. *Nature Rev. Drug. Discov.* 2002, 1; 300-308.

Lage A, Crombet T. Del nuevo producto biológico para el cáncer al impacto en la salud poblacional. *Rev. Cub. Sal. Pub.* 2012; 38 (5); 781-793.

Lledó EM, González I, Dorado, P, Pérez B. Calzadilla LR et al., Eating disorders symptoms and CYP2D6 variation in Cuban healthy Females: A report from the Iberoamerican Network of Pharmacogenetics. *Current Pharmacogenomics and Personalized Medicine.* 2012, 10, (4) 1-5.

Llerena A. Population pharmacogenetics and global health. *Drug Metabol. PErs.* Ther 2015 Editorial.

Malliepard M, Nofziger C. Papaluca M, Zineh I et al. Pharmacogenetics in the evaluation of new drugs: a multiregional regulatory perspective. *Nature reviews.* 2013; 12, 103-115.

Otsubo Y, Ishiguro A, Uyama Y. Regulatory perspective on remaining challenges for utilization of pharmacogenomics-guided drug developments. *Pharmacogenomics* 2013, 14 (2), 195-203.

Quiñones LA, Lavanderos MA, Cayun JP, Garcia-Martin E, Agundez JA et al. Perception of the usefulness of drug/gene pairs and barriers for pharmacogenomics in Latin America. Currents Drugs. *Metabolism,* 2014, 15, 202-8.

Ricci DS, Broderick ED, Techelet A et al., Global requirements for DNA sample collections: results of a survey of 204 ethics committees in 40 countries. *Clin. Pharmacol. Ther.* 2011, 89 (4), 554-561.

Rodeiro I, Remirez D, Garcia M, Dorado P, Llerena A and CEIBA, Pharmacogenetics in Latin American populations: regulatory aspects, application to herbal medicine, cardiovascular and psychiatric disorders. *Drug. Metab. Drug. Interact.* 2012, 27, (1) 57-60.

van Schie R, De Boer A, Van der Zee AH. Implementation of pharmacogenetics in clinical practice is challenging. *Pharmacogenomics* 2011, 12 (9), 1231-1233.

Warner AW, Bhathena A, Gilardi S et al. Challenges in obtaining adequate genetic sample sets in clinical trials: the perspective of the industry pharmacogenomics working group. *Clin. Pharmacol. Ther.* 2011, 89 (4), 529-536.

WHO, World Health Organization, *Technical Report Series* 937. 14 Reports, Geneva, 2006.

Zanger UM, Challenges and opportunities ahead. *Frontiers in Pharmacology.* 2010, (1), 1-.2.

In: Pharmacogenomics in Latin America
Editor: Luis A. Quiñones

ISBN: 978-1-53611-031-9

Chapter 7

PHARMACOGENOMICS IN PSYCHIATRIC PRACTICE: LATIN AMERICA INITIATIVES

Lina Ortiz*[1,*], *MD, MSc, Mauricio Moreno*[2§], *PhD and Luis A. Quiñones*[3,**], *PhD

[1]Department of Psychiatry, Clínica Las Condes, Santiago, Chile
[2]Laboratory of Oncology and Molecular Genetics, Clínica Las Condes, Santiago, Chile
[3]Laboratory of Chemical Carcinogenesis and Pharmacogenetics, Department of Basic-Clinical Oncology (DOBC), Faculty of Medicine, University of Chile, Santiago, Chile

ABSTRACT

Pharmacogenomics has had a good development in most of medical specialties, nevertheless in psychiatry has been particularly successful. Accordingly, it has been extremely useful in psychiatric patients considering how common is the use of therapeutic regimens that combine several drugs with significant interactions between them. Patients with complex pathologies such as bipolar affective disorder, major depression, psychotic depression, borderline personality disorder, organic brain damage with uncontrolled impulses, among others, have medical advice that is necessary to obtain their genotype profile. In some of these patients, the genotyping results may involve to withdraw some drugs, decrease doses, avoid certain combinations of drugs, or continue using high doses or complex combination therapies with greater confidence.

In this respect, CYP2D6 is a biotransformation enzyme particularly relevant in psychiatric drugs metabolism. Therefore, characterization of its variants in Latin American population is extremely important considering that only some few studies in the region have revealed ethnic differences.

Pharmacogenomics appears to be the main tool in psychiatry to select the right medicine and suitable dose for each patient.

Keywords: pharmacogenomics, pharmacogenetics, psychiatry, CYP2D6, Latin America

* Corresponding Author E-mail: Lina Ortiz, MD, MSc. E-mail: linaortizlobo@gmail.com.
§ E-mail: mmorenoc@clinicalascondes.cl.
** E-mail: lquinone@med.uchile.cl.

INTRODUCTION

The interest in individual variability in drug response has been present in medicine for more than 4 decades. In 1961, the study of plasma levels of active isoniazid and response to treatment, allowed to identify those patients with tuberculosis who were fast acetylators and needed higher doses of the drug, from slow acetylators, who most often showed toxic effects to the standard doses (Godeau, 2011).

In 1962, Werner Kalow at Karolinska Institute studied the plasma levels of tricyclic antidepressants in Europeans and Asians, showing very significant inter-ethnic differences that were linked to metabolic causes. At that time began to emerge Pharmacogenomics (Tillement, 2011), however the term had been already introduced by Fredrich Vogel in 1959 (Arribás, 2010).

At present, we know that the variation in the human genome is one of the most important causes of different response to drug therapy. Driven by advances in molecular biology, pharmacogenomics has become today one of the most active fields in applied biomedical research (Arribás, 2010). However, molecular genetics is an almost completely unknown map to some medical doctors mainly due to the use of a cryptic language, with abbreviations and acronyms that constitute rather a dialect (Mrazek, 2010a).

Therefore, it is a challenge of our times to create a bridge between these two worlds, translating the language of molecular geneticists to medical doctors, allowing the latter an access to the world of pharmacogenomics.

Although this discipline has had a good development in most of medical specialties, in psychiatry has been particularly successful. Indeed, pharmacogenomics is extremely useful in psychiatric patients considering the frequent use of therapeutic regimens that combine several drugs, with significant interactions between drugs. If these interactions are not considered, that could force an early discard of some drugs that might have been effective for a patient after adaptation of its posology according to the genotyping profile of this patient (Ortiz, 2012).

Moreover, the difficulty to objectify adverse effects of drugs has stigmatized for years patients who tolerate bad all sort of medications and in addition, we psychiatrists have often described as a placebo effect the improvement obtained with very low doses of sedatives and analgesics.

To determine what type of metabolizer is a given patient, even before prescribing any medication, will allow choosing a much more effective and efficient drug treatment for that individual, saving time and resources and more importantly, reducing the inherent risks of any pharmacotherapy.

PHARMACOGENETICS, PHARMACOGENOMICS AND PERSONALIZED MEDICINE

Personalized medicine consists in a tailored treatment to each patient based on the molecular and genetic profile of him/her, being this one of the most prominent aspects of modern medicine (Mrazek, 2010b). In this regard, a key element of personalized medicine is pharmacogenomics, discipline defined as the application of the study of genetic variability on the different ways of response to drug therapy in different individuals, due among other factors to the metabolic capacity of the subject (Arribás, 2010). This metabolic capacity varies depending on the presence of different polymorphisms for genes encoding enzymes responsible for drug metabolism.

It should be noted here the distinction between "mutation" and "polymorphism." A mutation is any nucleotidic change in DNA, which led to an altered function of the encoded protein and is present in less than 1% of general population. On the other hand, a polymorphism is a particular nucleotidic change in DNA that may or not result in an abnormal functionality of a given protein and is present in more than 1% of the population. While mutations are associated with diseases, polymorphisms may have a neutral effect or even a non-pathological phenotypic effect (change of hair color or height, for example) or be beneficial to people who bear it. The presence of these allelic variants will determine which enzymes are synthesized and whether they will have an increased, decreased or null activity (Arribás, 2010).

The ability to activate a drug to allow its therapeutic action, to keep it in the body long enough to exert its action and finally to remove it from the body, will determine that an individual has a good response, presents severe adverse effects or do not benefit from that drug. Especially considering that the therapeutic doses established for any particular drug were determined in clinical studies based on subjects with a "normal" metabolism.

Pharmacokinetics and pharmacodynamics will determine the drug metabolism from the time of administration until the therapeutic effect is achieved. Pharmacokinetics involves metabolism and bioavailability in the action site of the drug, while pharmacodynamics determines the effect of the drug in the action site, which is the interaction between the drug and its receptor. Inter-individual variability in the response to a drug can be attributed to the expression of this biological variability between individuals, which may be due to pharmacokinetic causes, which determine the different intensity and duration of response, or to pharmacodynamic causes (Arribás, 2010c). Each of these factors influences differently from one individual to another, due to genetic, environmental and/or pathological determinants.

There is a group of genes called pharmacogenes that are associated with drug safety or therapeutic efficacy and can be classified into four categories: pharmacokinetic genes, pharmacodynamics genes, modifiers of disease genes and neoplastic genes (Arribás, 2010a). These pharmacogenes will establish the final action of the drug and it has been established that they bear different polymorphisms that might influence the function of any particular drug. Accordingly, a genotyping of these genes would allow having the best performance for a drug in every patient.

Regarding the genetic determinants of the pharmacokinetics of drugs, these are present in all ADME process (absorption, distribution, metabolism and elimination). Likewise, genetic factors of the drug pharmacodynamics influence the dotation and structure of receptors, ion channels and other molecules, both with great variability among humans, which could explain the diversity of effects that we are able to see in the clinical practice (Arribás, 2010c).

Clinical Pharmacogenomics in Psychiatry

The clinical implementation of psychiatric pharmacogenomics only began in 2003; then, in 2004, the adoption of genotyping in clinical practice was greatly accelerated due to the FDA approval of the methodology established for testing the genes of two better studied cytochrome P450 enzymes, 2D6 and 2C19 (Mrazek, 2010b).

In psychiatric pharmacogenomics there are two main objectives applied to clinical practice: First, to use information about the structural genetic variants in order to minimize potential adverse effects of psychiatric drugs; and second, to have the ability of using genetic analysis to identify specifically psychotropic drugs that will be effective for a particular patient.

Among the pharmacogenetic biomarkers affecting the pharmacokinetics we can mention the Cytochrome P450 enzymes (CYPs) that are involved in drugs inactivation allowing them to be excreted, usually by renal pathway. The CYP450 genes are highly polymorphic in humans demonstrating the great variability on the metabolic capacity of our species and at the same time, present variability depending on ethnicity. Some of the main drug metabolizing enzymes belonging to CYP450 family are CYP2D6, 2C9, 2C19, 1A2, 3A4 and 3A5. However, other drug metabolizing enzymes such as N-acetyltransferase type 2 (NAT2), methyltransferases and UDP glucuronosyltransferases (UGT) family (e.g., UGT1A1, UGT1A4, UGT1A7, UGT1A9 and UGT2B7) are also important. Similarly, drug transporters (e.g., ABCB1, ABCC3), responsible for enabling drug molecules to cross biological membranes, have an essential role in the processes of absorption, distribution, metabolism and excretion of drugs.

Identification of pharmacodynamics genes and their polymorphisms involved in the phenotypes of response to drugs is a very complex task because it must include not only the target molecules of the drug and those involved in post-receptor events, but other related cellular pathways on which there is still little information available. However, some of them have been well studied and now they begin to be useful and even necessary in the clinical practice for therapeutic optimization of certain drugs. Among these, the most studied genes in psychiatry are those encoding the transporters of serotonin, dopamine and noradrenaline (SLC6A4, SLC6A3 and SLC6A2, respectively), serotonin receptors (HTR1A, HTR2A, HTR2C), dopamine receptors (DRD2, DRD3 and DRD4) and COMT (catechol-O-methyltransferase) (Ortiz, 2012).

Patients with complex pathologies such as bipolar affective disorder, major depression, psychotic depression, borderline personality disorder, organic brain damage with uncontrolled impulses, among others, have medical advice that is necessary to perform their genotyping for a proper therapeutic approach. In some of these cases, the result may withdraw some drugs, lower doses, avoid certain combinations of drugs, or continue using high doses or complex combination therapies with greater confidence and knowing that is the best option for that particular patient (Silva et al., 2007).

CYP2D6, THE KEY ENZYME IN BIOTRANSFORMATION OF PSYCHIATRIC DRUGS

Considering the relevance of CYP2D6 in biotransformation of psychiatric drugs, the characterization of its variants in Latin American population is extremely important. In this respect, some few studies have revealed ethnic differences. In Chile, Varela et al. (2015) reported the frequencies of CYP2D6 alleles (*2, *3, *4, *17) and gene duplication in 321 Chilean healthy volunteers. The frequencies are similar to those of the Spanish population likely attributable to the low Amerindian–Caucasian admixture of the studied group (18%). The lack of the *17 was expected since it is frequent among African populations (34%) but is typically not present among Caucasian populations. In this report, in order to analyze potential relationship between genotypes and CYP2D6 phenotype they performed an *in vivo* determination of CYP2D6 activity measuring the debrisoquine hydroxylation in 23 previously selected volunteers according to their genotypes, using the metabolic ratio 4-hydroxydebrisoquine/debrisoquine in urine samples by HPLC analyses. After determination of metabolic ratio (MR) and classification into metabolizer groups, they found a coincidence of 78.3% between expected and observed phenotypes, with exception of those subjects characterized as intermediate metabolizers (Roco et al., 2012; Varela et al., 2015). In Costa Rica the CYP2D6 variant alleles *2, *3, *4, *5, *6, *10, "17, *29, *35 and *41 were also determined. Thus, for the Costa Rican population, the frequency of PMs (poor metabolizer) and UMs (ultra-rapid metabolizer) was 6% and 6.5%, respectively. The percentage of UMs in the mestizo population was higher than in the Amerindian population. CYP2D6 UMs vary from 3.6% to 10.1% and PMs from 1.4% to 10.2% among three Costa Rican groups. The highest frequencies of UMs (10.1%) and PMs (10.2%) were found in the mestizo and Amerindian populations, respectively (Céspedes-Garro et al., 2014). Moreover, in Mexican population, a very low frequency of CYP2D6 PMs has been reported in Mexican-Amerindians (López-López et al., 2014). In a Brazilian sample, it was demonstrated that CYP2D6 is homogeneously distributed across different Brazilian regions and most of the differences can be attributed to inter-individual differences. The most frequent predicted metabolic status was the extensive metabolizers (EM) (83.5%) and the poor metabolizers and ultra-rapid metabolizers were 2.5% and 3.7%, respectively. The IM (intermediate metabolizer) predicted phenotype is associated with a higher proportion of African ancestry and a lower proportion of European ancestry in Brazilians. PM and UM classes did not vary among regions and/or ancestry proportions therefore the authors suggest a unique CYP2D6 testing guidelines for Brazilians to avoid ineffective or adverse events outcomes due to drug prescriptions (Friedrich et al., 2014). Finally, in an Argentinian population the frequency of the most common allelic variants and of CYP2D6 gUMs (>2 active genes) and poor metabolizers (0 active genes, gPMs) were studied. CYP2D6 alleles (*2, *3, *4, *5, *6, *10, *17, *35, *41 and multiple copies), genotypes and functional phenotype frequencies were determined. The frequencies of gUMs and gPMs in Ashkenazi Jews (AJ) from Argentina were 11.5% and 5.2%, respectively, whereas in multiethnic admixture Argentinians (GA), the frequencies of gUM and gPMs were 6.5% and 4.9%, respectively. The findings also support the interethnic variability of CYP2D6 genetic polymorphism in the overall Argentine population (Moya et al., 2016).

Chilean Clinical Applications of Pharmacogenomics in Psychiatry

Since 2011, a pioneer clinical application has been performed in Chile at Clínica Las Condes hospital, where a number of psychiatric patients have been genotyped and their pharmacotherapy was adapted according their genotype with interesting successful results. Table 1 shows results for CYP450 polymorphisms in a sample of the first fifteen patients studied in this medical center.

Conclusion

Even though medicine is, still far from knowing all the variables that determine the success of drug therapy for those patients who are perhaps not as significant in number. All the resources to find the right medication and the right dose for each of them will make a great difference in their quality of life and in that of their families.

Therefore, in this chapter, we wanted to bring clinical psychiatrists to an area in biomedical sciences under continuous development like pharmacogenomics. Its clinical application will allow designing customized or personalized drug treatments based on the genetic characteristics of drug metabolizing enzymes for each patient.

To the extent that the medical indication for this analysis is well understood and its demand increase the number of patients that can benefit from it will largely expand, because on the one hand, the cost will be less and on the other, we will have genetic data of different populations, enabling a more accurate interpretation of results.

In conclusion, while medicine is trying to know all the variables determining a successful drug therapy, particularly in psychiatric pharmacotherapy, where the individual variability of patients is highest, pharmacogenomics appear to be the main tool to find the right medicine and a suitable dose for each subject.

Table 1. Pilot pharmacogenomic study at Clínica Las Condes medical center in fifteen psychiatry patients

Polymorphism	Genotype														
	01	02	03	04	05	06	07	08	09	10	11	12	13	14	15
CYP2D6 Duplication *2 *3 *4	*1/*1	*1/*2	*1/*2	*2/*2	*1/*1	*2/*4	*1/*1	*2/*4	*1/*1	*1/*2	*1/*4	*2/*2	*1/*2	*1/*1	*2/*2
CYP2C9 *2	*1/*1	*1/*1	*1/*1	*1/*1	*1/*1	*1/*2	*1/*2	*1/*1	*1/*1	*1/*1	*1/*2	*1/*1	*1/*1	*1/*2	*1/*1
CYP2C19 *2	*1/*2	*1/*1	*1/*1	*1/*1	*1/*1	*1/*1	*1/*2	*1/*2	*1/*1	*1/*2	*1/*1	*1/*1	*1/*1	*1/*1	*1/*1
CYP1A2 *1F	*1F/*1F	*1/*1	*1/*1F	*1/*1	*1/*1	*1/*1F	*1/*1F	*1/*1F	*1/*1	*1/*1F	*1/*1F	*1/*1F	*1/*1F	*1F/*F	*1F/*F
CYP3A4 *1B	*1/*1	*1/*1	*1/*1	*1/*1	*1/*1	*1/*1	*1/*1	*1/*1	*1/*1	*1/*1B	*1/*1	*1/*1	*1/*1	*1/*1B	*1/*1
CYP3A5 *3	*1/*3	*1/*3	*1/*3	*1/*3	*3/*3	*3/*3	*3/*3	*3/*3	*3/*3	*3/*3	*3/*3	*3/*3	*3/*3	*3/*3	*3/*3

Adapted from Ortiz, 2012.

ACKNOWLEDGMENTS

Authors wanted to thank to the Academic Office at Clínica Las Condes for the financial support to set up the genotyping methods through the PI2012-DA012 Research Project granted to Lina Ortiz and all the patients who accept and consent to be part of the study.

REFERENCES

Alarcón R, Mrazek D. A.: Farmacogenómica psiquiátrica: actualización y perspectivas [Psychiatric pharmacogenomics: update and perspectives], En: Silva H., *Genética y Farmacogenómica en Psiquiatría.* Primera edición, Santiago [Genetics and Pharmacogenomics in Psychiatry. First Edition, Santiago]. Editorial C&C Ediciones, 2007: 59.

Alarcon R. Mental health and mental health care in Latin America. *World Psychiatry.* 2003 Feb; 2(1): 54-56.

Arribás IA. (a): Farmacogenética en Discurso Acto Recepción Académica. Academia de Farmacia "Reino de Aragón" [Pharmacogenetics in Speech Academic Reception Act. Academy of Pharmacy "Kingdom of Aragon"]. Zaragoza, 23 de Marzo 2010: 23-29.

Arribás IA. (b): Introducción en Discurso Acto Recepción Académica. Academia de Farmacia "Reino de Aragón" [Introduction in Discourse Acto Academic Reception. Academy of Pharmacy "Kingdom of Aragon"]. Zaragoza, 23 de Marzo 2010: 15-16.

Arribás IA. (c): Variabilidad inter individual en la respuesta a Medicamentos en Discurso Acto Recepción Académica. Academia de Farmacia "Reino de Aragón" [Interpersonal variability in the response to Medications in Speech Académica Académica. Academy of Pharmacy "Kingdom of Aragon"]. Zaragoza, 23 de Marzo 2010: 17-21.

Céspedes-Garro C, Jiménez-Arce G, Naranjo ME, Barrantes R, Llerena A Ethnic background and CYP2D6 genetic polymorphisms in Costa Ricans. *Rev. Biol. Trop.* 2014 Dec; 62(4): 1659-1671.

Friedrich DC, Genro JP, Sortica VA, Suarez-Kurtz G, de Moraes ME, Pena SD, dos Santos AK, Romano-Silva MA, Hutz MH. Distribution of CYP2D6 alleles and phenotypes in the Brazilian population. *PLoS One.* 2014 Oct. 20; 9(10): e110691.

Godeau, P: Introduction. En: Godeau P. *Pharmacogenetics and Pharmacogenomics.* Primera edición [first edition], France. Editorial Wolter Kluver/Lippincott Williams and Wilkins, 2011: 103-105.

Hernán Silva I. Farmacogenómica y psiquiatría [Pharmacogenomics and psychiatry]. *Rev. Chil. Neuro-Psiquiat.* 2007;45(2): 103-105.

Kohn R, Levav I, de Almeida JM, Vicente B, Andrade L, Caraveo-Anduaga JJ, Saxena S, Saraceno B. [Mental disorders in Latin America and the Caribbean: a public health priority]. *Rev. Panam. Salud Pública* [Rev. Panam. Public health]. 2005 Oct-Nov; 18(4-5): 229-240.

Lazarowski A1, Czornyj L. Potential role of multidrug resistant proteins in refractory epilepsy and antiepileptic drugs interactions. *Drug Metabol. Drug Interact.* 2011;26(1): 21-26.

López-López M, Peñas-Lledó E, Dorado P, Ortega A, Corona T, Ochoa A, Yescas P, Alonso E, Llerena A. CYP2D6 genetic polymorphisms in Southern Mexican Mayan Lacandones and Mestizos from Chiapas. *Pharmacogenomics*. 2014;15(15):1859-1865.

Moya G, Dorado P, Ferreiro V, Naranjo ME, Peñas-Lledó EM, Llerena A. High frequency of CYP2D6 ultrarapid metabolizer genotypes in an Ashkenazi Jewish population from Argentina. *Pharmacogenomics J*. 2016 Apr. 12 doi: 10.1038/tpj.2016.27. [Epub ahead of print].

Mrazek D.A. (a): The language of molecular genetics. In: Mrazek D. *Psychiatric Pharmacogenomics*. Primera edición [first edition], New York. Editorial Oxford University Press, 2010: 9-14.

Mrazek D.A. (b): Introduction. In: Mrazek D. A., *Psychiatric Pharmacogenomics*. Primera edición [first edition], New York. Editorial Oxford University Press, 2010: 3-8.

Ortiz L, Tabak R. Farmacogenómica en la práctica clinica [Pharmacogenomics in clinical practice], *Revista Médica Clínica Las Condes* [Medical Journal Clinic Las Condes], 2012 Sep, 23 (5): 616-621.

Roco A, Quiñones L, Agúndez JA, García-Martín E, Squicciarini V, Miranda C, Garay J, Farfán N, Saavedra I, Cáceres D, Ibarra C, Varela N. Frequencies of 23 functionally significant variant alleles related with metabolism of antineoplastic drugs in the chilean population: comparison with caucasian and asian populations. *Front. Genet.* 2012 Nov. 2; 3:229.

Silva H. Genética y Farmacogenómica en psiquiatría [Genetics and Pharmacogenomics in Psychiatry], editor: Dr. Hernán Silva, co-authors: Mónica Acuña, Renato Alarcón, Víctor Karpyak, Víctor Lermanda, David A. Mrazek, Fernando Novoa, Carlos Valenzuela y Hernán Silva, Ediciones de la Sociedad de Neurología, Psiquiatría y Neurocirugía de Chile [Editions of the Society of Neurology, Psychiatry and Neurosurgery of Chile], Santiago, Chile; 2007.

Tillement J.P.: Inter-ethnic, intra-ethnic and intraindividual variability in responsiveness to drugs. Godeau P. En: *Pharmacogenetics and Pharmacogenomics*. Primera edición, Francia [Pharmacogenetics and Pharmacogenomics. First Edition, France]. Editorial Wolter Kluver/Lippincott Williams and Wilkins, 2011: 106-107.

Varela N, Quiñones LA, Stojanova J, Garay J, Cáceres D, Cespedes S, Sasso J, Miranda C. Characterization of the CYP2D6 drug metabolizing phenotypes of the Chilean mestizo population through polymorphism analyses. *Pharmacol. Res.* 2015 Nov; 101:124-129.

In: Pharmacogenomics in Latin America
Editor: Luis A. Quiñones

ISBN: 978-1-53611-031-9

Chapter 8

CARDIOVASCULAR PHARMACOGENOMICS: CLINICAL APPLICATIONS IN LATIN AMERICA

Ángela M. Roco[1,2,*], Luis A. Quiñones[1,†], PhD and Carla E. Miranda[1,‡], PhD

[1]Laboratory of Chemical Carcinogenesis and Pharmacogenetics,
Department of Basic-Clinical Oncology (DOBC),
Faculty of Medicine, University of Chile, Santiago, Chile
[2]Departamento de Coordinación de la Red Asistencial,
Servicio de Salud Metropolitano Occidente, MINSAL, Santiago, Chile

ABSTRACT

Cardiovascular diseases (CVDs) are the number one cause of death globally. Most cardiovascular diseases can be prevented by addressing behavioral risk factors such as tobacco use, unhealthy diet and obesity, physical inactivity and harmful use of alcohol using population-wide strategies. Various factors help the occurrence of cardiovascular diseases. There are not-modifiable factors such as genetic inheritance and other modifiable such as smoking, alcohol intake, diet and physical activity risk factors. The overall level of risk of an individual is the one that determines the probability of cardiovascular disease, such as acute myocardial infarction, stroke, among others.

On the other hand, a number of medications, including: antiarrhythmics, anticoagulants, beta-blockers, calcium channel blockers, angiotensin receptor blockers, digitalis, diuretics, angiotensin converting enzyme (ACE) are the pharmacotherapeutic arsenal available. The drug of choice by the doctor must be in accordance with the characteristics of each patient and consider the recommendation of pharmacogenomic clinical guidelines.

Nowadays, the relationship between adverse reactions of drugs and genetically determined variations is a main focus of interest. Thus, pharmacogenomic studies are

* Corresponding Author: aroco@farmacogenetica.cl.

† lquinone@med.uchile.cl.

‡ cmiranda@farmacogenetica.cl.

required, especially in Latin American countries, where ethnic variability of pharmacotherapeutic response is not well understood.

The present chapter describes progress in understanding genomic variability in response to commonly used cardiovascular drugs.

Keywords: pharmacogenomics, pharmacogenetics, cardiovascular, variability, Latin America

INTRODUCTION

Cardiovascular diseases (CVDs) are the number one cause of death globally: more people die annually from CVDs than from any other cause. An estimated 17.5 million people died from CVDs in 2012, representing 31% of all global deaths. Of these deaths, an estimated 7.4 million were due to coronary heart disease and 6.7 million were due to stroke (WHO, 2015).

Table 1. Rate of mortality for cardiovascular disease in countries of America year 2012 (WHO, 2014)

	Age-standardized mortality rate by cause (/100 000 population)		
Countries	Cardiovascular diseases		
	Both sexes	Female	Male
Argentina	191.7	148.4	247.8
Bahamas	220.0	169.6	292.5
Barbados	128.1	102.6	159.8
Belize	190.7	180.8	201.6
Bolivia (Plurinational State of)	269.5	236.9	308.7
Brazil	214.2	177.7	258.9
Canada	88.6	68.1	112.2
Chile	115.1	90.4	145.2
Colombia	150.2	128.0	178.2
Costa Rica	140.1	118.4	163.0
Cuba	185.0	157.2	214.4
Dominican Republic	198.9	208.7	187.0
Ecuador	149.3	130.3	170.3
El Salvador	171.0	155.0	191.9
Guatemala	122.9	108.6	139.2
Guyana	544.8	451.0	709.7
Haiti	384.1	374.8	394.1
Honduras	200.5	164.4	240.1
Jamaica	232.6	204.3	265.5
Mexico	148.3	130.3	170.1
Nicaragua	227.8	197.8	262.0
Panama	151.3	125.3	179.4
Paraguay	219.7	179.7	261.7
Peru	122.6	105.3	143.3
Trinidad and Tobago	278.6	220.7	346.5
United States of America	136.0	107.8	169.5
Uruguay	147.4	110.1	197.3
Venezuela (Bolivarian Republic of)	187.3	152.1	226.3

Most cardiovascular diseases can be prevented using population-wide strategies aimed at modifying behavioral risk factors such as tobacco use, unhealthy diet and obesity, physical inactivity and harmful use of alcohol. People with cardiovascular disease or who are at high cardiovascular risk (due to the presence of one or more risk factors such as hypertension, risk of diabetes, hyperlipidemia or already with an established disease, need early detection and management using counselling and medicines, as appropriate (WHO, 2015)). In the Table 1 we show the rate of mortality for cardiovascular disease in countries of America (WHO, 2014).

Various factors help these cardiovascular diseases from occurring. There are not modifiable factors such as genetic inheritance and other modifiable ones such as smoking, alcohol consumption, diet and physical activity risk factors. The latter are crucial in the development of obesity which is one of the main triggers of other factors of greater risk, called physiological, such as diabetes, high blood pressure and blood cholesterol levels. When a person has more than one of these risk factors, the chance of developing a disease is increased. The overall level of risk of an individual is the one that determines the probability of cardiovascular disease, such as acute myocardial infarction, stroke, among others (Figure 1) (Pearson et al., 1993) complications, while recognizing that most cardiovascular events in a population occurs in people with average or slightly elevated risk factors levels (Escobar, 2012).

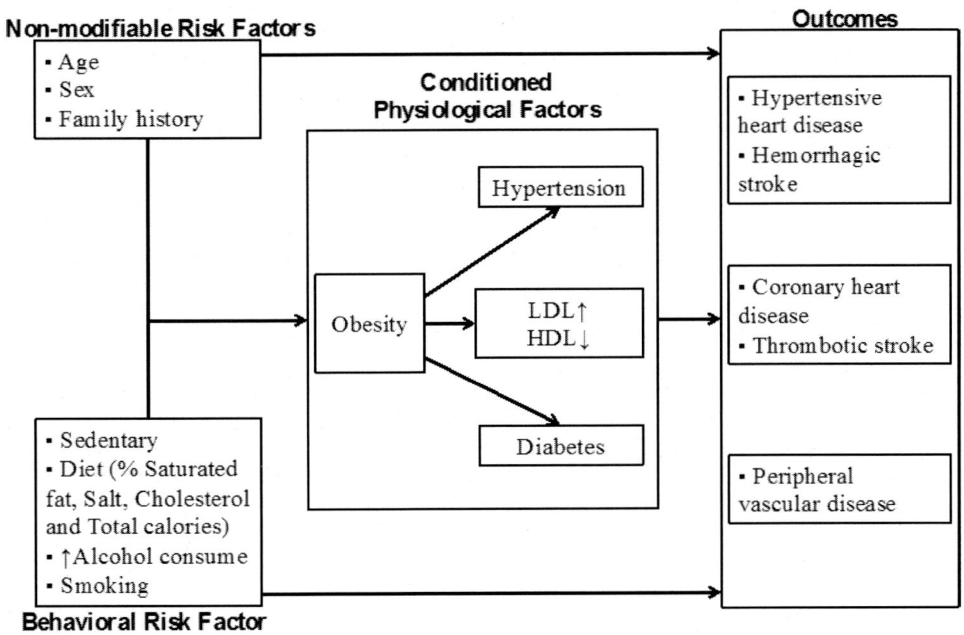

Figure 1. Relationship among general cardiovascular risk factors. (Adapted from Pearson et al. 1993).

We have presented evidence from three clinical studies, "Major Cardiovascular Risk Factors in Latin America: A Comparison with the United States. LASO 2013 "(Miranda et al., 2013)," The Global Burden of Disease Study (GBD) 2010 and Cardiovascular risk awareness, treatment, and monitoring in urban Latin America shows that one of the main factors prevalent in cardiovascular risk is high blood pressure, together with a high level of cholesterol and low HDL (Lim, 2012). In this regard, Chile has introduced new public policies in order to reduce cardiovascular events. These are mainly targeted preventive actions, which are directed to intervene in the general population (population strategy) (MINSAL, 2009, 2010a, 2010b, 2010d, 2011a) and patients (high-risk strategy) (MINSAL, 2011b), decreasing blood pressure, LDL cholesterol and increasing the HDL level. It is because of this, that the effective prevention and treatment of cardiovascular diseases require regular screening for risk factors, a high awareness of the disease, effective treatment of identified risk factors and adherence to prescribed treatment.

A number of medications, including: antiarrhythmics, anticoagulants, beta-blockers, calcium channel blockers, angiotensin receptor blockers, digitalis, diuretics, angiotensin converting enzyme (ACE) are the pharmacotherapeutic arsenal available (MINSAL 2010c). The drug of choice by the doctor must be in accordance with the characteristics of each patient and considered the recommendation of pharmacogenomic clinical guidelines.

PHARMACOGENOMICS

Pharmacogenetics – the study of how genes influences drug response – provides the opportunity to stratify patients into those likely to respond or not respond to therapy, or those likely to experience or not experience toxicity. The term "pharmacogenomics" is commonly used in the literature to define the broader field of genomics and genome-wide associations with drug response (Wilkinson, 2005; Xie & Frueh, 2005; Zhou et al., 2008; Patel, 2016).

The existence of interindividual heterogeneity in drug response, affecting both efficacy and toxicity, may be mediated through the altered pharmacokinetics and pharmacodynamics of drugs. These mechanisms of variability are shaped by genetic-environmental interaction. The contribution of each factor varies with each drug (Evans & McLeod, 2003; Wijnen et al., 2007).

The relationship between adverse reactions of drugs and genetically determined variations was demonstrated for the first time in the 50's. Friedrich Vogel was the first to use the term pharmacogenetics in 1959, but it was not until 1962 when pharmacogenetics was defined as the study of genetic variations that cause variability in response to drugs (Vesell, 2000). Pharmacogenetic studies are based on the investigation of genes from selected candidates for biological significance, either kinetic or their relationship in the pharmacological action; the ultimate goal is to identify individuals at risk of experiencing adverse or likely to be resistant to treatment effects.

The present chapter describes progress in understanding genomic variability in response to commonly used cardiovascular drugs.

APPLICATIONS OF PHARMACOGENOMICS AND PHARMACOGENETICS IN CLINICAL

After the success of the Human Genome Project, the International HapMap Project and the 1000 Genomes Project, our understanding of human genetic variation has increased sequentially. Concomitant extensive research has been carried out to find genetic biomarkers associated with susceptibility, diagnosis, prognosis and response to treatment techniques, candidates study genome-wide association ("Genome-Wide Association Studies" genes, GWAS) and new generation sequencing technologies.

It is interesting to note that studies of pharmacogenomics candidate genes have been substantially more successful in identifying common variants replicated appreciable effect size compared with investigations of candidate genes in the genetics of the disease. This is possibly due to a better understanding of the pharmacological pathways compared to disease processes (Johnson & Cavallari, 2013).

Moreover, while large-scale GWAS and subsequent meta-analysis (Ellinor et al., 2012; Schunkert et al., 2011; Smith et al., 2010) are now discovering associations genetic susceptibility to common cardiovascular disease, variant effect sizes are mostly lower than pharmacogenetic associations, particularly those related to adverse drug reactions (ADRs) (Kääb et al., 2012; Link et al., 2008; Roden, 2013; Yang et al., 2013).

However, despite high expectations, the transfer of genetic to clinical practice associations has been slow, having some notable exceptions, such as the identification of genotype HLA-B * 5701 before administering antiretroviral therapy abacavir, because it has been shown that the presence of this variation significantly increases the incidence of drug hypersensitivity (Mallal et al., 2008) syndrome. However, this is a phenotype security while in cardiovascular disease, most pharmacogenomic associations have focused on the efficacy endpoints, where the magnitude of effect is much smaller and therefore, even any association validated drug/gene.

Another notable exception is in the field of oncology, where there is a growing arsenal of genotype-dependent licensed therapies. For example, tamoxifen is indicated for the prevention of recurrence of the disease only in patients with estrogen receptor positive breast cancer, and predates any of the genomic advances that have occurred in this century. More recently vemurafenib inhibits BRAF E600 (positive mutation), but not wild-type (BRAF V600) has been approved for the treatment of unresectable or metastatic melanoma.

Pharmacogenetic studies in cardiology have focused heavily drug already licensed and widespread clinical use. This undoubtedly represents an additional obstacle, because change clinical practice accepted and therefore physician behavior is difficult, as it often requires a higher level of evidence.

Some pharmacogenomic efforts are described below.

ANTITHROMBOTICS

Warfarin

Warfarin and Acenocoumarol are an effective anticoagulant and have been applied as thrombosis prophylaxis in settings including atrial fibrillation, venous thromboembolic disease, and metallic prosthetic valves worldwide (Johnson et al., 2011). Warfarin acts by inhibiting vitamin K epoxide reductase (VKORC1), the enzyme responsible for maintaining vitamin K in its reduced state (Figure 2). It is under this condition that its catalytic property is preserved; in its oxidized state, it is unable to catalyze the gamma-carboxylation of the vitamin-k dependent clotting factors (II, VII, IX, X) and proteins C and S (Dandona, 2014).

Warfarin is metabolized by cytochrome P-450. Genome-wide association studies (GWAS) have subsequently identified rs2108622 in CYP4F2 to be associated with increased warfarin requirement; other SNPs have not met stringent genome-wide statistical thresholds. Warfarin and Acenocoumarol are administered as racemic mixtures consisting of 50% of each enantiomer. Although the mechanism of action of these drugs is similar, there are some important differences in their pharmacokinetics e.g., Warfarin has less activity than older acenocoumarol and RAMs (Gadisseur et al., 2002; Ufer, 2005).

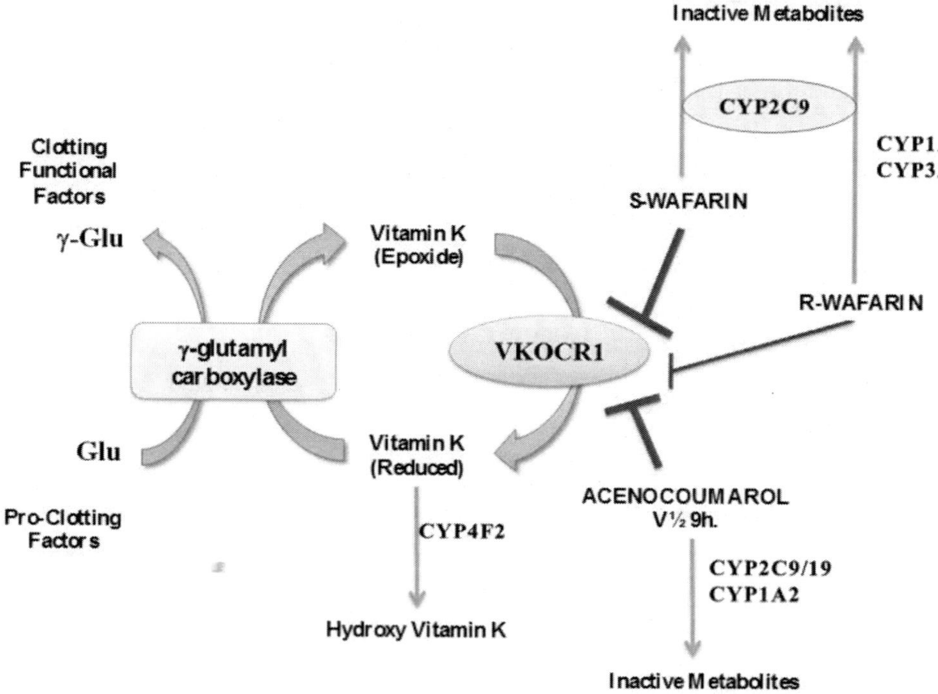

Figure 2. Mechanism of action and metabolism of Warfarin (Adapted of Miranda et al. 2011).

The enzyme Vitamin K Epoxide Reductase Subunit complex 1 (VKORC1), therapeutic target of these drugs, is responsible for the regeneration of reduced vitamin K, which is essential for glutamyl carboxylase cofactor. This enzyme is polymorphic, has a polymorphism of a single nucleotide noncoding (SNP) rs9923231 called (-1639G> A; G3673A), in which a binding site is altered in the promoter region of VKORC1 expression and produces a decrease (Johnson et al., 2011). As a result lower doses of warfarin (Takeuchi et al., 2009) are required. This has been confirmed in several populations including Caucasians and Africans, Asians (Lee & Klein, 2013). However, rs9923231 VKORC1 explains only ~ 20-25% of the variation in the maintenance dose of warfarin in Caucasian and Asian populations, and ~ 6% of the variability of the dose in African Americans, which is attributable to the lower frequency of alleles (Johnson et al., 2011; Johnson & Cavallari, 2013; Wang et al., 2008).

Several authors have shown that the dose of acenocoumarol is also influenced by VKORC1 genotype. Reitsma and his colleagues in 2005 had shown that the Dutch patients who carry one or two alleles polymorphism variants for 1173 require a dose 28% and 47% lower, respectively, compared to wild types (Reitsma, van der Heijden, Groot, Rosendaal, &

Büller, 2005). In Greek, heterozygous carriers of a variant allele require a dose 19% lower and 63% homozygous lower dose (Markatos et al., 2008). Similar percentages were found in populations of Germany, Austria, Serbia and Lebanon (Cadamuro et al., 2010; Esmerian et al., 2011; Kovac et al., 2010).

CYP2C9 P450 enzyme metabolizes more potent enantiomer of warfarin and S-30 allelic variants are recognized in this enzyme. CYP2C9 *2 (rs1799853) and CYP2C9 *3 (rs1057910) are the most frequent genetic variants of CYP2C9 in Caucasians, with frequencies of 0.13 and 0.07 respectively (Johnson et al., 2011). In Asians, CYP2C9 *2 is very rare and frequency of CYP2C9 * 3 is 0.04 (30). CYP2C9 *2 and CYP2C9 *3 encode proteins whose enzymatic activities are reduced by ~ 30-40% and ~ 80-90% respectively (Johnson et al., 2011). Accordingly, they are associated with a prolonged half-life warfarin, increasing the time to achieve therapeutic levels of INR, requiring a reduction in dose of warfarin (Johnson et al., 2011), and for patients with CYP2C9 *3, an increased risk of bleeding has been confirmed (Yang et al., 2013). Risk ratios reported by bleeding in patients with genotype CYP2C9 *1/*3, *3/*3 compared to the wild *1/*1 genotype is 2.05 (95% CI = 1.36 to 3 10) and 4.87 (95% CI 1.38 to 17.14 =), respectively (Yang et al., 2013). In general, CYP2C9 genotype accounts for ~ 7-10% of the variability in warfarin dose (Johnson & Cavallari, 2013).

Table 2. Warfarin doses according ethnicity and genotype (Wu et al., 2008)

Characteristics	Afroamerican	Caucasians	Spain	Asian
Average doses	5,2 mg/day	4,3 mg/day	4,0 mg/day	2,7 mg/day
CYP2C9*1	94%	74%	93%	95%
CYP 2C9*2	1%	19%	0%	0%
VKORC1 GG	82%	37%	32%	7%
VKORC1AA	6%	18%	27%	63%

The enzymes involved in the metabolism of acenocoumarol are CYP2C9, CYP1A2 and CYP2C19 (Gadisseur et al., 2002). Although little has been published on the CYP2C9 genotypes and acenocoumarol dose compared with warfarin, there are several studies that confirm the associations found with warfarin, genotypes and the risk of bleeding during acenocoumarol. The presence of a CYP2C9 * 3 allele reduces metabolism normally inactive S-acenocoumarol and therefore increases the average life of this enantiomer ((Thijssen, Drittij, Vervoort, & de Vries-Hanje, 2001). It means therefore that the patient requires 19 to 29% lower dose of acenocoumarol in carriers of this allele in wild genotypes (Schalekamp et al., 2004), but also 13-15% lower in carriers of * 2 allele (Tàssies et al., 2002; Visser et al., 2004). The risk of over-anticoagulation and severe bleeding is increased in patients with variant *3 (Schalekamp et al., 2004; Tàssies et al., 2002; Verstuyft et al., 2001; Visser et al., 2004).

Previous research to show that CYP2C9 acenocoumarol represents 14% of the interindividual variability in drug response (Gadisseur et al., 2002; Ufer, 2005), so it is not possible to establish a correlation between plasma concentrations of acenocoumarol and the level of prothrombin or INR. Notwithstanding the foregoing, preliminary results from our group show that the genetic variant CYP2C9 * 2, when present in homozygous way (*2/*2) is associated with variations in the plasma levels of acenocoumarol and other pharmacokinetic variables (Miranda et al., 2011). Therefore, the importance of CYP2C9 genetic variants in variability in response to acenocoumarol should not be underestimated.

The first warfarin dosing algorithms for incorporating CYP2C9 genotype were published in 2004 ((Brian F Gage et al., 2004; Hillman et al., 2004; Kamali et al., 2004). The algorithm by Gage et al. It was the largest and also CYP2C9 genotype, age, body surface area, sex, race, INR, the use of amiodarone and simvastatin included. The algorithm explained 39% of the variation in the daily dose of warfarin. Since then, more than 30 algorithms have been published on the basis of CYP2C9 and VKORC1 genotypes. Sconce et al. has published one of the first algorithms, CYP2C9 and VKORC1 including genotypes as well as the age and height (Sconce et al., 2005).

In 2008, Gage et al. published an updated algorithm including CYP2C9 and VKORC1 genotype, age, body surface area, the use of amiodarone, INR, race and smoking status (Gage et al., 2008). In a Caucasian population this algorithm explained 57% of the variation in the dose, but the predictive value was lower (31%) in African Americans. This type of algorithm has been adopted by the FDA and is currently recommends its use entity.

Wadelius et al. were able to explain almost 59% of the variation in a Swedish population, using the information for both genotypes, age, race, sex and number of interacting drugs that increase INR (Wadelius et al., 2009). R2 univariate CYP2C9 genotype was about 12% and 29% VKORC1. Warfarin Pharmacogenetics Consortium International (IWPC) created an algorithm in a more diverse population of 9 countries on 4 continents (Perera et al., 2013). 47% of the variation in dose by CYP2C9, VKORC1, age, height, weight, use of amiodarone, race and the number of CYP enzyme inducers explained.

For warfarin, many more algorithms have been published in different populations of several countries, most of these studies have included VKORC1 and CYP2C9 genotypes, but some have also included CYP4F2, CCCG and APOE genotypes. The formulas of these studies have allowed calculate a maintenance dose of warfarin. However, only a handful of studies have analyzed the algorithms for other types of doses of coumarin. When a patient starts a warfarin pharmacogenetics-guided dose is difficult to know how to adjust this dose after measurement of the INR (Verhoef et al., 2014).

Van Schie and colleagues developed a genotype-guided algorithm for acenocoumarol in a Dutch population (van Schie et al., 2011). The authors also provide loading dose related maintenance dose calculated and validated the algorithm acenocoumarol later, which explained 52.7% of variability (Lim et al., 2012).

Clopidogrel

STARS demonstrated the efficacy of dual antiplatelet therapy following coronary artery stenting. Studies such as CAPRIE have also demonstrated its efficacy as a single-agent therapy. The thienopyridines exert their effects by antagonizing the ADP receptor of the P2Y12 subtype. Through a series of oxidative steps, clopidogrel is metabolized to its active form—the first of which leads to formation of 2-oxo-clopidogrel and the second to the active metabolite. Studies have indicated that cytochromes P450 1A2, P450 2C9, and P450 2C19 are involved in the first step while cytochromes P450 3A4, P450 2C9, P450 2C19, and P450 2C19 are involved in the second. While cytochrome P450 2C19 is involved in both steps, cytochrome P450 3A4 is the major enzyme responsible for conversion to its active metabolite. There exists evidence that paraoxonase 1 may also be involved in transforming 2-oxo-clopidogrel to its active metabolite. Mega et al. hypothesized that patients taking clopidogrel who were also carriers of polymorphisms in cytochrome P450 carry an increased risk of ischemic events (Dandona, 2014; Weeke, 2014).

Meanwhile, the oral prodrug clopidogrel is a second generation thienopyridine whose active metabolite binds irreversibly to the membrane receptors purinergic platelet P2Y12 lifetime of a plate (~ 10 days) (Scott et al., 2013) and antagonizes platelet aggregation mediated ADP. Their metabolism is complex: ~ 85% is rapidly hydrolyzed to an inactive metabolite by hepatic carboxylesterase 1 (CES1) (Zhu et al., 2013), and the rest is subjected to two stages of sequential liver oxidation to the inactive metabolite intermediate (2-oxo first - clopidogrel) and the active metabolite (R-130964) by CYP1A2, CYP3A4/5, CYP2B6, CYP2C9 and CYP2C19 (Zhu et al., 2013).

There is substantial variability in platelet response to clopidogrel (Trenk & Hochholzer, 2014). A number of factors contribute to this variability, including the elderly (> 65 years), body mass index (BMI), drugs that inhibit CYP enzymes (statins, proton-pump inhibitor, erythromycin, etc.), diseases such as diabetes mellitus, renal failure and decreased left ventricular function, but together, all these factors explain only a small proportion of observed variability (Trenk & Hochholzer, 2014).

CYP2C19 is mainly responsible for the conversion of inactive clopidogrel to its active metabolite (Zhu et al., 2013). CYP2C19 *1 allele is wild-type, but more than 25 variants have been identified; most have reduced enzymatic activity and are rare, except for CYP2C19 * 2 (rs4244285, c.681G> A), which together with CYP2C19 * 3 are associated with a reduced level of circulating active metabolite of clopidogrel (Holmes et al., 2011).

To our knowledge, 13 meta-analyses have been published to date since 2010, which have evaluated the association between CYP2C19 genotypes and clinical outcomes. And robust consistent finding is that reducing the function of CYP2C19 (predominantly CYP2C19 * 2) alleles increases significantly the risk of thrombosis after percutaneous coronary intervention (PCI) compared to non-carriers. In addition, a gene dosage trend is clear: the association of CYP2C19 *2/*2 with risk of thrombosis is evident and significant (Mega et al., 2010).

On the other hand, the enzyme CES1, major enzyme responsible for the biotransformation of clopidogrel, 2-oxoclopidogrel and its active metabolite R-130964 to inactive compounds carboxylic acids, has 39 genetic variants that may contribute to interindividual variability in response to clopidogrel. Recent in vitro investigations have shown that G143E (rs71647871) variant isoform CES1A1 has completely diminished catalytic activity to metabolize clopidogrel and 2-oxo-clopidogrel (Zhu et al., 2013), which has been associated with higher levels of reduction active metabolite of clopidogrel and platelet aggregation stimulated by ADP later in patients with coronary disease. According to the above, the effect of G143E must be addressed as a genetic biomarker in anticoagulant treatment related cardiovascular pathologies.

Another interesting factor to consider is the ABCB1 gene (ATP-binding cassette (ABC) subfamily B (MDR/TAP) member 1), which encodes a P-glycoprotein, which is an efflux transporter that has a broad specificity, presenting a important role in removing substrates in the intestine, the urine and bile. A commonly studied ABCB1 variant is 3435C> T (rs1045642, Ile1145Ile). It has been observed that patients homozygous mutant (TT) has reduced the absorption of clopidogrel after a single oral dose compared to patients C/T and

CC, even though the results of other studies show controversies about (Su et al., 2012; Taubert et al., 2006).

Aspirin

The definition of aspirin resistance is variable, therefore estimates of its prevalence vary. Aspirin exerts its action by irreversible acetylation of cyclooxygenase-1 (COX-1), inhibiting its activity with a resultant reduction in the production of thromboxane A2. Sequence variation in COX-1 as it relates to aspirin response has been investigated, with studies yielding inconsistent data. Similar studies have been concluded with respect to SNP s that reside within the glycoprotein III a gene. These too have led to contradictory findings. In a large meta-analysis, however, it was concluded that in healthy subjects the PlA1/A2 variant is associated with aspirin resistance, potentially implying that the effect of this SNP in inhibiting aspirin-mediated platelet inhibition may be reduced by the coadministration of drugs that are commonly prescribed in the context of CAD. Relatively common side effects to aspirin include gastrointestinal hemorrhage and aspirin-induced urticaria. Studies of DNA sequence variants that may alter the frequency of such endpoints have been investigated with variable results (Dandona, 2014).

CHOLESTEROL-LOWERING THERAPY

Variability in Statin Response

Statins, the most commonly prescribed drug class worldwide, are indicated for primary and secondary prevention of cardiovascular disease. Their main mechanism of action is the reduction of LDL and cholesterol by competitive inhibition of the enzyme 3-hydroxy-3-methylglutaryl-coenzyme A (HMG-CoA) reductase, an enzyme limiting the de novo synthesis of cholesterol. Genetic variation in lipid-lowering efficacy of statins has been widely investigated and more than 40 candidate genes have been described (Verschuren et al., 2012). Results of these studies have been identified as relevant pharmacogenomic factor to SLCO1B1 gene (Solute Carrier Organic Anion Transporter Family Member 1B1), particularly genetic variants rs4363657 and rs4149056 (521T> C, V174A; SLCO1B1 * 5) relating mainly to the statin-induced muscle toxicity. The frequency of myopathy and statin-induced rhabdomyolysis is estimated at ~ 1/1000 ~ 1/100,000, respectively (Link et al., 2008; Ramsey et al., 2014; Wilke et al., 2012). Studies have reported that there is a strong association between the variant and the presence of severe myopathy. The association between the genetic variant and adverse reactions to statins has been particularly shown with simvastatin. There is a lack of supporting documentation about their participation in treatment with pravastatin, rosuvastatin and atorvastatin (Carr et al., 2013; Danik et al., 2013; de Keyser et al., 2014).

In 2012 (Wilke et al., 2012) and subsequently ratified in 2014 (Ramsey et al., 2014), the CPIC (Clinical Pharmacogenetics Implementation Consortium) issued consensus guidelines for SLCO1B1 *5 and its relationship with myopathy simvastatin induced, including consideration of dose reductions or use an alternative for patients presenting with one or two variant alleles statin. However, this is not widely practiced today.

In 2015, Pardo et al., assessed single nucleotide polymorphisms (SNPs) in the SLCO1B1 gene and their effect on atorvastatin response. Essay included 129 Chilean hypercholesterolemic patients undergoing 10 mg/day of atorvastatin therapy during 4 weeks. Lipid profile was determined before and after drug administration. Genotyping of SLCO1B1 rs4149056 (c.521T>C) SNP was performed with allele-specific polymerase chain reaction, whilst polymerase chain reaction-restriction fragment length polymorphism (PCR-RFLP) was used for genotyping the SLCO1B1 rs2306283 (c.388A>G) variant. After statin therapy, concentrations of TC, LDL-C and TG decreased from baseline ($p < 0.05$). Also, HDL-C levels increased ($p < 0.05$). Minor allele frequencies for the rs2306283 and rs4149056 variants were 0.547 and 0.136, respectively. LDL-C response to atorvastatin was not associated with the SLCO1B1 rs4149056 nor the rs2306283 polymorphisms ($p > 0.05$). However, the latter SNP was associated with HDL-C variability after atorvastatin medication ($p = 0.02$). Indicating that LDL-C reduction following atorvastatin therapy is not influenced by the SNPs evaluated. In addition, the polymorphism rs2306283 at the SLCO1B1 gene determines greater HDL-C concentrations in response to atorvastatin medication in Chilean hypercholesterolemic subjects (Pardo et al., 2015).

ApoE Gene and Statin Response

Ambiguous data exists with respect to the epsilon2 variant of the apolipoprotein (apo) e gene and statin response (Utermann, 1987; Nieminen, 2008) a metaanalysis of three GWAS results showed that a SNP in the calmin gene was associated with the response to statin therapy, yet this remains to be confirmed. DNA sequence variation in apoC1, adjacent to apoe, was also associated with the response to statin therapy (Barber, 2010).

β-Blockers

Two common nonsynonymous polymorphisms in the β-1-adrenergic receptor gene (ADBR1), resulting in S49G (rs1801252) and R389G (rs1801253), are associated with the clearest evidence for modulating β-blocker action. In vitro, G49 is more susceptible to agonist-promoted downregulation than S49, and the R389 form of the receptor couples more efficiently to G protein than does the G389 variant. In vivo, one study reported that homozygous carriers of the R389 genotype experienced greater improvements in left ventricular ejection fraction following β-blocker therapy (carvedilol and metoprolol) than did individuals with other genotypes. Improved outcome in R389 homozygotes was also reported in the β-Blocker Evaluation of Survival Trial (BEST), a large study of bucindolol in heart failure patients. As a result, a superiority trial designed to assess the safety and efficacy of bucindolol in~3,200 homozygous R389 heart failure patients is planned. Improved antihypertensive response to β-blockers was also reported among homozygous R389 carriers (Weeke, 2014).

The β-2-adrenergic receptor is encoded by ADBR2. Two common ADBR2 polymorphisms, R16G (rs1042713) and Q27G (rs1042714), are resistant to agonist-mediated downregulation. Associations between common ADRB2 polymorphisms and altered clinical cardiovascular outcomes have been reported but have not been replicated (Weeke, 2014).

CYP2D6 metabolizes some commonly used β-blockers (e.g., propranolol, timolol, and metoprolol) and propafenone, an antiarrhythmic with β-blocking properties. There are many loss-of-function variants in the gene, and individuals who carry two loss-of-function alleles, ~7% of Caucasians and Africans, are termed poor metabolizers. Rarer individuals carry multiple functional copies of the gene and are termed ultrarapid metabolizers, and the remainder are extensive metabolizers. Poor metabolizers have higher metoprolol and propafenone concentrations than extensive metabolizers (Rau, 2002), a difference associated with increased risk for bradyarrhythmias or bronchospasm. There is some evidence that the poor metabolizers may be at increased risk for ADRs (Bijl, 2009), and the FDA has added a statement to the metoprolol and carvedilol labels to this effect.

Some other genetic variants related to the influence of other non-metabolizing genes of drugs for cardiovascular but also relevant use have been studied by our group and establish the importance of genetic variability in cardiovascular diseases of coagulation factors II and V, converting enzyme (ACE), the carrier protein cholesteryl ester (CETP), apolipoprotein E (ApoE), the plasminogen activator inhibitor (PAI-1) and methylenetetrahydrofolate reductase (MTHFR) (Roco et al., 2012).

Accordingly, the approach of using molecular biomarkers panels genomic-pharmacogenómicos openly posed as the area of future development for assessing susceptibility to cardiovascular events and response to drug therapy.

Conclusion

Despite an increasing number of studies and partnerships between drug response and metabolism genes drugs (pharmacogenomics), most of cardiovascular research of this type is in early stages, as researchers have found difficulties to identify and validate associations, which is largely due to the heterogeneity of patient populations and their phenotypes, or the difficulty of obtaining adequate sample sizes. The creation of consortium study groups have addressed these constraints. Progress towards normalization of the pharmacogenomic research, the best use of financial resources involved, conducting larger studies, assessment of associations pharmacogenomic in different ethnic groups, performing meta-analysis to validate the associations found, the determination of minimum requirements on the evidence for genetic associations and proposing consensus clinical guidelines are required. In this regard, several pioneering centers have initiated genomic drugs programs (Manolio et al., 2013). An example is the Medical Center at Vanderbilt University, USA, where patients scheduled for coronary angiography are preemptively genotyped on a platform with 184 variants, including CYP2C19. Recommendations based on genotype are automatically provided electronically so that doctors have access when they require antiplatelet therapy prescribed. Clinical use of this pharmacogenomic program has enabled Vanderbilt University to develop solutions to logistical, financial and knowledge barriers and execution, along with other programs has generated consensus frameworks.

A more advanced proposal in this regard is the recent suggestion to develop dosing algorithms, as has already been done for warfarin, in order to avoid excessive exposure to cardiovascular drugs use (Kimmel et al., 2013). The authors propose considering clinical and demographics (gender, age, body mass index, ethnicity, dose and time of the last dose), genetic (genetic variants in CYP2C9, SLCO1B1 and ABCG2) and metabolic (4β-hydroxycholesterol) to formulate dosing algorithms that define the response to rosuvastatin and atorvastatin. The first results show that these algorithms predict the response of approximately 50% of patients taking higher doses of standard clinical practice, systemic exposure to statin exceeds the 90th percentile (DeGorter et al., 2013). However, the global clinical utility of these algorithms need to be validated and several knowledge, logistical and financial barriers to the widespread application of cardiovascular pharmacogenomics in Latin America need to be overcome (Quiñones et al., 2014). In the same way, considering the ethical issues in pharmacogenomic analysis procedures it should be included as a requirement in the doctor-patient relationship for these effects.

Looking ahead, there is a clear need for better guidance on how biomarkers should be qualifying, what kind of evidence are acceptable, and further harmonization among regulatory agencies worldwide and clinical centers. This will provide clearer routes for reimbursement and application in clinical practice. It is important that researchers are cautious in their recommendations in the discovery phase, and reproduction of any applicable biomarker in various patient populations.

In Chile some isolated practices have been carried out, backed by our research group in various hospitals and clinical centers, where they are genotyping variants to explain the interindividual variation of drugs for depression and cancer.

Finally, this chapter has focused on genomics/pharmacogenomics variation, although there are other "omics" technologies also interesting (epigenomic, transcriptomics, proteomics, metabolomics and metagenomics), more distance clinical application. We have also focused our presentation on the state of the art in those areas of cardiovascular drugs use and related genes have more scientific evidence.

In conclusion, although the cardiovascular pharmacogenomics are still in early stages and results in many cases are even contradictory, it is our expectation that pharmacogenomics of cardiovascular drugs can offer a real benefit to the patient, surpassing the obstacles mentioned above. Slowly but surely, with dedication and hard work the cardiovascular pharmacogenomics is positioning itself as a mainstream tool in clinical practice, although much remains to be done.

References

Barber MJ, Mangravite LM, Hyde CL, Chasman DI, Smith JD, McCarty CA, et al. Genome-wide association of lipid-lowering response to statins in combined study populations. *PLoS One.* 2010 Mar 22; 5(3): e9763.

Bijl MJ, Visser LE, van Schaik RH, et al. Genetic variation in the CYP2D6 gene is associated with a lower heart rate and blood pressure in beta-blocker users. *Clin. Pharmacol. Ther.* 2009; 85:45– 50.

Cadamuro J, Dieplinger B, Felder T, Kedenko I, Mueller T, Haltmayer M, et al. Genetic determinants of acenocoumarol and phenprocoumon maintenance dose requirements. *Eur J Clin Pharmacol.* 2010; 66:253–60.

Carr D, O'Meara H, Jorgensen A, Campbell J, Hobbs M, McCann G, et al. SLCO1B1 genetic variant associated with statin-induced myopathy: a proof-of-concept study using the clinical practice research datalink. *Clin Pharmacol Ther.* 2013; 94:695–701.

Dandona S. Cardiovascular Drugs and the Genetic Response. *Methodist DeBakey Cardiovascular Journal*. 2014;10(1):13-17.

Danik J, Chasman D, MacFadyen J, Nyberg F, Barratt B, Ridker P. Lack of association between SLCO1B1 polymorphisms and clinical myalgia following rosuvastatin therapy. *Am Heart J.* 2013; 165:1008–14.

De Keyser C, Peters B, Becker M, Visser L, Uitterlinden A, Klungel O, et al. The SLCO1B1 c.521T>C polymorphism is associated with dose decrease or switching during statin therapy in the Rotterdam Study. *Pharmacogenet Genomics.* 2014; 24:43–51.

DeGorter M, Tirona R, Schwarz U, Choi Y-H, Dresser G, Suskin N, et al. Clinical and pharmacogenetic predictors of circulating atorvastatin and rosuvastatin concentrations in routine clinical care. *Circ Cardiovasc Genet.* 2013; 6:400–8.

Ellinor P, Lunetta K, Albert C, Glazer N, Ritchie M, Smith A, et al. Meta-analysis identifies six new susceptibility loci for atrial fibrillation. *Nat Genet.* 2012;44:670–5.

Escobar M. Prevención del Riesgo Cardiovascular: Políticas Chilenas. *Rev Med Clin Condes.* 2012; 23(6):651–5.

Esmerian M, Mitri Z, Habbal M-Z, Geryess E, Zaatari G, Alam S, et al. Influence of CYP2C9 and VKORC1 polymorphisms on warfarin and acenocoumarol in a sample of Lebanese people. *J Clin Pharmacol.* 2011; 51:1418–28.

Evans W, McLeod H. Pharmacogenomics-drug disposition, drug targets, and side effects. *N Engl J Med.* 2003;348:538–49.

Gadisseur A, van der Meer F, Adriaansen H, Fihn S, Rosendaal F. Therapeutic quality control of oral anticoagulant therapy comparing the short-acting acenocoumarol and the long-acting phenprocoumon. *Br J Haematol.* 2002; 117:940–6.

Gage B, Eby C, Johnson J, Deych E, Rieder M, Ridker P, et al. Use of pharmacogenetic and clinical factors to predict the therapeutic dose of warfarin. *Clin Pharmacol Ther.* 2008; 84:326–31.

Gage B, Eby C, Milligan P, Banet G, Duncan J, McLeod H. Use of pharmacogenetics and clinical factors to predict the maintenance dose of warfarin. *Thromb Haemost.* 2004; 91:87–94.

Hillman M, Wilke R, Caldwell M, Berg R, Glurich I, Burmester J. Relative impact of covariates in prescribing warfarin according to CYP2C9 genotype. *Pharmacogenetics.* 2004;14: 539–47.

Holmes M, Perel P, Shah T, Hingorani A, Casas J. CYP2C19 genotype, clopidogrel metabolism, platelet function, and cardiovascular events: a systematic review and meta-analysis. *JAMA.* 2011; 306:2704–14.

Johnson J, Cavallari L. Pharmacogenetics and cardiovascular disease-implications for personalized medicine. *Pharmacol Rev.* 2013; 65:987–1009.

Johnson J, Gong L, Whirl-Carrillo M, Gage B, Scott S, Stein C, et al. Clinical Pharmacogenetics Implementation Consortium Guidelines for CYP2C9 and VKORC1 genotypes and warfarin dosing. *Clin Pharmacol Ther.* 2011; 90:625–9.

Kääb S, Crawford D, Sinner M, Behr E, Kannankeril P, Wilde A, et al. A large candidate gene survey identifies the KCNE1 D85N polymorphism as a possible modulator of drug-induced torsades de pointes. *Circ Cardiovasc Genet.* 2012;5:91–9.

Kamali F, Khan T, King B, Frearson R, Kesteven P, Wood P, et al. Contribution of age, body size, and CYP2C9 genotype to anticoagulant response to warfarin. *Clin Pharmacol Ther.* 2004; 75: 204–12.

Kaufman, A. L., Spitz, J., Jacobs, M., Sorrentino, M., Yuen, S., Danahey, K., O'Donnell, P. H. Evidence for Clinical Implementation of Pharmacogenomics in Cardiac Drugs. *Mayo Clinic Proceedings* 2015, 90(6), 716–729.

Kimmel S, French B, Kasner S, Johnson J, Anderson J, Gage B, et al. A pharmacogenetic versus a clinical algorithm for warfarin dosing. *N Engl J Med.* 2013; 369: 2283–93.

Kimmel S, French B, Kasner S, Johnson J, Anderson J, Gage B, et al. A pharmacogenetic versus a clinical algorithm for warfarin dosing. *N Engl J Med.* 2013; 369: 2283–93.

Kovac M, Maslac A, Rakicevic L, Radojkovic D. The c.-1639G>A polymorphism of the VKORC1 gene in Serbian population: retrospective study of the variability in response to oral anticoagulant therapy. *Blood Coagul Fibrinolysis.* 2010; 21:558–63.

Lee M, Klein T. Pharmacogenetics of warfarin: challenges and opportunities. *J Hum Genet.* 2013; 58:334–8.

Lim S, Vos T, Flaxman A, Danaei G, Shibuya K, Adair-Rohani H, et al. A comparative risk assessment of burden of disease and injury attributable to 67 risk factors and risk factor clusters in 21 regions, 1990-2010: A systematic analysis for the Global Burden of Disease Study 2010. *Lancet.* 2012; 380: 2224–60.

Link E, Parish S, Armitage J, Bowman L, Heath S, Matsuda F, et al. SLCO1B1 variants and statin-induced myopathy-a genomewide study. *N Engl J Med.* 2008; 359:789–99.

Mallal S, Phillips E, Carosi G, Molina J-M, Workman C, Tomazic J, et al. HLA-B*5701 screening for hypersensitivity to abacavir. *N Engl J Med.* 2008; 358:568–79.

Manolio T, Chisholm R, Ozenberger B, Roden D, Williams M, Wilson R, et al. Implementing genomic medicine in the clinic: the future is here. *Genet Med. American College of Medical Genetics and Genomics;* 2013; 15: 258–67.

Markatos C, Grouzi E, Politou M, Gialeraki A, Merkouri E, Panagou I, et al. VKORC1 and CYP2C9 allelic variants influence acenocoumarol dose requirements in Greek patients. *Pharmacogenomics.* 2008; 9: 1631–8.

Mega J, Simon T, Collet J-P, Anderson J, Antman E, Bliden K, et al. Reduced-function CYP2C19 genotype and risk of adverse clinical outcomes among patients treated with clopidogrel predominantly for PCI: a meta-analysis. *JAMA.* 2010; 304: 1821–30.

MINSAL. Aprueba Garantias Explicitas de Salud del Regimen General de Garantias Explicitas en Salud. Decreto No1, 6.01.2010. Publicado en el Diario oficial el 27.02.2010. 2010.

MINSAL. Estrategia Nacional de Salud 2011-2020. 2011. Available from: http://web.minsal.cl/portal/url/item/c4034eddbc96ca6de0400101640159b8.pdf.

MINSAL. Estrategia para la Reducción del Consumo de Sal en Chile. Departamento de Alimentos y Nutricion. Division de Politicas Publicas Saludables y Promocion. 2010.

MINSAL. Hipertensión Arterial Primaria o Esencial en personas de 15 años y más. Hipertensión Arterial Primaria o Esencial en personas de 15 años y más. 2010. p. 27–47. Available from: http://web.minsal.cl/portal/url/item/7220fdc4341c44a9e04001011f0113b9.pdf.

MINSAL. Implementacion del Enfoque de Riesgo en el Programa Salud Cardiovascular. 2009. Available from: http://www.redcronicas.cl/index. php?option=com_.

MINSAL. Mortalidad por algunas causas de Chile 2000 a 2011. Available from: www.deis.cl/wp-content/uploads/2014/04/0-Chile.xlsx.

MINSAL. Norma Tecnica de Vigilancia de Enfermedades No Transmisibles y sus Factores de Riesgo. Departamento de Epidemiologia, División de Planificación Sanitaria. 2011. Available from: http://epi.minsal. cl/epi/0notransmisibles/vent/NormaTecnicaVENT.pdf.

MINSAL. Objetivos Sanitarios de la década 2000-2010. Evaluación final del período. 2010.

Miranda C, Roco Á, Garay J, Squicciarini V, Tamayo E, Agúndez J, et al. Determinación del polimorfismo de CYP2C9*2 y su relación con la farmacocinética de acenocoumarol en voluntarios sanos. *Rev Chil Cardiol.* 2011; 30:218–24.

Miranda J, Herrera V, Chirinos J, Gómez L, Perel P, Pichardo R, et al. Major cardiovascular risk factors in Latin America: a comparison with the United States. The Latin American Consortium of Studies in Obesity (LASO). *PLoS One*. 2013; 8:e54056.

Nieminen T, Kähönen M, Viiri LE, Grönroos P, Lehtimäki T. Pharmacogenetics of apolipoprotein E gene during lipidlowering therapy: lipid levels and prevention of coronary heart disease. *Pharmacogenomics.* 2008 Oct; 9(10): 1475-86.

Patel J. Cancer pharmacogenomics, challenges in implementation, and patient-focused perspective, *Pharmgenomics Pers Med.* 2016; 9:65-77.

Pearson T, Jamison D, Trejo-Gutiérrez J. Cardiobascular Diseases. In: Jamison D, Measham A, Mosely W, Bobadilla J, editors. Disease Control Priorities in Developing Countries. Washington DC: The World Bank, Oxford University Press; 1993. p. 577–94.

Perera M, Cavallari L, Limdi N, Gamazon E, Konkashbaev A, Daneshjou R, et al. Genetic variants associated with warfarin dose in African-American individuals: a genome-wide association study. *Lancet.* 2013; 382: 790–6.

Prado, Y.1., Saavedra, N., Zambrano, T., Lagos, J., Rosales, A., Salazar, L.A. (2015) SLCO1B1 c.388A>G Polymorphism Is Associated with HDL-C Levels in Response to Atorvastatin in Chilean Individuals. *Int J Mol Sci.* 2015 Aug 31; 16(9): 20609-19.

Quiñones, L., Roco, A., Miranda, C. Farmacogenómica: Aplicaciones cardiovasculares. *Revista Médica Clínica Las Condes*, 2015, 26(2): 198-209.

Quinones, L.A., Lavanderos, M.A., Cayun, J.P., Garcia-Martin, E., Agundez, J.A., Caceres, D.D., Roco, A.M., Morales, J.E., Herrera, L., Encina, G., Isaza, C.A., Redal, M.A., Larovere, L., Soria, N.W., Eslava-Schmalbach, J., Castaneda-Hernandez, G., Lopez-Cortes, A., Magno, L.A., Lopez, M., Chiurillo, M.A., Rodeiro, I., Castro, D.E., Guerra, D., Teran, E., Estevez-Carrizo, F., Lares-Assef, I. Perception of the usefulness of drug/gene pairs and barriers for pharmacogenomics in Latin America. *Curr Drug Metab* 2014, Feb;15 (2):202-8.

Ramsey L, Johnson S, Caudle K, Haidar C, Voora D, Wilke R, et al. The clinical pharmacogenetics implementation consortium guideline for SLCO1B1 and simvastatin-induced myopathy: 2014 update. *Clin Pharmacol Ther.* 2014; 96:423–8.

Rau T, Heide R, Bergmann K, et al. Effect of the CYP2D6 genotype on metoprolol metabolism persists during long-term treatment. *Pharmacogenetics.* 2002; 12: 465–472.

Reitsma P, van der Heijden J, Groot A, Rosendaal F, Büller H. A C1173T dimorphism in the VKORC1 gene determines coumarin sensitivity and bleeding risk. *PLoS Med.* 2005; 2:e312.

Roco A, Quiñones L, Sepúlveda P, Donoso H, Lapostol C, Alarcón R, et al. Cardiovascular related-polymorphisms profile in a mestizo Chilean population. *Acta Cardiol.* 2015 Oct; 70(5): 528-35.

Roden D. Cardiovascular pharmacogenomics: the future of cardiovascular therapeutics? *Can J Cardiol.* 2013; 29:58–66.

Schalekamp T, van Geest-Daalderop J, de Vries-Goldschmeding H, Conemans J, Bernsen M, de Boer A. Acenocoumarol stabilization is delayed in CYP2C93 carriers. *Clin Pharmacol Ther.* 2004; 75:394–402.

Schunkert H, König I, Kathiresan S, Reilly M, Assimes T, Holm H, et al. Large-scale association analysis identifies 13 new susceptibility loci for coronary artery disease. *Nat Genet.* 2011; 43:333–8.

Sconce E, Khan T, Wynne H, Avery P, Monkhouse L, King B, et al. The impact of CYP2C9 and VKORC1 genetic polymorphism and patient characteristics upon warfarin dose requirements: proposal for a new dosing regimen. *Blood.* 2005;106: 2329–33.

Scott S, Sangkuhl K, Stein C, Hulot J-S, Mega J, Roden D, et al. Clinical Pharmacogenetics Implementation Consortium guidelines for CYP2C19 genotype and clopidogrel therapy: 2013 update. *Clin Pharmacol Ther.* 2013; 94: 317–23.

Smith N, Felix J, Morrison A, Demissie S, Glazer N, Loehr L, et al. Association of genome-wide variation with the risk of incident heart failure in adults of European and African ancestry: a prospective meta-analysis from the cohorts for heart and aging research in genomic epidemiology (CHARGE) consortium. *Circ Cardiovasc Genet.* 2010; 3: 256–66.

Su J, Xu J, Li X, Zhang H, Hu J, Fang R, et al. ABCB1 C3435T polymorphism and response to clopidogrel treatment in coronary artery disease (CAD) patients: a meta-analysis. *PLoS One.* 2012;7: e46366.

Takeuchi F, McGinnis R, Bourgeois S, Barnes C, Eriksson N, Soranzo N, et al. A genome-wide association study confirms VKORC1, CYP2C9, and CYP4F2 as principal genetic determinants of warfarin dose. *PLoS Genet.* 2009; 5: e1000433.

Tàssies D, Freire C, Pijoan J, Maragall S, Monteagudo J, Ordinas A, et al. Pharmacogenetics of acenocoumarol: cytochrome P450 CYP2C9 polymorphisms influence dose requirements and stability of anticoagulation. *Haematologica.* 2002; 87:1185–91.

Taubert D, von Beckerath N, Grimberg G, Lazar A, Jung N, Goeser T, et al. Impact of P-glycoprotein on clopidogrel absorption. *Clin Pharmacol Ther.* 2006;80:486–501.

Thijssen H, Drittij M, Vervoort L, de Vries-Hanje J. Altered pharmacokinetics of R- and S-acenocoumarol in a subject heterozygous for CYP2C9*3. *Clin Pharmacol Ther.* 2001; 70:292–8.

Trenk D, Hochholzer W. Genetics of platelet inhibitor treatment. *Br J Clin Pharmacol.* 2014; 77:642–53.

Ufer M. Comparative pharmacokinetics of vitamin K antagonists: warfarin, phenprocoumon and acenocoumarol. *Clin Pharmacokinet.* 2005; 44:1227–46.

Utermann G. Apolipoprotein E polymorphism in health and disease. *Am Heart J.* 1987 Feb;113(2 Pt 2): 433-40.

Van Schie R, Wessels J, le Cessie S, de Boer A, Schalekamp T, van der Meer F, et al. Loading and maintenance dose algorithms for phenprocoumon and acenocoumarol using patient characteristics and pharmacogenetic data. *Eur Heart J.* 2011; 32:1909–17.

Verhoef T, Redekop W, Daly A, Van Schie R, De Boer A, Maitland-Van Der Zee AH. Pharmacogenetic-guided dosing of coumarin anticoagulants: Algorithms for warfarin, acenocoumarol and phenprocoumon. *Br J Clin Pharmacol.* 2014; 77:626–41.

Verschuren J, Trompet S, Wessels J, Guchelaar H-J, de Maat M, Simoons M, et al. A systematic review on pharmacogenetics in cardiovascular disease: is it ready for clinical application? *Eur Heart J.* 2012; 33:165–75.

Verstuyft C, Morin S, Robert A, Loriot M, Beaune P, Jaillon P, et al. Early acenocoumarol overanticoagulation among cytochrome P450 2C9 poor metabolizers. *Pharmacogenetics.* 2001; 11:735–7.

Vesell E. Advances in pharmacogenetics and pharmacogenomics. *J Clin Pharmacol.* 2000; 40:930–8.

Visser L, van Vliet M, van Schaik R, Kasbergen A, De Smet P, Vulto A, et al. The risk of overanticoagulation in patients with cytochrome P450 CYP2C9*2 or CYP2C9*3 alleles on acenocoumarol or phenprocoumon. *Pharmacogenetics.* 2004;14: 27–33.

Wadelius M, Chen L, Lindh J, Eriksson N, Ghori M, Bumpstead S, et al. The largest prospective warfarin-treated cohort supports genetic forecasting. *Blood.* 2009; 113: 784–92.

Wang D, Chen H, Momary KM, Cavallari L, Johnson J, Sadée W. Regulatory polymorphism in vitamin K epoxide reductase complex subunit 1 (VKORC1) affects gene expression and warfarin dose requirement. *Blood.* 2008; 112:1013–21.

Weeke P, Roden DM. Applied Pharmacogenomics in Cardiovascular Medicine. *Annual Review of medicine*. 2014; 65:81-94.

WHO, 2014 available in http://apps.who.int/gho/data/node.main.A865CARDIOVASCULAR?lang=en/(Accessed on September 18, 2016).

WHO, 2016, available in http://www.who.int/mediacentre/factsheets/fs317/en/ (Accessed on September 18, 2016).

WHO. Cardiovascular diseases mortality: age-standardized death rate per 100 000 population, 2000-2012. Available from: http://gamapserver.who.int/ gho/interactive_charts/ncd/mortality/cvd/atlas.html (accessed on October 1st, 2016).

Wijnen P, Op den Buijsch R, Drent M, Kuijpers P, Kuipers P, Neef C, et al. The prevalence and clinical relevance of cytochrome P450 polymorphisms. *Aliment Pharmacol Ther.* 2007; 26:211–9.

Wilke R, Ramsey L, Johnson S, Maxwell W, McLeod H, Voora D, et al. The clinical pharmacogenomics implementation consortium: CPIC guideline for SLCO1B1 and simvastatin-induced myopathy. *Clin Pharmacol Ther.* 2012; 92:112–7.

Wilkinson G. Drug metabolism and variability among patients in drug response. *N Engl J Med.* 2005; 352:2211–21.

Wu AH, Wang P, Smith A, Haller C, Drake K, Linder M, et al. Dosing algorithm for warfarin using CYP2C9 and VKORC1 genotyping from a multi-ethnic population: comparison with other equations. *Pharmacogenomics* 2008;9:169-78.

Xie H-G, Frueh F. Pharmacogenomics steps toward personalized medicine. *Per Med.* 2005; 2:325–37.

Yang J, Chen Y, Li X, Wei X, Chen X, Zhang L, et al. Influence of CYP2C9 and VKORC1 genotypes on the risk of hemorrhagic complications in warfarin-treated patients: a systematic review and meta-analysis. *Int J Cardiol.* 2013; 168:4234–43.

Zhou S, Di Y, Chan E, Du Y, Chow V, Xue C, et al. Clinical pharmacogenetics and potential application in personalized medicine. *Curr Drug Metab.* 2008; 9:738–84.

Zhu H-J, Wang X, Gawronski B, Brinda B, Angiolillo D, Markowitz J. Carboxylesterase 1 as a determinant of clopidogrel metabolism and activation. *J Pharmacol Exp Ther.* 2013; 344:665–72.

In: Pharmacogenomics in Latin America
Editor: Luis A. Quiñones
ISBN: 978-1-53611-031-9

Chapter 9

CANCER PHARMACOGENOMIC STUDIES IN LATIN AMERICA

Andrés López-Cortés[1,*], Santiago Guerrero[2] and María Ana Redal[3]

[1]Centro de Investigación Genética y Genómica, Facultad de Ciencias de la Salud, Universidad Tecnológica Equinoccial, Quito, Ecuador
[2]Gene Regulation, Stem Cells and Cancer Programme, Centre for Genomic Regulation (CRG), Barcelona, Spain
[3]Instituto de Fisiopatología y Bioquímica Clínica, Facultad de Farmacia y Bioquímica, Universidad de Buenos Aires, Centro de Diagnóstico Molecular, MEDgenomica, Buenos Aires, Argentina

ABSTRACT

For more than 50 years it has been proven that the genetic differences among people contribute to interindividual differences on the response to drugs commonly used in cancer treatments.

In this century all drugs developed for the treatment of cancer are "Biological Drugs" forward molecular targets and its effect mainly depends on genetic variants that may be present in the tumor.

Pharmacogenomics makes it possible to identify genetic variations that may predict patients' response to different types of chemotherapy more efficiently. The genetic variations significantly change among ethnic groups, and the assessment of the haplotypes may generate results that are highly correlated to the phenotype.

Latin America is a region where its populations have different phenotypic characteristics due to the great inter-ethnic mixing. Consequently, determines an important genetic flow leading to the appearance of complex characteristics influenced by given geographic and environmental factors that allow individuals to get adapted to the region where they live. These evolving changes, most of them subtle, establish a

[*] Corresponding Author E-mail: aalc84@gmail.com.

profile that could help to develop pharmacogenomic therapies on populations and individuals in order to take control of diseases, toxicity.

Pharmacogenomics allows for improving the investment in public and private health in the Latin American countries, saving time and resources that doctors and patients need, finding addequate treatments based on "trial and error". An additional benefit has to do with the improvement of drug dosification used in the different treatment plans against cancer, starting from the genetic chart of each patient rather than their age and weight.

Keywords: cancer, pharmacogenomics, pharmacogenetics, Latin America, SNPs

INTRODUCTION

Pharmacogenetics and Pharmacogenomics

For more than 50 years it has been proven that the genetic differences among people contribute to interindividual differences on the response to drugs commonly used in cancer treatments. Pharmacogenetics is the science that explains how drug response is affected by the inheritability process. Pharmacogenomics is a rapidly growing field that makes it possible to elucidate the genetic basis for interindividual differences in drug response and to use this genetic information to predict drug safety, toxicity, and efficiency in individuals and populations. The term pharmacogenomics was associated with the Human Genome Project (HGP). According to the HGP, the 99.9 percent of the information found in around 23,000 human genes is identical among individuals, whereas the remaining 0.1 percent of genes is specific to each individual. This difference causes no problems to body development but it may be influential in the susceptibility to develop any type of cancer or to determine how an individual reacts to different treatments and how drugs are metabolized (Carr et al., 2014; Relling et al., 2015).

The term pharmacogenetics comes from the combination of two words: pharmacology and genetics. Pharmacology studies how drugs act on the body and genetics studies how characteristics resulting from the action of one or several genes acting together are inherited and how they work in the body cells (Johnson et al., 2013). Pharmacogenetics starts with an unexpected drug response result and tries to determine a genetic cause. It focuses on the role played by the genetic variation in pharmacokinetics, such as drug absorption, distribution, metabolism, and excretion; as well as in pharmacodynamics, such as drug-response proteins, receptors, channels, and transporters (Carr et al., 2014; Relling et al., 2015; Abedon et al. 2014). On the other hand, pharmacogenomics is seeking the genetic differences in the population that explain certain observed responses to drugs or susceptibility to a health problem. The human genome is made up of 3.1 billion nucleotide bases. Each person inherits two copies of most of the genes; one from each parent. Variants that are found in more than 1 percent of the population are single nucleotide polymorphisms (SNPs), deletions, insertions, and tandem repeats (Nuchnoi et al., 2011). These variants are found in genes that codify proteins. The alteration of the DNA sequencing may affect protein coding and consequently, changes may occur in the phenotype of individuals.

Single Nucleotide Polymorphisms (SNPs)

During the 90's after digesting DNA sequences, leading them to a single nucleotide, the existence of variations in the cutting sites that exactly belonged to a single nucleotide was found. Later it has been observed that there are approximately 84.7 million nucleotide variants in the human genome (dbSNP). Likewise, the variants can be found both in coding sequences called exons and non-coding sequences called introns, and can be responsible for a higher or lower tendency to develop illnesses. The SNPs may or may not cause changes in the essential information of nucleotides; and therefore, the gene, but regardless of the case, their relation to pathologies, such as different types of cancer, is becoming clearer (Paz-y-Miño et al., 2014).

The SNPs in drug-metabolizing enzymes, transporters, and receptors have relevant effects in the efficiency and toxicity of some drugs (Wiwanitkit et al., 2008; Katara et al., 2014). Consequently, science and technology make progress everyday in order to create drugs that can be used in personalized treatments for patients suffering from different types of cancer. Despite the fact that environmental factors, age, type of nutrition, and health condition may be influential in the response to the pharmacological treatment, the genomic information is the key to creating personalized drugs with greater efficacy and safety. The SNPs are the most common variation in the DNA sequence, whereas mutations are uncommon variations, but the main cause of genetic disorders (Kumar et al., 2011). From the point of view of evolution, the SNPs are interesting to be analyzed. First, the frequency of SNPs in exons and introns is very similar: 1/346 base pairs (bp) and 1/354 bp, respectively. The SNPs of exons could be related to illnesses, whereas the SNPs of introns, especially all the perigenetics, are related to variations in the alternative splicing and non-expression sites for miRNAs. When comparing SNPs between chimpanzees and humans, little variations in number (0.6%) has been found. After analyzing their distribution in the genome the difference is of some 32%. Additionally, it has been discovered that the SNPs vary among populations. For instance, African American people and African people have more SNPs than Europeans and Asians (93:17). The studies focused on the genome estimate that out of 84.7 million SNPs found in the human genome, 500,000 are non-coding SNPs, 200,000 are silent coding SNPs, and 200,000 are replacement coding SNPs (Halushka MK, et al., 1999; Huang T, et al., 2015). A person would have from 24,000 to 40,000 SNPs in heterozygosis and some 82% of the SNPs would be polymorphics (Paz-y-Miño et al., 2014).

Polymorphisms in Drug Transporters, Drug Targets, and Drug-Metabolizing Enzymes

Pharmacogenomics makes it possible to identify the inherited genetic variations that may predict patients' response to different types of chemotherapy more efficiently. The genetic variations significantly change among ethnic groups, and the assessment of the haplotypes may generate results that are highly correlated to the phenotype (Huang et al., 2015).

Drug Transporters

Considering the polymorphisms in drug transporters, the MDR1 gene codifies the P-glycoprotein (PGP) protein which is the most known ATP-binding cassette transporter. The PGP transports hydrophobic drugs, including cytotoxic chemotherapeutic agents, hormones, and carcinogens (Borst et al., 1993; Schinkel et al., 1997). The PGP membrane transporter is also found in the normal liver, kidney, small intestine, colon, adrenal glands, and brain tissue (Cordon-Cardo et al., 1989; Cordon-Cardo et al., 1987). Genetic variants in the MDR1 gene have been correlated to drug exposure; drugs, such as digoxin and fexofenadine. The association of polymorphisms of the MDR1 gene in haplotypes differs according to the racial background, generating differences in chemotherapy pharmacokinetics and drug response (Eichelbaum et al., 2004; Marzolini et al., 2003). For example, the C3435T variant found in the exon 26 has a frequency of 80% in African people, but a frequency of 45% in individuals from Europe and Asia (Kim et al., 2001).

Drug Targets

As for the polymorphisms in drug targets, the mechanism of action of the 5-fluorouracil (5-FU) consists of the inhibition of the thymudylate synthase (TS) by FdUMP. The TS is precursor of the thymudine triphosphate, required for DNA synthesis and repair (Grem et al., 2000) Therefore, the inhibition of TS is an important target for 5-FU as well as other folate-based antimetabolites. The resistance to the TS-targeted agents has been associated with the overexpression of TS in tumors (Leichman et al., 1997; Johnston et al., 1995). The TS expression levels are regulated by polymorphic tandem repeats in the TS enhancer region (TSER); the more repeats, the more enzyme activity. Therefore, three tandem repeats (TSER*3) have higher mRNA expression levels in the tumor tissue unlike TSER*2 and that is correlated to a lower response reported to 5-F (Pullarkat et al., 2004). These results suggest that the TSER genotyping is essential to select patients capable of responding to a treatment with 5-FU (Mandola et al., 2003).

Currently, 5-FU based chemotherapy has been recognized as the first line regimen and is utilized for adjuvant and/or neoadjuvant treatment of CRC patients. The recent incorporation of molecularly targeted drugs (Benson et al., 2013) such as anti-EGFR monoclonal antibodies, into the traditional 5-FU-based chemotherapeutic regimen (FOLFOX and FOLFIRI) improves efficacy and is now a pivotal component in the treatment of metastatic colorectal cancer (mCRC); (Grothey et al., 2012). However, the EGFR-targeted therapies accomplish the partial response or stabilization of disease only in a subgroup of patients (Adams et al., 2008). Moreover, the tumor's mutation status, especially in the *Kirsten ras* (*KRAS*) gene, is a predictive marker for response of anti-EGFR antibody therapies in patients with mCRC. Several clinical trials have clearly shown that only mCRCs with wild-type KRAS respond to anti-EGFR treatment. The *KRAS* is member of the *ras* gene family (H-, K-, and N-ras), which encodes highly similar membrane-localized G proteins with molecular weights of 21 kDa (Amado et al., 2008) All three different known proteins are capable of binding and hydrolyzing GTP and participate in a signal transmission pathway from the cytoplasm to the nucleus (Karapetis et al., 2008). Members of the *ras* gene family have been recognized as key targets in tumorigenesis due to their participation in controlling multiple pathways affecting cell growth, differentiation, and apoptosis by interacting with a series of coordinators and effectors (Barbacid et al., 1987) as an essential component of the EGFR signaling cascade. In particular, *KRAS* is involved in the pathogenesis of many different malignant tumors, including lung cancer, pancreatic cancer, and colon cancer (Macara et al., 1996; Cárdenas-Ramos et al., 2014) Activating mutations of the KRAS gene, resulting in EGFR- independent activation of the mitogen-activated protein kinase pathway (MAPK). *Kirsten ras* can acquire activating mutations in exon 2, codons 12 and 13 (Rodenhuis et al., 1987). The most frequent alterations are detected in codon 12 (approximately 77% of all reported KRAS mutations) and codon 13 (approximately 23%). Mutations in other positions, such as codon 61, have also been reported. However, these alterations account for a minor proportion (1–4%) of KRAS mutations, and their clinica relevance in CRC still remains unclear. The prevalence of *KRAS* mutations varies greatly amongst different human tumors. Previous studies support that the frequency of mutation is around 30–40% in CRC and we reported 32% of mutations (Zocche et al., 2015). These results are similar across different ethnic groups (Cárdenas-Ramos et al., 2014; Sameer et al., 2009; Elsamany et al., 2014). Identifying the status of *KRAS* in each patient is important in order to determine the best therapy: patients with the wild type (WT) could receive monoclonal antibodies against EGFR (Schubbert et al., 2007) while *KRAS* mutated patients have been associated with no-response to targeted therapies and poor prognosis in different studies (De Roock et al., 2011; Douillard et al., 2013).

Drug-Metabolizing Enzymes

There are more than 30 families of drug metabolising enzymes in humans, and all of them have genetic variants causing functional changes in the encoded proteins, and thereby the metabolism of drugs changes. The 6-mercaptopurine (6-MP) is a purine antimetabolite used to treat leukemia. The antitumor action of 6-MP consists of the inhibition of the formation of nucleotides that are essential for DNA and RNA synthesis. The thiopurine methyltransferase (TPMT) catalyzes the S-methylation of 6-MP to form inactive metabolites (Lee et al., 2005). Patients with the TPMT*2, TMPT*3A, and TPMT*3C polymorphisms risk having hematologic toxicities when treated with 6-MP (Evans et al., 1991, Lennard et al., 1993). Each one of these mutant alleles encodes TPMT proteins that are rapidly degradated, generating enzyme deficiency. The frequency of the TPMT alleles differ among ethnic groups (Tai et al., 1996, Collie-Duguid et al., 1995). Consequently, an adequate molecular diagnosis of TPMT deficiency can assist with determining a safe starting dose for 6-MP therapy on patients with acute lymphatic leukemia (Yates et al., 1997). Irinotecan is a drug requiring metabolic activation by carboxylesterase to form the active metabolite 7-ethyl-10-hydroxycamptothecin (SN-38), which inhibits topoisomerase-I (Rothenberg et al., 1993). Irinotecan is a popular chemotherapy agent since its antitumoral activity is strong. The clinical pharmacogenetics of irinotecan is associated with the presence of polymorphisms in UDP-glucuronosyltransferase 1A1 (UGT1A1), the enzyme responsible for glucuronidation of SN-38 to form the least toxic, inactive metabolite SN38G (Gupta et al., 1994). The presence of seven repeats TA in the UGT1A1 gene promoter generates reduced enzyme expression and activity (Bosma et al., 1995, Innocenti et al., 2004). The allele frequencies of UGT1A1*28 reach up to 35% in Caucasian and African American populations, whereas the frequency in

Asian populations is much lower. The cytochrome P450 enzymes are an important family of drug metabolising enzymes since they catalyze metabolism of more medications than other enzyme families. Debrisoquin hydroxylase (CYP2D6) is the most typical polymorphism of the P450 enzymes worldwide. Subsequently, > 30 drugs were found to be substrates for CYP2D6. The polymorphisms of the CYP1A1 gene are considered as possible risk factors in the development of breast cancer since they act as mediators in the tumorigenesis caused by the metabolism of estrogens, metabolic pathway where the enzyme encoded by this gene is involved because it catalyzes several steps in the biosynthesis of steroid hormones, such as estrogen. Its derivative metabolites have an important antiproliferative and antiangiogenic activity, whereas other products of the metabolism of estrogen may join the DNA and damage it, suggesting that estrogen and the intermediary products of its metabolism may turn into potential carcinogens (Evans et al., 2003).

Genotyping the Latin American populations with Cancer

It is known that some genetic markers (characteristics of proteins, enzymes, chromosomes, immunology) are related to different types of cancer. This means that a person with a specific genetic marker is more likely to develop a given illness than another person without the same marker.

It should also be consider that in this century all drugs developed for the treatment of cancer are "targeted drugs" forward molecular targets and its effect mainly depends on genetic variants that may be present in the tumor.

Latin America is a region where its populations have different phenotypic characteristics due to the great interracial mixing. Population mixing; consequently, determines an important genetic flow leading to the appearance of complex characteristics influenced by given geographic and environmental factors that allow individuals to get adapted to the region where they live. These evolving changes, most of them subtle, establish a profile that could help to develop pharmacogenomic therapies on populations and individuals in order to take control of diseases, toxicity, and economic investment (Paz-y-Miño et al., 2014).

Table 1. Genotypes' reports on the cancer patients in Latin America

Country	Genes	Disease	Study	Year
Colombia	BRCA1/2	Breast cancer/Ovarian cancer	Descriptive	2014
Chile	CYP1A1, CYP2E1, GSTM1	Lung cancer	Case - control	2001
Chile	CYP1A1, GSTM1	Prostate cancer	Case - control	2003
Chile	CYP1A1, GSTM1	Larynx cancer	Case - control	2013
Chile	CYP1A1, GSTM1	Oral cancer	Case - control	2010
Chile	TP53	Lung cancer	Case - control	2009
Chile	CYP1A1, GSTM1	Gastric cancer	Case - control	2006
Chile	CDKN2A, MC1R	Melanoma	Descriptive	2015
Chile	BRCA1/2	Breast cancer/Ovarian cancer	Descriptive	2011 2006
Cuba	BRCA1/2	Breast cancer/Ovarian cancer	Descriptive	2008
Ecuador	GPX1, MnSOD	Bladder cancer	Case - control	2010
Ecuador	MTHFR, MTR,	Prostate cancer	Case - control	2013

Country	Genes	Disease	Study	Year
	MTRR			
Ecuador	hRAD54	Chronic myelogenous leukemia	Case - control	2011
Ecuador	MTHFR, MTR, MTRR	Breast cancer	Case - control	2015
Ecuador	EGFR	Lung cancer	Case - control	2010
Ecuador	CCND1	Colorectal cancer	Case - control	2015
Ecuador	hMSH2	Lymphoma and Leukemia	Case - control	2003
Ecuador	RB1	Retinoblastoma	Case - control	2003
Ecuador	SRD5A2	Prostate cancer	Case - control	2009
Venezuela	IL-1	Gastric cancer	Case - control	2014
Venezuela	TP53	Gastric cancer	Case - control	2009
Venezuela	WNT pathway	Gastric cancer	Descriptive	2015
Venezuela	8q24 region	Gastric cancer	Case - control	2015
Venezuela	BRCA1/2	Breast cancer/Ovarian cancer	Descriptive	2015
Puerto Rico	BRCA1/2	Breast cancer/Ovarian cancer	Descriptive	2012 2015
Peru	BRCA1/2	Breast cancer/Ovarian cancer	Descriptive	2015
Mexico	ABCB1, ABCC5, XO	Acute lymphoblastic leukemia	Descriptive	2015
Mexico	CDKN2A, MC1R	Melanoma	Descriptive	2015
Mexico	BRCA1/2	Breast cancer/Ovarian cancer	Descriptive	2015
Argentina	BRCA1/2	Breast cancer/Ovarian cancer	Case-control	2011
Argentina	MTHFR, GST, NQO1	Bladder cancer	Case - control	2004
Argentina	TP53	Colorectal cancer	Case - control	2012
Argentina	TNFα	Cervical cancer	Case - control	2012
Argentina	CDKN2A, MC1R	Melanoma	Descriptive	2015
Brazil	CYP1A1, CYP2E1	Lung cancer	Case - control	1995
Brazil	CYP1A1	Lung cancer	Case - control	2009
Brazil	GSTA1, GSTM1, GSTT1, GSTP1	Prostate cancer	Case - control	2014
Brazil	TP53	Cervical cancer	Descriptive	2004
Brazil	IL-8	Gastric cancer	Case - control	2012
Brazil	CDKN2A, MC1R	Melanoma	Descriptive	2015
Brazil	BRCA1/2	Breast cancer/Ovarian cancer	Descriptive	2007
Brazil, Uruguay, Argentina	MLH1, MLH2	Colorectal cancer (Lynch syndrome)	Case - control	2012
Uruguay	CDKN2A, MC1R	Melanoma	Descriptive	2015
Uruguay	BRCA1/2	Breast cancer/Ovarian cancer	Descriptive	2011
The Bahamas	BRCA1/2	Breast cancer/Ovarian cancer	Descriptive	2014

Scientists from different research, health centers, and hospitals in Latin America have published dozens of scientific articles in indexed magazines. These articles focus on the population studies of different genes involved in the risk to develop different types of cancer. Among the most distinguished research, in the Chilean population the BRCA1/2, CYP1A1, CYP2E1, GSTM1, and TP53 genes in breast cancer, lung cancer, prostate cancer, larynx cancer and oral cancer have been studied *(Quiñones* et al. *2001, Gallardo* et al., 2006). As for the Ecuadorian population, the GPX-1, MnSOD, MTHFR, MTRR, MTR, hRAD54, EGFR, CCND1, hMSH2, RB1, and SRD5A2 genes in bladder cancer, prostate cancer, chronic myelogenous leukemia, breast cancer, lung cancer, colorectal cancer, lymphoma, and retinoblastoma have been analyzed (Pérez et al., 2006; Larre Borges et al., 2009). Concerning the Venezuelan population, the IL-1, TP53 genes, the 8q24 chromosome region, and the WNT pathway in gastric cancer have been analyzed (Puig et al., 2015; Sugimura et al., 1995). The ABCB1, ABCC5, and XO genes were studied in the Mexican population with acute lymphoblastic leukemia *(Zaruma-Torres* et al., 2015). The MTHFR, GST, NQO1, TP53, and TNFα genes were analyzed in Argentinean patients with bladder cancer, colorectal cancer, and cervical cancer (Moore LE, et al., 2004; Badano I, et al., 2012). Regarding the Brazilian population, the CYP1A1, CYP2E1, GSTA1, GSTM1, GSTT1, GSTP1, TP53, and IL-8 genes in patients with lung cancer, prostate cancer, cervix cancer, and gastric cancer have been analyzed (Sugimura et al., 1995; Felipe et al., 2012). Finally, the MLH1 and MLH2 genes in people with colorectal cancer (Lynch syndrome) from Brazil, Uruguay, and Argentina were studied. Concerning melanoma, Puig et al. (Puig et al., 2015) recently showed that Latin American families had CDKN2A mutations more frequently than Spanish ones and presented a higher prevalence of MC1R variants compared with Spanish patients. In breast and ovarian cancer, genetic alterations in tumor suppressor genes BRCA1 and BRCA2 have been studied in Argentina et al., 2012), Brazil (Gomes et al., 2007), Chile (Gonzalez-Hormazabal et al., 2011; Gallardo et al., 2006), Colombia (Hernández et al., 2014), Cuba (Rodriguez et al., 2008), Mexico (Villarreal-Garza et al., 2015), Venezuela (Lara et al., 2012), Puerto Rico (Dutil et al., 2015; Dutil et al., 2012), Peru (Abugattas et al., 2015), The Bahamas (Akbari et al., 2014), and Uruguay (Delgado et al., 2011). All this research have determined the association of different genetic variants with the highest risk to develop different types of cancer in the populations from Latin America. These results make it possible to understand the genome both at population and individual level in the best possible pathway, turning this into a relevant step for the development of drugs in a directed treatment plan (Table 1).

CONCLUSION

Barriers and Benefits of Pharmacogenomics in Latin America

The implementation of pharmacogenomics in health policies conveys many benefits to patients who suffer from different types of cancer. Nevertheless, according to a research conducted by Quiñones et al., there are important barriers to implement the use of pharmacogenomics testing in clinical practice. Some of the barriers that can be found in Latin America in order from highest to lowest relevance are the following: Need for clear guidelines for the use of pharmacogenomics in clinical practice, insufficient awareness about pharmacogenomics among clinicians, absence of a regulatory institution that facilitates the use of pharmacogenetic tests, fragmentation of healthcare systems, insufficient pharmacogenomic characterisation of the target population, insufficient characterization of pharmacogenetic variability in Latin America, insufficient use of electronic records information of patients, healthcare system do not promote pharmacogenomics use, concerns about test costs, need for implementation of gene/drug pairs, lack of clear information about mutations actually has functional relevance, need for demonstration of clinical validity and utility of pharmacogenomics test, reluctance of clinicians to use genetic biomarkers as markers of clinical response, insufficient definition of the clinical impact of SNP on specific drugs, and ethical, legal, and social implications (Quiñones et al., 2014).

However, overcoming the obstacles previously mentioned with planning will make it possible to get several benefits. Pharmacogenomic tests are capable of improving patient safety; in other words, individuals who are likely to experience dangerous reactions to drugs could be identified, leading to the adjustment of drug doses in an individual manner. Pharmacogenomics allows for improving the investment in public and private health in the Latin American countries, saving time and resources that doctors and patients need, finding adequate treatments based on "trial and error". An additional benefit has to do with the improvement of drug dosification used in the different treatment plans against cancer, starting from the genetic chart of each patient rather than their age and weight (Johnson et al., 2013).

Pharmacology of the future intends to conduct individualized pharmacotherapeutic treatment for the manifestation of a disease and the appropriate dose for the therapeutic effect in a given patient, minimizing the risk of adverse reactions. In order to implement successful pharmacogenomics tests in clinical practice at the hospitals in Latin America, it is important to understand the interethnic and intraethnic genetic variability of its populations (Innocenti et al., 2004, Delgado et al., 2011). Likewise, these analyses should include ethnic comparison of pharmacogenomic profiles, gene expression, and regulation, the impact of polymorphism on phenotype, metabolic profiles of patients with a given drug and relevant environmental factors that influence drug response. Therefore, the main idea is to accomplish the five "R" for drug therapy: "the Right dose of the Right drug for the Right indication in the Right patient at the Right time" (Quiñones et al., 2014).

REFERENCES

Abedon ST. Phage Therapy: Eco-Physiological Pharmacology. Scientifica. 2014;2014. doi:10.1155/2014/581639.

Abugattas J, Llacuachaqui M, Allende YS, Velásquez AA, Velarde R, Cotrina J, et al. Prevalence of BRCA1 and BRCA2 mutations in unselected breast cancer patients from Peru. *Clin Genet.* 2015;88: 371–375. doi:10.1111/ cge.12505.

Acevedo C, Opazo JL, Huidobro C, Cabezas J, Iturrieta J, Quiñones Sepúlveda L. Positive correlation between single or combined genotypes of CYP1A1 and GSTM1 in relation to prostate cancer in Chilean people. *The Prostate.* 2003;57: 111–117. doi:10.1002/ pros.10274.

Adams R, A. Meade, H.Wasan, G. Griffiths, T. Maughan, Cetuximab therapy in first-line metastatic colorectal cancer and intermittent palliative chemother- apy: review of the COIN trial, Expert Rev. *Anticancer Ther.* 2008, 8: 1237–1245.

Akbari MR, Donenberg T, Lunn J, Curling D, Turnquest T, Krill-Jackson E, et al. The spectrum of BRCA1 and BRCA2 mutations in breast cancer patients in the Bahamas. *Clin Genet.* 2014;85: 64–67. doi:10.1111/ cge.12132.

Amado R. G., Wolf M., Peeters M., Van Cutsem E., Siena S., Freeman D. J., et al. Wild-type KRAS is required for panitumumab efficacy in patients with metastatic colorectal cancer. *J. Clin. Oncol.* 2008, 26 1626–1634.

Badano I, Stietz SM, Schurr TG, Picconi AM, Fekete D, Quintero IM, et al. Analysis of TNFα promoter SNPs and the risk of cervical cancer in urban populations of Posadas

(Misiones, Argentina). *J Clin Virol Off Publ Pan Am Soc Clin Virol.* 2012;53: 54–59. doi:10.1016/j.jcv.2011.09.030.

Barbacid M. Ras genes. Annu. Rev. Biochem. 1987, 56 779–827.

Benson A., Bekaii-Saab C. E., Choti M., Cooper H., Engstrom P., Enzinger P., et al. (2013). Clinical Practice Guidelines in Oncology: Colon Cancer. Fort Washington, PA: Network National Comprehensive Cancer Network.

Borst P, Schinkel AH, Smit JJ, Wagenaar E, Van Deemter L, Smith AJ, et al. Classical and novel forms of multidrug resistance and the physiological functions of P-glycoproteins in mammals. *Pharmacol Ther.* 1993;60: 289–299.

Bosma PJ, Chowdhury JR, Bakker C, Gantla S, de Boer A, Oostra BA, et al. The genetic basis of the reduced expression of bilirubin UDP-glucuronosyltransferase 1 in Gilbert's syndrome. *N Engl J Med.* 1995; 333: 1171–1175. doi:10.1056/NEJM199511023331802.

Brenna SMF, Silva IDCG da, Zeferino LC, Pereira J, Martinez EZ, Syrjänen KJ. Prevalence of codon 72 P53 polymorphism in Brazilian women with cervix cancer. *Genet Mol Biol.* 2004;27: 496–499. doi:10.1590/S1415-47572004000400005.

Cáceres DD, Quiñones LA, Schroeder JC, Gil LD, Irarrázabal CE. Association between p53 codon 72 genetic polymorphism and tobacco use and lung cancer risk. Lung. 2009;187: 110–115. doi:10.1007/s00408-008-9133-3.

Cañas M, Morán Y, Camargo ME, Rivero MB, Bohórquez A, Villegas V, et al. Polimorfismo del codón 72 de TP53 y riesgo de cáncer gástrico: estudio caso-control en individuos de la región centroccidental de Venezuela. *Investig Clínica.* 2009;50: 153–161.

Cárdenas-Ramos S. G., Alcázar-González G., Reyes-Cortés L. M., Torres-Grimaldo A. A., Calderón-Garcidueñas A. L., Morales-Casas J. The frequency and type of K-RAS mutations in Mexican patients with colorectal cancer. *Am. J. Clin. Oncol.* 2004, Oct 20. [Epub ahead of print].

Carr DF, Alfirevic A, Pirmohamed M. Pharmacogenomics: Current State-of-the-Art. Genes. 2014;5: 430–443. doi:10.3390/genes502043.

Chiurillo MA. Role of gene polymorphisms in gastric cancer and its precursor lesions: current knowledge and perspectives in Latin American countries. *World J Gastroenterol.* 2014;20: 4503–4515. doi:10.3748/wjg.v20. i16.4503.

Chiurillo MA. Role of the Wnt/β-catenin pathway in gastric cancer: An in-depth literature review. *World J Exp Med.* 2015;5: 84–102. doi:10.5493/wjem.v5.i2.84.

Collie-Duguid ES, Pritchard SC, Powrie RH, Sludden J, Collier DA, Li T, et al. The frequency and distribution of thiopurine methyltransferase alleles in Caucasian and Asian populations. *Pharmacogenetics.* 1999;9: 37–42.

Cordero K, Espinoza I, Caceres D, Roco A, Miranda C, Squicciarini V, et al. Oral cancer susceptibility associated with the CYP1A1 and GSTM1 genotypes in Chilean individuals. *Oncol Lett.* 2010;1: 549–553. doi:10.3892/ol_00000097.

Cordon-Cardo C, O'Brien JP, Casals D, Rittman-Grauer L, Biedler JL, Melamed MR, et al. Multidrug-resistance gene (P-glycoprotein) is expressed by endothelial cells at blood-brain barrier sites. *Proc Natl Acad Sci U S A.* 1989;86: 695–698.

Cordon-Cardo C, O'Brien JP, Casals D, Rittman-Grauer L, Biedler JL, Melamed MR, et al.Cellular localization of the multidrug-resistance gene product P-glycoprotein in normal human tissues. *Proc Natl Acad Sci* U S A. 1987;84: 7735–7738.

De Roock W., De Vriendt V., Normanno N., Ciardiello F., Tejpar S. KRAS, BRAF, PIK3CA, and PTEN mutations: implications for targeted therapies in metastatic colorectal cancer. *Lancet Oncol.* 2011, 12 594–603.

Delgado L, Fernández G, Grotiuz G, Cataldi S, González A, Lluveras N, et al. BRCA1 and BRCA2 germline mutations in Uruguayan breast and breast-ovarian cancer families. Identification of novel mutations and unclassified variants. *Breast Cancer Res Treat.* 2011;128: 211–218. doi:10.1007/ s10549-010-1320-2.

Douillard J. Y., Olineret K. S., Siena S., Tabernero J., Burkes R., Barugel M., et al. Panitimumab-FOLFOX4 treatment and Ras mutations in colorectal cancer. *N. Engl. J. Med.* 2013, 369 1023–1034.

Dutil J, Colon-Colon JL, Matta JL, Sutphen R, Echenique M. Identification of the prevalent BRCA1 and BRCA2 mutations in the female population of Puerto Rico. *Cancer Genet.* 2012;205: 242–248. doi:10.1016/j.cancergen. 2012.04.002.

Dutil J, Golubeva VA, Pacheco-Torres AL, Diaz-Zabala HJ, Matta JL, Monteiro AN. The spectrum of BRCA1 and BRCA2 alleles in Latin America and the Caribbean: a clinical perspective. *Breast Cancer Res Treat.* 2015;154: 441. doi:10.1007/s10549-015-3629-3.

Eichelbaum M, Fromm MF, Schwab M. Clinical aspects of the MDR1 (ABCB1) gene polymorphism. *Ther Drug Monit.* 2004;26: 180–185.

Elsamany S. A., Alzahrani A. S., Mohamed M. M., Elmorsy S. A., Zekri J. E., Al-Shehri A. S., et al. Clinico-pathological patterns and survival outcome of colorectal cancer in young patients: Western Saudi Arabia experience. *Asian Pac. J. Cancer Prev.* 2014, 15 5239–5243.

Evans W. Pharmacogenomics: marshalling the human genome to individualise drug therapy. *Gut.* 2003;52: ii10–ii18. doi:10.1136/gut.52.suppl_2.ii10.

Evans WE, Horner M, Chu YQ, Kalwinsky D, Roberts WM. Altered mercaptopurine metabolism, toxic effects, and dosage requirement in a thiopurine methyltransferase-deficient child with acute lymphocytic leukemia. *J Pediatr.* 1991;119: 985–989. doi:10.1016/S0022-3476(05)83063-X.

Felipe AV, Silva TD, Pimenta CA, Kassab P, Forones NM. Interleukin-8 gene polymorphism and susceptibility to gastric cancer in a Brazilian population. *Biol Res.* 2012;45: 369–374. doi:10.4067/S0716-97602012 000400007.

Fojo AT, Ueda K, Slamon DJ, Poplack DG, Gottesman MM, Pastan I. Expression of a multidrug-resistance gene in human tumors and tissues. *Proc Natl Acad Sci U S A.* 1987;84: 265–269.

Gallardo M, Silva A, Rubio L, Alvarez C, Torrealba C, Salinas M, et al. Incidence of BRCA1 and BRCA2 mutations in 54 Chilean families with breast/ovarian cancer, genotype-phenotype correlations. *Breast Cancer Res Treat.* 2006;95: 81–87. doi:10.1007/s10549-005-9047-1.

Gomes MCB, Costa MM, Borojevic R, Monteiro ANA, Vieira R, Koifman S, et al. Prevalence of BRCA1 and BRCA2 mutations in breast cancer patients from Brazil. *Breast Cancer Res Treat.* 2007;103: 349–353. doi:10.1007/s10549-006-9378-6.

Gonzalez-Hormazabal P, Gutierrez-Enriquez S, Gaete D, Reyes JM, Peralta O, Waugh E, et al. Spectrum of BRCA1/2 point mutations and genomic rearrangements in high-risk breast/ovarian cancer Chilean families. *Breast Cancer Res Treat.* 2011;126: 705–716. doi:10.1007/s10549-010-1170-y.

Grem JL. 5-Fluorouracil: forty-plus and still ticking. A review of its preclinical and clinical development. *Invest New Drugs.* 2000;18: 299–313.

Grothey A., Allegra C. J. Antiangiogenesis therapy in the treatment of metastatic colorectal cancer. *Ther. Adv. Med. Oncol.* 2012, 4 301–319.

Gupta E, Lestingi TM, Mick R, Ramirez J, Vokes EE, Ratain MJ. Metabolic fate of irinotecan in humans: correlation of glucuronidation with diarrhea. *Cancer Res.* 1994;54: 3723–3725.

Halushka MK, Fan JB, Bentley K, Hsie L, Shen N, Weder A, et al. Patterns of single-nucleotide polymorphisms in candidate genes for blood-pressure homeostasis. *Nat Genet.* 1999;22: 239–247. doi:10.1038/10297.

Hernández JEL, Llacuachaqui M, Palacio GV, Figueroa JD, Madrid J, Lema M, et al. Prevalence of BRCA1 and BRCA2 mutations in unselected breast cancer patients from medellín, Colombia. *Hered Cancer Clin Pract.* 2014;12: 11. doi:10.1186/1897-4287-12-11.

Honma HN, Capitani D, Mello E, Barbeiro A de S, Costa DB, Morcillo A, et al. Polymorphism of the CYP1A1*2A gene and susceptibility to lung cancer in a Brazilian population. *J Bras Pneumol.* 2009;35: 767–772. doi:10.1590/S1806-37132009000800008.

Huang T, Shu Y, Cai Y-D. Genetic differences among ethnic groups. *BMC Genomics.* 2015;16: 1093. doi:10.1186/s12864-015-2328-0.

Innocenti F, Undevia SD, Iyer L, Chen PX, Das S, Kocherginsky M, et al. Genetic variants in the UDP-glucuronosyltransferase 1A1 gene predict the risk of severe neutropenia of irinotecan. *J Clin Oncol Off J Am Soc Clin Oncol.* 2004;22: 1382–1388. doi:10.1200/JCO.2004.07.173.

Johnson JA, Cavallari LH. Pharmacogenetics and Cardiovascular Disease—Implications for Personalized Medicine. *Pharmacol Rev.* 2013;65: 987–1009. doi:10.1124/pr.112.007252.

Johnston PG, Lenz HJ, Leichman CG, Danenberg KD, Allegra CJ, Danenberg PV, et al. Thymidylate synthase gene and protein expression correlate and are associated with response to 5-fluorouracil in human colorectal and gastric tumors. *Cancer Res.* 1995;55: 1407–1412.

Karapetis C. S., Khambata-Ford S., Jonker D. J., O'Callaghan C. J., Tu D., Tebbutt N. C., et alK-Ras mutations and benefit from cetuximab in advanced colorectal cancer. N. *Engl. J. Med.* 2008, 359 1757–1765.

Katara P. Single nucleotide polymorphism and its dynamics for pharmacogenomics. *Interdiscip Sci Comput Life Sci.* 2014;6: 85–92. doi:10.1007/s12539-013-0007-x.

Kim RB, Leake BF, Choo EF, Dresser GK, Kubba SV, Schwarz UI, et al. Identification of functionally variant MDR1 alleles among European Americans and African Americans. *Clin Pharmacol Ther.* 2001;70: 189–199. doi:10.1067/mcp.2001.117412.

Kumar GM. Computational Analysis of SNPs in 10 kb Region of Human Chromosome 1. *J Comput Sci Syst Biol.* 2011;04. doi:10.4172/jcsb. 1000073.

Labrador L, Torres K, Camargo M, Santiago L, Valderrama E, Chiurillo MA. Association of common variants on chromosome 8q24 with gastric cancer in Venezuelan patients. *Gene.* 2015;566: 120–124. doi:10.1016/j.gene. 2015.04.081.

Lara K, Consigliere N, Pérez J, Porco A. BRCA1 and BRCA2 mutations in breast cancer patients from Venezuela. *Biol Res.* 2012;45: 117–130. doi:10.4067/S0716-97602012000200003.

Larre Borges A, Borges AL, Cuéllar F, Puig-Butillé JA, Scarone M, Delgado L, et al. CDKN2A mutations in melanoma families from Uruguay. *Br J Dermatol.* 2009;161: 536–541. doi:10.1111/j.1365-2133.2009.09242.x.

Lee K, Cáceres D, Varela N, Csendes D A, Ríos R H, Quiñones S L. Allelic variants of cytochrome P4501A1 (CYP1A1), glutathione S transferase M1 (GSTM1) polymorphisms and their association with smoking and alcohol consumption as gastric cancer susceptibility biomarkers. *Rev Médica Chile.* 2006;134: 1107–1115. doi:/S0034-98872006000900004.

Lee W, Lockhart AC, Kim RB, Rothenberg ML. Cancer pharmacogenomics: powerful tools in cancer chemotherapy and drug development. *The Oncologist.* 2005;10: 104–111. doi:10.1634/theoncologist.10-2-104.

Leichman CG, Lenz HJ, Leichman L, Danenberg K, Baranda J, Groshen S, et al. Quantitation of intratumoral thymidylate synthase expression predicts for disseminated colorectal cancer response and resistance to protracted-infusion fluorouracil and weekly leucovorin. *J Clin Oncol Off J Am Soc Clin Oncol.* 1997;15: 3223–3229.

Lennard L, Gibson BE, Nicole T, Lilleyman JS. Congenital thiopurine methyltransferase deficiency and 6-mercaptopurine toxicity during treatment for acute lymphoblastic leukaemia. *Arch Dis Child.* 1993;69: 577–579.

Leone PE, Vega ME, Jervis P, Pestaña A, Alonso J, Paz-y-Miño C. Two new mutations and three novel polymorphisms in the RB1 gene in Ecuadorian patients. *J Hum Genet.* 2003;48: 639–641. doi:10.1007/s10038-003-0092-5.

López-Cortés A, Echeverría C, Oña-Cisneros F, Sánchez ME, Herrera C, Cabrera-Andrade A, et al. Breast cancer risk associated with gene expression and genotype polymorphisms of the folate-metabolizing MTHFR gene: a case-control study in a high altitude Ecuadorian mestizo population. *Tumour Biol J Int Soc Oncodevelopmental Biol Med.* 2015;36: 6451–6461. doi:10.1007/s13277-015-3335-0.

López-Cortés A, Jaramillo-Koupermann G, Muñoz MJ, Cabrera A, Echeverría C, Rosales F, et al. Genetic polymorphisms in MTHFR (C677T, A1298C), MTR (A2756G) and MTRR (A66G) genes associated with pathological characteristics of prostate cancer in the Ecuadorian population. *Am J Med Sci.* 2013;346: 447–454. doi:10.1097/MAJ.0b013e3182882578.

Macara I. G., Lounsbury K. M., Richards S. A., McKiernan C., Bar-Sagi D. The Ras superfamily of GTPases. *FASEB J.* 1996, 10 625–630.

Mandola MV, Stoehlmacher J, Muller-Weeks S, Cesarone G, Yu MC, Lenz H-J, et al. A novel single nucleotide polymorphism within the 5' tandem repeat polymorphism of the thymidylate synthase gene abolishes USF-1 binding and alters transcriptional activity. *Cancer Res.* 2003;63: 2898–2904.

Marsh S, McLeod HL. Thymidylate synthase pharmacogenetics in colorectal cancer. *Clin Colorectal Cancer.* 2001;1: 175–178; discussion 179–181. doi:10.3816/CCC.2001.n.018.

Marzolini C, Paus E, Buclin T, Kim RB. Polymorphisms in human MDR1 (P-glycoprotein): recent advances and clinical relevance. *Clin Pharmacol Ther.* 2004;75: 13–33. doi:10.1016/j.clpt.2003.09.012.

Moore LE, Wiencke JK, Bates MN, Zheng S, Rey OA, Smith AH. Investigation of genetic polymorphisms and smoking in a bladder cancer case-control study in Argentina. *Cancer Lett.* 2004;211: 199–207. doi:10.1016/j.canlet.2004.04.011.

Nuchnoi P, Nantakomol D, Chumchua V, Plabplueng C, Isarankura-Na-Ayudhya C. The Identification of Functional Non-Synonymous SNP in Human ATPBinding Cassette (ABC), Subfamily Member 7 Gene: Application of Bioinformatics Tools in Biomedicine. *J Bioanal Biomed.* 2011;03. doi:10.4172/1948-593X.1000039.

Paz-y-Miño C, Fiallo BF, Morillo SA, Acosta A, Giménez P, Ocampo L, et al. Analysis of the polymorphism [gIVS12-6T > C] in the hMSH2 gene in lymphoma and leukemia. *Leuk Lymphoma.* 2003;44: 505–508. doi: 10.1080/1042819021000047038.

Paz-y-Miño C, López-Cortés A, Muñoz MJ, Cabrera A, Castro B, Sánchez ME. Incidence of the L858R and G719S mutations of the epidermal growth factor receptor oncogene in an Ecuadorian population with lung cancer. *Cancer Genet Cytogenet.* 2010;196: 201–203. doi:10.1016/ j.cancergencyto.2009.10.007.

Paz-y-Miño C, López-Cortés A, Muñoz MJ, Castro B, Cabrera A, Sánchez ME. Relationship of an hRAD54 gene polymorphism (2290 C/T) in an Ecuadorian population with chronic myelogenous leukemia. *Genet Mol Biol.* 2010;33: 646–649. doi:10.1590/S1415-47572010005000095.

Paz-y-Miño C, López-Cortés A. *Genética Molecular y Citogenética Humana: Fundamentos, aplicaciones e investigaciones en el Ecuador*. First edition. Quito-Ecuador: Yachay EP Editorial; 2014. [Molecular Genetics and Human Cytogenetics: Fundamentals, applications and research in Ecuador].

Paz-y-Miño C, Muñoz MJ, López-Cortés A, Cabrera A, Palacios A, Castro B, et al. Frequency of polymorphisms pro198leu in GPX-1 gene and ile58thr in MnSOD gene in the altitude Ecuadorian population with bladder cancer. Oncol Res. 2010;18: 395–400.

Paz-y-Miño C, Salazar C, Zurita T, López-Cortés A, Hidalgo R, Rosales F, Montalvo A, Leone PE. Positive Association between the Polymorphic Variant CCND1 A870G and Colorectal Cancer in Ecuadorian Mestizo Population. J Cancer Res Updat. 2015;4: 163–170. doi:10.6000/1929-2279.2015.04.04.4.

Paz-y-Miño C, Witte T, Robles P, Llumipanta W, Díaz M, Arévalo M. Association among polymorphisms in the steroid 5alpha-reductase type II (SRD5A2) gene, prostate cancer risk, and pathologic characteristics of prostate tumors in an Ecuadorian population. Cancer Genet Cytogenet. 2009;189: 71–76. doi:10.1016/j.cancergencyto.2008.09.012.

Pérez LO, Abba MC, Dulout FN, Golijow CD. Evaluation of p53 codon 72 polymorphism in adenocarcinomas of the colon and rectum in La Plata, Argentina. World J Gastroenterol. 2006;12: 1426–1429.

Puig S, Potrony M, Cuellar F, Puig-Butille JA, Carrera C, Aguilera P, et al. Characterization of individuals at high risk of developing melanoma in Latin America: bases for genetic counseling in melanoma. Genet Med Off J Am Coll Med Genet. 2015; doi:10.1038/gim.2015.160.

Pullarkat ST, Stoehlmacher J, Ghaderi V, Xiong YP, Ingles SA, Sherrod A, et al. Thymidylate synthase gene polymorphism determines response and toxicity of 5-FU chemotherapy. *Pharmacogenomics J.* 2001;1: 65–70.

Quiñones L, Lucas D, Godoy J, Cáceres D, Berthou F, Varela N, et al. CYP1A1, CYP2E1 and GSTM1 genetic polymorphisms. The effect of single and combined genotypes on lung cancer susceptibility in Chilean people. *Cancer Lett.* 2001;174: 35–44.

Quiñones LA, Lavanderos MA, Cayun JP, García-Martín E, Agúndez JA, Cáceres DD, Roco AM, Morales JE, Herrera L, Encina G, Isaza CA, Redal MA, Larovere L, Soria NW, Eslava-Schmalbach J, Castaneda-Hernandez G, López-Cortés A, Magno LA, López M,

Chiurillo MA, Rodeiro I, Castro de Guerra D, Terán E, Estévez-Carrizo F, Lares-Assed I. Perception of the usefulness of drug/gene pairs and barriers for pharmacogenomics in Latin America. *Curr Drug Metab.* 2014; 15(2):202-208.

Rahal E M, J H, José M, Quiñones S L, Farfán T N, Cáceres L D, et al. Frecuencia de los polimorfismos CYP1A1*2A y deleción del gen GSTM1 en pacientes con carcinoma de células escamosas de laringe en relación al hábito tabáquico: Estudio piloto en Chile. *Rev Otorrinolaringol Cir Cabeza Cuello.* 2013;73: 7–16. doi:10.4067/S0718-48162013000100002.

Relling MV, Evans WE. Pharmacogenomics in the clinic. *Nature.* 2015;526: 343–350. doi:10.1038/nature15817.

Rodenhuis S., Wetering M., Mooi W., Evers S., Zandwijk N., Bos J. Mutational activation of the K-Ras oncogene. N. Engl. J. Med. 1987, 317 929–935.

Rodriguez RC, Esperon AA, Ropero R, Rubio MC, Rodriguez R, Ortiz RM, et al. Prevalence of BRCA1 and BRCA2 mutations in breast cancer patients from Cuba. *Fam Cancer.* 2008;7: 275–279. doi:10.1007/s10689-008-9187-7.

Rothenberg ML, Kuhn JG, Burris HA, Nelson J, Eckardt JR, Tristan-Morales M, et al. Phase I and pharmacokinetic trial of weekly CPT-11. *J Clin Oncol Off J Am Soc Clin Oncol.* 1993;11: 2194–2204.

Så RA de, Moreira ADS, Cabello PH, Ornellas AA, Costa EB, Matos C da S, et al. Human glutathione S-transferase polymorphisms associated with prostate cancer in the Brazilian population. *Int Braz J Urol Off J Braz Soc Urol.* 2014;40: 463–473.

Sameer A. S., Chowdhri N. A., Abdullah S., Shah Z. A., Siddiqi M. A. Mutation pattern of K-Ras gene in colorectal cancer patients of Kashmir: a report. *Indian J. Cancer* 2009, 46 219–225.

Schinkel AH. The physiological function of drug-transporting P-glycoproteins. *Semin Cancer Biol.* 1997;8: 161–170. doi:10.1006/scbi.1997.0068.

Schubbert S., Shannon K., Bollag G. Hyperactive Ras in developmental disorders and cancer. *Nat. Rev. Cancer* 2007, 7: 295–308.

Solano AR, Aceto GM, Delettieres D, Veschi S, Neuman MI, Alonso E, et al. BRCA1 And BRCA2 analysis of Argentinean breast/ovarian cancer patients selected for age and family history highlights a role for novel mutations of putative south-American origin. *SpringerPlus.* 2012;1: 20. doi:10.1186/2193-1801-1-20.

Sugimura H, Hamada GS, Suzuki I, Iwase T, Kiyokawa E, Kino I, et al. CYP1A1 and CYP2E1 polymorphism and lung cancer, case-control study in Rio de Janeiro, Brazil. *Pharmacogenetics.* 1995;5 Spec No: S145–148.

Tai HL, Krynetski EY, Yates CR, Loennechen T, Fessing MY, Krynetskaia NF, et al. Thiopurine S-methyltransferase deficiency: two nucleotide transitions define the most prevalent mutant allele associated with loss of catalytic activity in Caucasians. *Am J Hum Genet.* 1996;58: 694–702.

Valentin MD, Da Silva FC, Santos EMM, Da Silva SD, De Oliveira Ferreira F, Aguiar Junior S, et al. Evaluation of MLH1 I219V polymorphism in unrelated South American individuals suspected of having Lynch syndrome. *Anticancer Res.* 2012;32: 4347–4351.

Villarreal-Garza C, Alvarez-Gómez RM, Pérez-Plasencia C, Herrera LA, Herzog J, Castillo D, et al. Significant clinical impact of recurrent BRCA1 and BRCA2 mutations in Mexico. *Cancer.* 2015;121: 372–378. doi:10.1002/cncr.29058.

Wiwanitkit V. Possible Single Nucleotide Polymorphism (SNP) in the Nucleic Sequence of A-kinase-anchoring Protein 9. *J Proteomics Bioinform.* 2008;01: 227–229. doi:10.4172/jpb.1000027.

Yates CR, Krynetski EY, Loennechen T, Fessing MY, Tai HL, Pui CH, et al. Molecular diagnosis of thiopurine S-methyltransferase deficiency: genetic basis for azathioprine and mercaptopurine intolerance. *Ann Intern Med.* 1997;126: 608–614.

Zaruma-Torres F, Lares-Asseff I, Reyes-Espinoza A, Loera-Castañeda V, Chairez-Hernández I, Sosa-Macías M, et al. Association of ABCB1, ABCC5 and xanthine oxidase genetic polymorphisms with methotrexate adverse reactions in Mexican pediatric patients with ALL. *Drug Metab Pers Ther.* 2015;30: 195–201. doi:10.1515/dmpt-2015-0011.

Zocche D, Ramirez C,Fontao F, Costa L, and Redal M.Global impact of KRAS mutation patterns in FOLFOX treated metastatic colorectal cancer. *Front Genet.* 2015; 6: 116.

In: Pharmacogenomics in Latin America
Editor: Luis A. Quiñones
ISBN: 978-1-53611-031-9

Chapter 10

PHARMACOGENOMICS OF ANTIRETROVIRAL THERAPY IN LATIN AMERICA

***Nelson M. Varela*[1,*] *and Fernando Bernal*[2]**
[1]Laboratory of Chemical Carcinogenesis and Pharmacogenetics, Department of Basic-Clinical Oncology (DOBC), Faculty of Medicine, University of Chile
[2]Department of Infectious Disease, San Juan de Dios Hospital, Santiago, Chile

ABSTRACT

AIDS is caused by infection with human immunodeficiency virus (HIV), which when untreated produces a critical decline in $CD4^+$ T cells, triggering a progressive dysfunction of the immune system and the development of opportunistic infections and/or malignancies leading to death. Currently, there are more than 20 anti-retrovirals (ARVs) approved for commercial use in Latin America, and a large number of new ARV studies. These are divided into 6 classses: nucleos(t)ide analogue reverse transcriptase inhibitors (NRTIs), non-nucleoside reverse transcriptase inhibitors (NNRTIs), protease inhibitors (PI), fusion inhibitors (FIs), co-receptor antagonists (CCR5-antagonists) and integrase inhibitors (INSTI). Nevertheless, the high inter-individual variability in the response and the adverse effects of these drugs has been the main explanation for the lack of adherence to treatment. In Latin America several studies have been conducted to evaluate the frequency of the polymorphisms in proteins related to pharmacotherapeutic response to ARV treatment both in patients living with HIV and/or in the general population. The results show variable frequencies between the different countries, regions and/or ethnicities.

Despite international evidence on the importance of these polymorphisms to the success of ARV therapy, findings are controversial, since most of the studies conducted are focused only on one genetic variant and just a single drug, without addressing the complexity of multidrug treatment currently used in patients, and particularly in patients from multi-ethnic backgrounds.

Keywords: pharmacogenomics, pharmacogenetics, antiretroviral, AIDS, Latin America

---

[*] Corresponding Author E-mail: nvarela@med.uchile.cl.

INTRODUCTION

The acquired immunodeficiency syndrome (AIDS) is one of the major global public health problems worldwide, it has been estimated that approximately 35 million people are living with HIV. The steady increase in the number of new cases has led to position itself as one of the leading causes of death (1.5 million in 2013), especially in younger, individuals and in low and middle income countries (UNAIDS, 2015).

AIDS is a disease caused by infection with human immunodeficiency virus (HIV). When untreated, HIV produces a profound decline in $CD4^+$ T cells, triggering a progressive dysregulation of the immune system and the development of opportunistic infections and/or malignancies leading to death. AIDS is characterized by a $CD4^+$ lymphocytes count lower than 200cells/mm^3, or one of the CDC/WHO characterized opportunistic infections or opportunistic malignancies associated with profound immunosuppression. (Richman et al., 2009; Maartens et al., 2014).

HIV is transmitted through exposure to infected sexual fluids, blood or breast milk. The main routes of transmission are sexual, parental (intravenous drug or needlestick) and vertical (during pregnancy, childbirth and breastfeeding) (Maartens et al., 2014).

The mechanism of action of HIV infection is characterized by intense viral replication in cells expressing CD4 receptor, such as lymphocytes, macrophages and dendritic cells. In early stages of the disease, a balance exists between the neutralization of new virions and generation of new immune cells, resulting in an asymptomatic clinical presentation. In early stages of infection, HIV is characterized by an initial burst of viremia; although anti-HIV-1 antibodies are undetectable, HIV-1 RNA or p24 antigen are present. Recent infection generally is considered the phase up to 6 months after infection during which anti-HIV-1 antibodies are detectable. An estimated 40% to 90% of patients with acute HIV-1 infection will experience symptoms of acute retroviral syndrome, such as fever, lymphadenopathy, pharyngitis, skin rash, myalgia, arthralgia, and other symptoms. However, because the self-limiting symptoms are similar to those of many other viral infections, such as influenza and infectious mononucleosis, primary care clinicians often do not recognize acute HIV-1 infection. Acute infection can also be asymptomatic (Rosenberg et al. 2000). In next stage of disease a balance exists between the neutralization of new virions and generation of new immune cells, resulting in an asymptomatic clinical presentation. However, after a variable period of time – in overage 10 years- , the viral load begins to increase and the counts of $CD4^+$ T cells decline gradually, until very advanced stage defined clinically as AIDS (Deeks and Philips, 2009).

In 2010 the WHO determined that more than 7,000 people were infected with HIV daily, totaling about 3 million new cases of the disease worldwide per year; by the end of 2015, it is estimated that 36.7 million people are living with HIV globally. It was estimated in 2015 there were 2.1 million new infections worldwide, of which 150,000 were children (UNAIDS, 2016). Although new infections annually have declined by 35% since 2000, the number of infected persons has increased, partly due to access to antiretroviral treatment (ART). As of mid-2016 there were 18.2 million people in treatment, and 2015 coverage was 46%. (UNAIDS, 2016).

The core project developed by UNAIDS 2015 has a "rapid response approach" to meet specific, time-bound targets, the 90-90-90 goals. This targets refer to the pathway by which a person is tested, linked and retained in HIV care, and initiates and adheres to antiretroviral drugs (ARVs). One of these key objectives is to suppress the viral load of 90% of people on ARV treatment. If these goals are achieved, it is estimated that the number of new HIV infections annually would fall to fewer than 200,000 by 2030. This would also be predicted to be the end of the HIV epidemic as a public health threat.

This 90-90-90 objectives are anticipated to be expensive, whit a cost of 9 billion dollars worldwide, in order to reach the goals to 2020. Over the next five years, the AIDS response requires innovative investments, as well as mechanisms and alliances to avoid non-discrimination. To this end, pharmacogenomics has the potential to contribute significantly to 90-90-90 metrics by allowing optimization of ART choices using observation regarding genetic predictors of response and toxicity.

In Latin America, the number of new HIV infections in 2014 was 17% lower than in 2000 (2000: 100,000; 2014: 87,000 approx.), a fall that was lower than that observed in other regions of the world for the same years: sub-Saharan Africa (41%), the Caribbean (50%), and Asia and the Pacific (31%). However, other regions showed an increase in new infections by 2014: Middle East and North Africa (26%), and Eastern Europe and Central Asia (30%). With regard to the number of AIDS-related deaths, Latin America managed to decrease by 31% in 2014 (41,000) compared to 2000 (60,000), a favorable situation it shares with the Caribbean (50% reduction), sub-Saharan Africa (34%), and Western and Central Europe and North America (12%). This compares with the increase observed in Asia and the Pacific (11%), and in the Middle East, North Africa, Eastern Europe and Central Asia, where deaths have more than tripled (UNADIS, 2015).

Pharmacology of HIV

The HIV replication cycle (Figure 1) is occurs in CD4$^+$ lymphocytes and macrophages, using as cellular entry pathways chemokine receptors CCR5 and CXC4 (Alkhatib et al., 1996). Virus binding to CD4 receptors causes a conformational change in the membrane glycoprotein gp120, which mediate increase interactions between the virus and the cell membrane, facilitating their entry (Berger et al., 1999). After entry, it releases two capsid viral RNA molecules in the cytoplasm, together with a number of other proteins required for its replication and integration. The reverse transcription, initially uses one RNA molecule to synthesize a single-stranded DNA, which is then used as a template to produce a double-stranded DNA (dsDNA). Then the dsDNA is associated with a pre-integration complex and migrates to the nucleus to bind irreversibly to random cellular chromatin. The integration of the viral DNA into the host cell's genome is carried out by another viral enzyme called integrase. This integrated viral DNA may then lie dormant, in the latent stage of HIV infection (Sloan et al., 2011). The synthesis of viral RNA depends on the cellular transcriptional machinery. The mRNA is transported to the cytoplasm through nuclear pores, similar to what happens with normal mRNA. Protein synthesis is mainly mediated by Tat protein, which increases transcription of mRNA and Rev, an accessory protein that mediates transport of complete RNA from the nucleus to the cytoplasm (Cullen, 2003). After the RNA and viral proteins have been accumulated in the cytoplasm, the formation of the viral particles occurs by a protease, thus favoring virion maturation and release to the extracellular space (Evans et al., 2010).

There is still no sterilizing treatment effecting a "cure" to established HIV infection, because the virus causes "genomic reservoirs" in early stages of infection that persist despite the durable suppression of the plasma viral load of the patient. To accomplish durable virologic suppression, anti-retroviral therapy (ART) with 3 drugs is, at present, the standard treatment for adults and children living with HIV. Its effectiveness can suppress viral replication and keep viral load undetectable, almost always accompanied by immune reconstitution – sometimes to pre-infection levels of CD4+ lymphocytes, and reducing immune-compromise-associated morbility and mortality. The tests used most commonly in the UK/USA have a lower limit of detection of either 40 or below 20 copies/ml. Virologic suppression and its attendant immune reconstitution improves patient's quality of life (individual goal of therapy) and reduces the risk of sexual transmission (public health goal of therapy) when the virologic suppression is achieved (Cohen M et al. 2016). However, the effectiveness of this therapy can be reduced by late start in the course of infection (importance of timely diagnosis) and/or medication toxicity, which cannot always be corrected with changes in therapeutic regimens, making it relevant to point towards the individualization of therapy initiation (Gupta et al., 2011; MINSAL 2013a; Suarez-Kurtz, 2010). Unfortunately late presentation to care, defined as firs CD4 count below 200 cells/mm^3, has been reported previously between 38% and 45% by PAHO, CCASAnet and the Latin-American Workshop Group with significant differences among countries, suggesting that late presentation to care is a direct consequence of insufficient testing in Latin America. (Celi AP 2016)

Currently, there are more than 20 anti-retrovirals (ARVs) approved for commercial use in Latin America, and a large number of new ARV studies. These are divided into 6 classes: nucleos(t)ide reverse transcriptase inhibitors (NRTIs), non-nucleoside reverse transcriptase inhibitors (NNRTIs), protease inhibitors (PI), fusion inhibitors (FIs), co-receptors antagonists (CCR5) and integrase inhibitors (INSTI), see Figure 1 (Michaud et al, 2012; Hass and Tarr, 2015).

The Latin American guideline supports as first-line regimen combining 2 NRTIs with: one NNRTIs (usually efavirenz or nevirapine), or 1 PI (usually Atazanavir/Ritonavir, Lopinavir/Ritonavir and Darunavir in some case), or 1 INSTI (e.g., Raltegravir). The most frequently used in the initial treatment are: Zidovudine (AZT), Abacavir (ABC), Tenofovir disoproxil fumarate (TDF), emtricitabine (FTC) and lamivudine (3TC). In this regard, it is important to note that there some NRTIs are available as co-formulated fixed-dose combination tablets (FDC), including TDF/FTC, ABC(3TC and AZT/3TC. The Antiretroviral drugs stavudine (d4T), indinavir (IDV) and nelfinavir (NFV) are not recommended in the Chilean HIV/AIDS Clinical Guidelines (MINSAL 2013a).

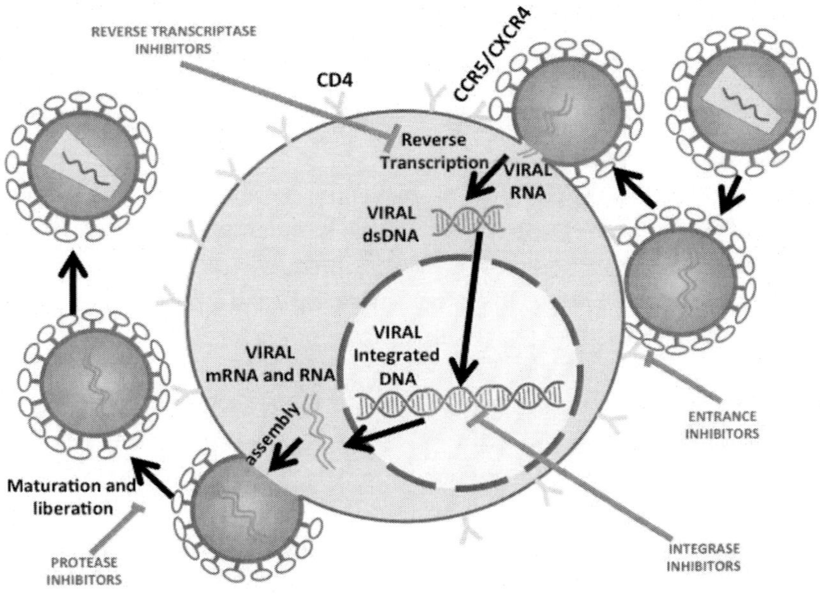

Figure 1. HIV replication cycle and molecular targets of antiretroviral drugs. Modified Michaud et al., 2012.

When initiating ART, is important to consider the clinical evidences and the adverse events profile of the regimen. The generally accepted formula for a potent antiretroviral regimen includes 2 NRTIs + a third agent. When considering NRTI's, thymidine analogues (AZT [or d4T]) may produce mitochondrial toxicity, dyslipidemia, insulin resistance, anemia, myopathy and neutropenia. ABC can cause a hypersensitivity reaction, the reaction can be avoided if the agent is not used in individuals whit the polymorphism HLA-B * 5701, the major allele associated with such reaction. Clinical studies have shown that the TDF/FTC FDC is more effective than AZT/3TC, as those treated with the latter combination had higher rate of discontinuation for lipoatrophy and anemia (Pozniak et al., 2006). The third drug to be incorporated into the regimen is most commonly an NNRTI, PI or INSTI. National and international evidences show that Efavirenz (EFV) has a greater efficacy and less adverse reactions than nevirapine (NVP) (van Leth et al., 2004), with lower failure rate than other treatment regimens (Llibre and Podzamczer, 2012), although several studies have confirmed that EFV can cause rashes, lipoatrophy, altered lipid profile and CNS toxicity (see Table 1) that have been associated with high plasma levels of the drug (Mathiesen et al., 2006; Lowenhaupt et al., 2007). Protease inhibitors that avaible in Chile include Lopinavir (LPV), Atazanavir (ATV) and Darunavir (DRV). Atazanavir/ritonavir (ATV/r) has presented similar efficacy to efavirenz (Molina et al., 2010). These are frequently co-administered with a potent inhibitor of CYP3A4 and P-glycoprotein, Ritonavir (r), which serves to increase plasma levels of the co administered PI improving the pharmacokinetic parameters of PI. Among the adverse events of PI's are dyslipidemia, glucose intolerance and central fat accumulation, increased cardiovascular risk, being these events the main limitation of its ARVs (Table 1).

A table of commonly used ART initial treatment regimen in patients without prior ARV exposure, and the recommended changes for adverse events, can be seen in Table 2 and 3. In general, and according to cohort studies in Latin America, a second line regimen is defined as that containing one of the following drugs: darunavir, etravirine, enfuvirtide, maraviroc or raltegravir (Cesar et al, 2014).

Globally, increased use of ART has dramatically decreased the progression of HIV to AIDS, and accounts for the increase by 17.7% in the number of people living with HIV in the world from 2001 to 2012, despite the rates of new infections diagnosed being 33% higher in 2001 than in 2012 (UNAIDS 2014). In Latin America, Brazil's public health system was the pioneer in ensuring free access to ARV treatment, beginning in the 1990s.

Table 1. Major toxicities of antiretroviral drugs

ARVs	Principal toxicity	Other toxicities
Zidovudine (AZT)	Anemia-Neutropenia MetabolicLipoatrophy	Gastrointestinal-headache Exanthema-Lactic acidosis-Myopathy
Lamiduvine (3TC)	--	Gastrointestinal-headache
Abacavir (ABC)	Hypersensitivity Reaction	Gastrointestinal
Tenofovir Disoproxil Fumarate (TDF)	Kidney-Osteopenia	Gastrointestinal
Efavirenz (EFV)	Central nervous system (CNS) Fat accumulation-Metabolic	Exanthema, Hepatotoxicity
PI (except Atazanavir)	Fat accumulation-Metabolic	Hepatotoxicity-Gastrointestinal Osteonecrosis
INSTI	Myopathy	Hypersensitivity

(Adapted from the Clinic Guide AUGE, HIV/AIDS, MINSAL Chile, 2013).

Nevertheless, the high inter-individual variability in the response and the adverse effects of these drugs has been the main explanation for the lack of adherence to treatment (Akshaya et al., 2012), and the latter the main cause, putting at high risk the ART effectiveness (ability to suppress viral load). In Chile between 16.7% and 31.0% of patients require ART change because of their toxicity (see Table 1), explaining about half of switches from first-line ART (Bernal et al., 2013). In general, national and international guidelines recommend switch of the treatment when high grade toxicities appear. A Chilean study by Bernal et al. (2013) in 92 patients who started ARV treatment at the *San Juan de Dios* Hospital, reported the presence of adverse effects in 75% of subjects. 85.9% of the notifications were graded according to their severity: 34.1% grade 1 toxicity; 32.9% grade 2; 9.4% grade 3 and grade 4, 3.5% 31.8% (22/69) of the patients required a change in treatment, within a week of initiation. The most frequent causes were: anemia due to AZT (45.4%; n = 10) and diarrhea associated with the use of lopinavir/ ritonavir (27.3%; n = 6).

In previous international studies reasons for regimen discontinuation include skin irritation, hyperbilirubinemia, hepatotoxicity, hypersensitivity to neurological impairment that can lead to death of the patient (Hawkins, 2010). In Chile, the major causes of regimen discontinuation/switching are hematologic toxicity (anemia and/or neutropenia) gastrointestinal (vomiting and/or diarrhea), and hypersensitivity.

Table 2. Changes in ARV scheme, recommended and usually applied in Chile and Latin America. (MINSAL-Chile 2013; Cesar et al., 2014)

Initial regimen (examples)	Recommended Change (examples)
2 NRTI (tenofovir/emtricitabine o abacabir/lamiduvine) + 1 NNRTI (efavirenz)	2 NRTI + 1 PI/r (atazanavir/ritonavir o lopinavir/ritonavir)
2 NRTI (tenofovir/emtricitabine o abacabir/lamiduvine) + 1 PI/r (atazanavir/ritonavir o lopinavir/ritonavir)	2 NRTI + 1 NNRTI (efavirenz)
	2 NRTI + 1 PI alternative/r
	1 NRTI + 1 NNRTI + 1 PI alternative/r
2 NRTI (tenofovir/emtricitabine o abacabir/lamiduvine) + 1 INSTI (raltegravir)	

A study that included 5 countries in Latin America (Argentina, Brazil, Honduras, Mexico and Peru), observed 5.3% of patients require a second line regimen and, only 0.8% of the patients who started ART required a third line regimen, with a mean follow-up of 3.5 years. However, this rate increases to 6% when evaluated at 5 years. (Cesar et al., 2014).

Currently the WHO recommendations have been recently updated, recommending as a preferential regimen for adults the start of 2 NRTI + 1 INSTI or NNRTI. The INSTI recommended is dolutegravir. This recommendation is based mainly on the safety profile, high barrier to resistance, and low potential for pharmacokinetic interactions. (WHO, 2016) (Table 3).

Adverse events diminish may adherence to ART, and on the other hand, are the most common cause of treatment switches. The toxicity of ART is the leading cause of poor adherence to treatment, which reaches 47% in the first months of therapy. While it is true there is no consensus on what does it mean adherence to ART, it could be defined as "the patient's ability to start and correctly decide on therapy, in order to suppress viral replication" (OPS, 2011). Therefore, it is considered non-adherence to that which is insufficient to achieve the therapeutic goals, for instance, if the patient does not fulfill at least 95% of the prescription (MINSAL 2013a). Non-adherence is the leading cause of treatment failure, disease progression and increased mortality (Lima et al., 2009), even, it is one of the factors that lead to development resistance to antiretroviral drugs (Nieuwkerk and Oort, 2005). The change of antiretroviral drug due to toxicity, in a scheme in failure, involves sequential monotherapy and facilitates the development of resistance (Cozzi-Lepri et al., 2008).

Table 3: First-line ART regimens for adults, pregnant or breastfeeding women and adolescents. (WHO, Recommendation 2016)

First-line ART	Preferred first-line	Alternative first-line regimen
Adults	TDF + 3TC(or FTC) + EFV	AZT + 3TC + EFV(or NVP) TDF + 3TC(or FTC) + DTG TDF + 3TC(or FTC) + EFV TDF + 3TC(or FTC) + NVP
Pregnant or breastfeeding women	TDF + 3TC(or FTC) + EFV	AZT + 3TC + EFV(or NVP) TDF + 3TC(or FTC) + NVP
Adolescents	TDF + 3TC(or FTC) + EFV	AZT + 3TC + EFV(or NVP) TDF (or ABC) + 3TC(or FTC) + DTG TDF (or ABC) + 3TC(or FTC) + EFV TDF (or ABC) + 3TC(or FTC) + NVP

One of the main criteria used to evaluate failure of the high activity antiretrovial therapy (HAART) is viral load (VL), which must be undetectable and sustainable over time. Patients who fail to sustained suppression of viral replication are more exposed to immune failure, clinical progression and death. There is no consensus on the level of detectable VL defining virological failure. However, Clinics Guides recommends consider, virologic failure, (1) HIV-1 RNA level never dropped below 400 copies/ml after 6 months of therapy, (2) HIV-1 RNA level dropped below 400 copies/ml but then there were two consecutive values >400 copies/ml (without regards to time between measurements), (3) HIV-1 RNA level dropped below 400 copies/ml but then there was a single measurement >1000 copies/ml (Cesar et al., 2014)

The inter and intra individual variability observed in response to ART can be explained largely by different pharmacokinetic patients patterns against homologous dose (Suarez-Kurtz et al, 2010), which may be due for a number of factors such as the quality of the drug, anthropometric patient characteristics, co-medication, and environmental agents and individual genetics; the latter factor accounts for between 20% to 90% variability in pharmacokinetics, which may explain the failure of suboptimal treatment drug, or otherwise, toxicity increased in plasma levels. This variation was mainly due to the presence of polymorphisms in metabolizing enzymes and/or transporters related drugs (Evans and Relling, 1999; Michaud et al., 2012; Hass and Tarr, 2015).

The long-term survival of HIV patients after initiating highly active ART has not been fully and adequately described in Latin America and the Caribbean compared to other regions. Considering that the HIV epidemic in Latin America is unique, since it has a wide and varied geography where different ethnic, socioeconomic and cultural conditions coexist.

A recent study described the incidence of mortality, loss of follow-up (LTFU) and associated risk factors for 16,996 patients included in the Caribbean, Central and South America Network (CCASAnet), belonging to Hospital Fernández and Centro Médico Huésped in Buenos Aires, Argentina (HF/CMH-Argentina); Instituto de Nacional de Infectologia Evandro Chagas, Fundaçao Oswaldo Cruz in Rio de Janeiro, Brazil (FIOCRUZ-Brazil); Fundación Arriarán in Santiago, Chile (FA-Chile); Le Groupe Haïtien d'Etude du Sarcome de Kaposi et des Infections Opportunistes in Port-au-Prince, Haiti (GHESKIO-Haiti); Instituto Hondureño de Seguridad Social and Hospital Escuela in Tegucigalpa, Honduras (IHSS/HE-Honduras); El Instituto Nacional de Ciencias Médicas y Nutrición Salvador Zubirán in Mexico City, Mexico (INNSZ-Mexico); and Instituto de Medicina Tropical Alexander von Humboldt in Lima, Peru (IMTAvH-Peru). The patients ART initiators were followed for a median of 3.5 years (interquartile range (IQR): 1.6-6.2), median age at ART initiation 36 years (IQR: 30-44), predominantly male (63%), median CD4 count was 156 cells/mL (IQR: 60-251) and 26% of subjects had clinical AIDS prior to starting ART. Initial ARTs were mostly based on a non-nucleoside reverse transcriptase inhibitor (86%). In general, it shows an adequate response from Latin America to the requirements of ART against the HIV epidemic. However, LTFU rates turn out to be very varied, highlighting the high incidence of LTFU in Argentina versus the good follow-up of patients in Chile and Brazil (Carriquiry et al., 2015).

This first large long-term study achieved very heterogeneous global estimates of mortality, where countries such as Chile and Brazil have a probability of survival similar to those of Europe and the United States, versus the reality of Haiti and Honduras, where the socioeconomic situation and policy clearly affects the health system by influencing mortality rates. In general, the risk factors associated with mortality were low CD4 count, advanced age and clinical AIDS at the start of ART (Carriquiry et al., 2015). In addition, it emphasizes the importance of evaluating adherence to ART, which would allow better follow-up of patients, improve clinical outcomes (efficacy and safety) and favor the quality of epidemiological data. It is precisely one of the objectives of the personalized medicine that the pharmacogenetics in the HAART points to is to ensure an adequate prescription in patients who initiate their treatment.

Pharmacogenomics in the Antiretroviral Therapy (ART)

The discipline that studies how individual genetic factors affect and predispose the response to a specific drug therapy in terms of efficacy, safety and toxicity is called pharmacogenomics (Tozzi, 2010; Michaud et al., 2012.). Thanks to the Human Genome Project, research in this area has been advancing at a fast pace to detect the efficacy of a treatment, and most importantly, the ability to customize drug therapy, by changing the classical dosage medicine and finding other more suitable drugs for a particular patient, personalized pharmacology (Phillips and Mallal, 2008).

The application of personalized medicine in the chronic treatment of people living with HIV is essential because it allows improving tolerability, avoiding adverse effects, which favors adherence to treatment. Therapeutic drug monitoring has incorporated the evaluation of hereditary genetic factors that affect patient response to treatment and are characterized by interindividual variability, and in the case of population studies many of these show ethnic patterns to consider.

The ART used in patients living with HIV meets all criteria for the application of pharmacogenetics:

- It is a chronic use therapy
- It considers, for the choice of therapy, a battery with more than 25 drugs divided into at least 6 families.
- It usually includes the use of two or more drugs that may share routes of metabolization or where a drug may be inducing or inhibiting the pathway of metabolizing another drug included in the ART or of a drug used in the treatment of a concomitant pathology (e.g., other infections)
- It has high interindividual variability, both in the incidence of adverse effects and in the effectiveness achieved
- It is of worldwide use, therefore, it is applied in different ethnic groups.

It has been observed high intra- and inter-subject variability in the response to ART. There are reports of studies that have shown a high interindividual variation in plasma concentrations after a standard dose of ART (Cressey and Lallemant, 2007; Barreiro et al., 2014.). These variations are mainly attributed to genetic polymorphisms in metabolic enzymes responsible for both phase I and II, and cellular carriers involved (Table 5), explaining the wide variability in plasma levels and thus in therapy response (efficacy and toxicity).

The benefits of the comprehensive and correct application of pharmacogenetics criteria to ART are shown in Figure 2.

The Human Leukocyte Antigen (HLA)-B*57:01 Polymorphism

Abacavir, a NRTI candidate for first-line treatment, may produce a hypersensitivity reaction (HRS), usually within six weeks of initiating treatment. This reaction is explained by the secretion of TNF-α and IFN-γ by CD8 + T lymphocytes, which are activated by HLA-B*57:01, mediated by the presentation of antigens in MHC-I context (Martin et al., 2004). In this case, it is advisable to perform the determination of the HLA-B * 5701 polymorphism in all ART naive patients including Abacavir (Hughes, et al., 2004), considering that patients without the allele are highly unlikely to develop an immunological hypersensitivity to Abacavir, but only about half of those with the allele will develop HRS (CPIC Abacavir, 2012 y 2014).

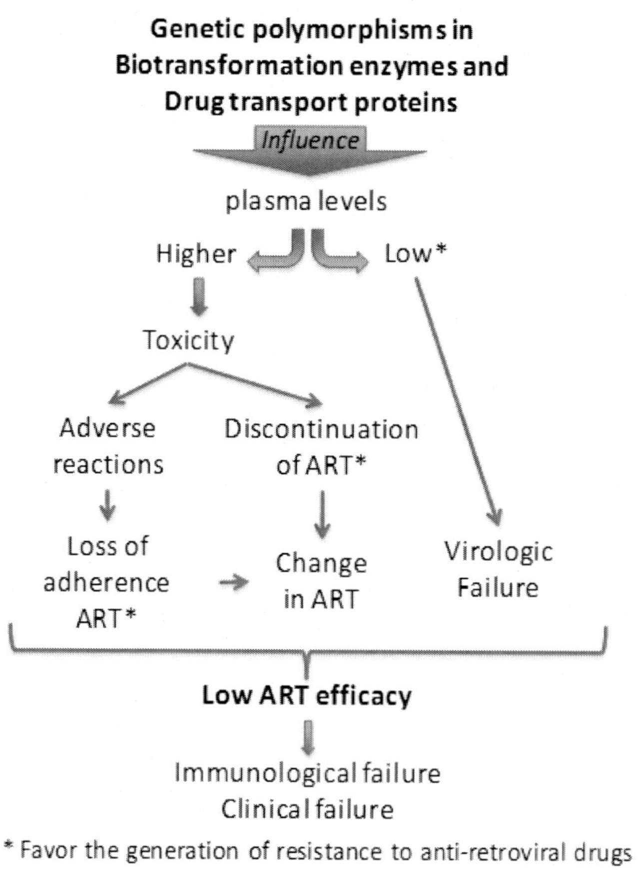

Figure 2. Schematic hypothetical, importance of pharmacogenetics in the ART.

HLA-B*57:01 allele occurs at approximately 5% frequency in European populations, 1% in Asian populations, and less than 1% in African populations, is known ethnic origin of source is caucasians.

In Latin America (mainly in Chile, Brazil, Costa Rica and Argentina) studies have been conducted to evaluate the frequency of this allele in patients living with HIV and/or in the general population, the results show quite variable frequencies between the different countries, regions and/or ethnicities. Ranging from less than 2% (Chile) to 4,9% (Argentina). Table 4 shows the results obtained in these studies and data for the frequency of HLA-B*57:01 in other studies associated with evaluation of population variability and/or characterization of stem cell banks (www.allelefrequencies.net).

Table 4. Frequency of the HLA-B*57:01 allele in different Latin American populations

Country/City or Region	Population	Rare allele frequency	n	Reference
Argentina/Buenos aires	Caucasian	0.025	1,216	www.allelefrequencies.net
Argentina/Cuyo (Mendoza, San Juan y San Luis)	Caucasian	0.018	420	www.allelefrequencies.net
Argentina/central region	HIV Patients	0.049	1,646	Moragas et al., 2015
Bolivia	Amerindian (Quechua)	0.007	80	Martinez-Laso et al., 2006
Brazil (Parana)	Caucasian	0.031	2,775	Ruiz et al., 2005
Brazil (Piaui)	Mixed	0.027	21,943	www.allelefrequencies.net
Northeastern Brazil/Recife, Pernambuco	Mixed African (44%) Caucasian (34%) Amerindian (22%)	0.034	234	Alves-Silva et al., 2000 Crovella et al., 2011
Brazil	HIV Patients	0.031	96	Crovella et al., 2011
Chile	Amerindian (Mapuches)	0.028	104	Rey et al., 2013
Chile/Santiago	Mixed	0.019	920	www.allelefrequencies.net
Chile	Mixed	0.020	300	Poggi et al., 2010.
Costa Rica/Valle Central	Mestizo	0.038	130	Arrieta-Bolaños et al., 2010
Costa Rica/Valle Central	Healthy Volunteers	0.025	200	Arrieta-Bolaños et al., 2014
Cuba	Mixed	0.027	189	Sierra et al., 2007
Cuba	Mulato	0.000	42	Williams et al., 2001
Guatemala	Amerindian (Mayan)	0.009	132	www.allelefrequencies.net
Perú/Arequipa	Mestizo	0.003	168	de Pablo et al., 2000.
Venezuela/Caracas	Mestizo	0.010	50	Gendzekhadze et al., 2003
Venezuela/Valencia and Maracaibo	Mixed	0.026	96	www.allelefrequencies.net

Cytochrome P450 (CYP)

CYP is a family of enzymes that protect the body through the transformation of fat-soluble molecules in water-soluble molecules. The main families (CYP1, CYP2 and CYP3) are involved in most Phase I biotransformation drug reactions ARV (Table 5) where several agents are included, constituting the largest metabolizing system NNRTIs (e.g., Efavirenz and Nevirapine, by CYP2B6) and protease inhibitors (e.g., atazanavir, lopinavir and ritonavir, by CYP3A4 and CYP3A5). The presence of certain genetic polymorphisms in CYP450 enzymes significantly impacts the inter- and intra-individual variability against the drugs clearance and thereby the efficacy and safety (toxicity) of these drugs.

CYP2B6 Metabolism Efavirenz (EFV) and Nevirapine (NVP)

CYP2B6 is highly polymorphic, and so far, it has beed described about 30 allelic variants (CYP ALLELE Nomenclature Committee). Two polymorphisms were considered relevant in response to NNRTIs: CYP2B6*6 and CYP2B6*18. The CYP2B6*18 (983T>C) variant, is relatively abundant in black populations (see Table 4), this allele produces an amino acid change (T328I), causing a decrease in the enzyme activity and thus an increase plasma concentration of drug metabolizing (Dhoro et al., 2015). Moreover, the polymorphism CYP2B6*6 (516G>T; 785A>G), cause a reduction in the catalytic ability of this enzyme and in its expression (amino acid change: Q172H), which causes a considerable increase in the efavirenz plasma concentration (Tsuchiya et al., 2004). *In vitro* studies (conducted in human microsomes) have shown variation of up to 44 times the activity of efavirenz and wherein said variability was significantly correlated with the presence of the allelic variant CYP2B6*6 (Desta et al., 2007). Pharmacokinetic studies in patients treated with efavirenz, have shown that the presence of the allelic variant could explain about 27% to 31% of the differences in the clearance of efavirenz (Cabrera et al., 2009; Arab-Alameddine et al., 2009). Accordingly with this, another study found significant association of allele CYP2B6*6 with the occurrence of adverse CNS effects during the first week of therapy (Haas et al., 2004), and liver damage (Yimer et al., 2012). These facts turn out to be radical when searching for an explanation for the large interindividual variability observed in plasma concentrations of efavirenz (Stahle et al., 2004).

A study in a court of Swiss patients showed that the homozygous presence of the alleles *6 and *18, with the presence of polymorphisms associated with reduced activity in the CYP2A6 and/or CYP3A4 gene, were associated with an increased risk of discontinue therapy with efavirenz during the first year of an initial or first-line regimen (Lubomirov et al., 2011).

In 2010, Carr et al., published a study of 219 Chilean patients treated with efavirenz (214 mestizos and 5 Amerindians), in which they sought to associate different haplotypes of the CYP2B6 gene with plasma concentrations of the drug. They were able to establish 11 SNPs significantly associated with efavirenz levels and determined 3 representative SNPs (rs10403955, rs2279345 and rs8192719). It is important to note that rs2279345 (g.18492) is located at a locus very close to rs2279343 (g.18053), this latter SNP is characteristic of the allele CYP2B6*6, *13 and *19. Another Chilean study in the same cohort of patients published by Carr et al. (2010), sought association with the pharmacokinetic parameters of efaviranz with pharmacogenetic variants in CYP2B6, CYP2A6, UGT2B7 and CAR (androstane constituent receptor), the analysis of 208 patients showed a significant association with the CYP2B6 516G> T SNPs and with rs2307424 from CAR (Cortes et al., 2013). These studies did not incorporate clinical variables such as adverse reactions and/or discontinuation of treatment, and are the same authors that conclude the need for future research to clinically assess the functionality of such SNPs. Another important aspect to consider in studies of pharmacogenetic correlation v/s pharmacokinetics is the phenomenon of metabolic adaptation, since efavirenz can induce its own metabolism (Zhu et al., 2009). Therefore, when patients who started treatment taking efavirenz doses for 2 weeks with a median duration of therapy were 3.6 years (interquartile range of 1.6-5.8 years), the plasma levels obtained in these patients could present fluctuations expected after an induction process, which in patients of this study, probably not yet started. For this reason, it is essential to associate the presence of genetic polymorphisms with plasma levels in patients who initiate treatment for the first time, and where the collection of inter-subject blood plasma samples is performed in time-limited periods after treatment initiation, in addition, to considering the measurement of plasma levels several months (3 to 6 months) after the start of treatment, according to pre-established protocols.

Table 5. Metabolizing enzymes and transporters, drugs most commonly used

ARV	Type	Metabolizing enzymes	Membrane Transporter
Zidovudine (AZT)	NRTI	UGT2B7	ABCC4
Lamivudine (3TC)	NRTI	NA	ABCC4
Abacavir (ABC)	NRTI	UGT1A1	ABCB1 ABCC4
Tenofovir (TDF)	NRTI	NA	ABCB1 ABCC2 ABCC4
Emtricitabine (FTC)	NRTI	NA	ABCC1
Efavirenz (EFV)	NNRTI	CYP2B6* CYP3A4 UGT2B7	ABCB1 ABCC1 ABCC2
Nevirapine (NVP)	NNRTI	CYP2B6* CYP3A4 CYP3A5	ABCB1
Etravirine (ETR)	NNRTI	CYP3A4* CYP2C9 CYP2C19	NA
Rilpivirine (RPV)	NNRTI	CYP3A4	NA
Atazanavir (ATV)	PI	CYP3A4 CYP3A5 UGT1A1	ABCB1 ABCC1 ABCC2
Lopinavir (LPV)	PI	CYP3A4 CYP3A5	ABCB1 ABCC1 ABCC2
Darunavir (DRV)	PI	CYP3A4	SLCO1A2, SLCO1B1
Ritonavir (r)	PI	CYP3A4 CYP3A5 CYP2D6	ABCB1 ABCC1 ABCC2
Raltegravir (RAL)	INSTI	UGT1A1	ABCB1
Elvitegravir (EVG)	INSTI	UGT1A1/3 CYP3A4*	ABCB1
Dolutegravir (DTG)	INSTI	UGT1A1* CYP3A	NA

NA: It lacks metabolism Phase I and II described *more relevant
(Adapted from Michaud et al., 2012).

A multinational study (SMART, FIRST and ESPRIT), which included 758 patients (9% from South American countries), shows that the high pharmacogenetic risk of discontinuing treatment with efavirenz is statistically significant when characterizing a group of SNPs in CYP2A6 (rs28399433), CYP2B6 (rs28399499, rs35303484, rs35979566, rs3745274), and CYP3A4 (rs4646437) (Cummins et al., 2015).

Another intrinsic CYP2B6 SNP (g.15582C > T, which affects splicing) has been associated with lower levels of efavirenz, suggesting its incorporation in future pharmacogenetics studies, considering its high frequency in Hispanics (0.57), Asian (0.39) and Caucasian (0.31) compared to South African (0.08) and Cameroonian (0.06). This SNP may be relevant in several Latin American populations (Evans et al., 2015).

CYP2B6 is also responsible for the metabolism of nevirapine (Erickson et al., 1999), and previous data have demonstrate association of allele *6, significant reduction in clearance of nevirapine (Mahungu et al., 2009), and *18 high plasma levels of nevirapine in black patients (Wyen et al., 2008).

In light of this background, it is essential to evaluate the frequency of both polymorphisms, in the Latin American population, as in the sub-population of patients with HIV, and even more essential is to assess its possible impact on the effectiveness and safety associated with the ART, which includes NNRTIs such as efavirenz or nevirapine. This national research project is further strengthened, considering that international studies have shown that setting low dose of efavirenz based on the presence of allele CYP2B6*6 reduce the symptoms associated with adverse CNS effects (Mathiesen et al., 2006; Damronglerd et al., 2015; Hui et al., 2016) while maintaining efficiency regarding virologic suppression (Gatanaga et al., 2007) and further studies to validate future translational approaches is suggested (Zanger and Klein, 2013; Martin et al., 2014; Hass and Tarr, 2015).

CYP3A4/5 NNRTIs and PI Metabolism

Another family of enzymes important in NNRTIs and PI metabolism is CYP3A4/5. CYP3A4 and CYP3A5 have high similarity (85%) in their amino acid sequences (Ortiz de Montellano, 2005). CYP3A4 is the most abundant P450 liver enzyme (up to 50% of total content of CYP450) and is involved in the metabolism of nearly 50% of all drugs (Evans and Relling, 1999). The catalytic activity of CYP3A4 differs widely and is explained in large part by being a highly inducible gene (Gibson et al., 2002). In regards to drug ARV metabolism, CYP3A4/5 is involved primarily in the metabolism of PI, and the concomitant use of ritonavir and PI is explained by its ability to inhibit the CYP3A4/5 generating a "booster" amplifier effect or other levels of PI (e.g., atazanavir and lopinavir). In the context of triple therapy, it is important to consider that some NNRTIs are able to induce expression of CYP3A4/5, affecting plasma levels of other drugs used in the HAART (Abel et al., 2008).

The main polymorphism known for CYP3A4 is a substitution A>G at position -392 in the 5' region promoter, termed CYP3A4*1B. It is postulated that this polymorphism decreases the affinity of transcription factors, phenotypically with a decrease of enzyme activity (Cavalli et al., 2001). The relevance of this polymorphism in HAART has been widely studied with a few concordant results, due to the inductive nature of some drugs HAART expression of CYP3A4 (Michaud et al., 2012; Hass and Tarr, 2015).

For CYP3A5, the main SNP characterized is a substitution A>G at 6986 position in intron 3 of the gene, results in site of alternative splicing by insertion of an alternate 3B exon of exon 3, changing the reading frame, which produce a premature end codon after amino acid 102, an abnormal protein folding, and hence reduction or complete elimination of the enzymatic activity of CYP3A5 (Josephson et al., 2007). This allele, called CYP3A5*3 is the most common wild-type allele, CYP3A5*1, most stocks except African Americans, and has been associated with a decrease in the clearance of several PI (Anderson et al., 2009), while the *1 allele is associated with increased clearance compared to patients carrying allele *3 (Josephson et al., 2007). Anderson et al. (2009) showed that plasma levels of atazanavir (ATV) were significantly lower in patients carrying the allele *1 compared to patients homozygous for the allele *3. A study in Brazilian patients treated with Lopinavir/ritonavir showed that the CYP3A5 genotype did not affect the plasma levels of these drugs, suggesting that the inhibitory effect of ritonavir could generate a phenotypic masking effect on the genotype of this gene (Estrela et al., 2008).

Glucuronyl Transferase (UGT)

Glucuronidation Phase II biotransformation plays an important role in the removal of endogenous compounds (bilirubin, bile and steroid hormones) and some ARV as abacavir, zidovudine (NRTI), Efavirenz (NNRTIs), atazanavir (PI) and raltegravir, dolutegravir (INSTI) (Table 5). These reactions are catalyzed by UDP-glucuronyl transferases (UGTs). The UGTs have been divided into two subfamilies (UGT1 and UGT2) based on their sequence identity and a large interindividual variation in expression observed (Court, 2010).

UGT1A1 and UGT2B7 in Phase II Drug Metabolism ARV

UGT2B7 is the major isoform involved in glucuronidation of zidovudine and efavirenz, and UGT2B7*1C allelic variant (c.735A>G) has been associated with a high expression of the enzyme which directly affects the efavirenz concentration (Kwara et al., 2009).

One of the most common adverse effects observed in patients treated with atazanavir is jaundice, associated with an increase of unconjugated bilirubin (Bissio and Lopardo, 2013). This effect exerted a noncompetitive inhibition by atazanavir on UGT1A1 (responsible for the conjugation of bilirubin). The allelic variant UGT1A1*28 (more than one TA repeats in the promoter region of the gene) is associated with Gilbert's syndrome. It has been observed that patients treated with atazanavir and carrying a homozygous genotype for this polymorphism, present jaundice with higher frequency (90%) (Park et al., 2010). In agreement with this, the study published by Lubomirov et al. (2011) correlated the presence of allelic variants of UGT1A1 gene and discontinuity of treatment toxicity associated with atazanavir.

ABC Transporters

One of the most studied families are the ABC transporters (ATP-binding cassette), given its importance in contribution to the cell molecules flow. These transporters are found in many epithelial, endothelial and liver cells, participating in the absorption and excretion of many drugs (Hollenstein et al., 2007).

Another postulate that seeks to explain variability in response to ART, is the generation of a sub-therapeutic drug concentration in target cells, given mainly by the performance of these cellular carriers. These transporters modulate the response to HAART in two ways: changing their bioavailability via intestinal and hepatic carriers as modifying molecules access to target cells (Sankatsign et al., 2004).

ABCB1 Polymorphisms in Genes ABCC4 and Its Influence on the ARV Transport

Gene ABCB1 (ABC subfamily B, member 1) gives rise to P-glycoprotein in human MDR1, is the carrier most studied in HIV+ patients since their high affinity for PI (Zastre et al., 2009) and because its expression observed on B and T lymphocytes (Turriziani et al., 2008). The main carrier of this polymorphism is caused by a C>T substitution at position 3435, resulting in decreased affinity for its substrates (Kimchi-Sarfaty et al., 2007).

In a Latin American population, a Brazilian study in 113 patients, who found no association between the presence of exon polymorphisms, 1236C> T, 2677G> T/A and 3435C> T and their corresponding haplotypes, in the ABCB1 gene with the levels of Lopinavir and ritonavir in blood, semen and saliva (Estrela et al., 2009).

In general, polymorphisms in the ABCB1 gene are widely studied for pharmacogenetics associations with ART, however, the results obtained to determine their influence on both adverse reactions and their therapeutic effectiveness remain contradictory (Michaud et al., 2012).

Another member of the ABC transporter family that could play a key role in the distribution of antiretroviral agents, is ABCC4. This transporter is expressed at higher levels in $CD4^+$ cells (Hollenstein et al., 2007). ABCC4 is involved in the transport of various ARV, such as zidovudine and lamivudine. The A3463G variant of this gene has been associated with an increase in tenofovir in HIV patients with predisposition to kidney damage (Kiser et al., 2008). So far, there are no conclusive reports on the possible impact of genetic polymorphisms in ABCC2 and ABCC1 conveyors.

In Table 6, the allelic frequencies reported for each of the polymorphisms raised in this chapter, both in the Chilean population and other populations are summarized below.

Table 6. Allele frequencies of genetic polymorphisms associated with ART, in different populations

Gene SNP ID	Chilean population Rare Allele frequencies (n) *(Reference)*	Other populations Rare Allele frequencies (n) *(Reference)*	dbSNP Rare Allele Frequencies*
CYP2B6*6 rs3745274	0.35 (n = 219) *(Carr* et al., *2010)*	Japanese: 0.17 (n = 442) *(Gatanaga* et al., *2007)* Caucasians: 0.28 (n = 135) *(Jacob* et al., *2004)* African: 0.58 (n = 180) *(Dhoro* et al., *2015)* Mongolians: 0.21 (n = 100) *(Davaalkham* et al., *2009)*	Caucasians: 0.24 – 0.32 African: 0.35 – 0.38 Asian: 0.15 – 0.20
CYP2B6*18 rs28399499	ND	African: 0.16 (n = 185) *(Dhoro* et al., *2015)*	African: 0.05 - 0.12
CYP3A4*1B rs2740574	0.06 (n = 253) *(Roco* et al., *2012)*	Caucasians: 0.04 (n = 116) African Americans: 0.55 (n = 116) Asian : 0.00 (n = 80) *(Roco* et al., *2012)*	Caucasians: 0.02 – 0.03 Hispanics: 0.10 African: 0.50 Spanish: 0.04
CYP3A5*3 rs776746	0.76 (n = 253) *(Roco* et al., *2012)*	Caucasians: 0.93 (n = 154) Asian: 0.75 (n = 68) *(Roco* et al., *2012)*	Caucasians: 0.98 Hispanics: 0.59 – 0.84 African: 0-15 – 0.35 Asian: 0.69
UGT2B7*1C rs28365062	ND	---	Caucasians: 0.15 Multiple origins: 0.12 – 0.17
UGT1A1*28	ND	Japanese: 0.11 (n = 134) *(Takeuchi* et al., *2004)* Caucasians: 0.38 (n = 71) Asiáticos: 0.16 (n = 47) African: 0.43 (n = 101) *(Beutler* et al., *1998)*	
ABCC4 (G3463A) rs1751034	ND	---	Caucasians: 0.15 African: 0.17 – 0.25 Asian: 0.20-0.40
ABCB1 (C3435T) rs1045642	ND	---	Caucasians: 0.37-0.53 Hispanics: 0.45 African: 0.85 Asian: 0.47-0.63

*Data were extracted from dbSNP http://www.ncbi.nlm.nih.gov/SNP

ND: no data reported

CONCLUSION

Despite international evidence on the importance of these polymorphisms in the ART, they are still contradictory, since most of the studies conducted are focused only on one genetic variant and just a single drug, without addressing the complexity of treatment currently used in patients. On the other hand, the genotype frequencies of some polymorphisms have been not studied in the Latin American populations and even worst, its potential association with the pharmacological response to ARV treatment. In this sense, more importantly, it is unknown how these polymorphisms are related to plasma levels and consequent clinical response, specifically the CD4$^+$ cell count, viral load and adverse reactions; considering that they are very frequent, essentially influencing adherence to treatment, and therefore in effectiveness of treatment (Figure 2).

REFERENCES

Abel, S; Jenkins, TM; Whitlock, LA; Ridgway, CE; Muirhead, GJ. Effects of CYP3A4 inducers with and without CYP3A4 inhibitors on the pharmacokinetics of maraviroc in healthy volunteers. *Br J Clin Pharmacol*, 2008, 65, 38–46.

Akshaya, B; Chandra Babru, S; Harlokesh Narayan y Sunil Kumar, J. Incidence of Adverse Drug Reactions in Human Deficiency Virus-Positive Patients Using Active Antiretroviral Therapy. *J adv Pharm Technol Res.*, 2012, 3(1), 62 -67.

Alkhatib, G; Combadiere, C; Broder, CC; Feng, Y; Kennedy, PE; Murphy, PM; Berger, EA. CC CKR5: a RANTES, MIP-1alpha, MIP-1beta receptor as a fusion cofactor for macrophage-tropic HIV-1. *Science*, 1996, 272, 1955–1958.

Alves-Silva, J; da Silva Santos, M; Guimaraes, PE; Ferreira, AC; Bandelt, HJ; Pena, SD; et al. The ancestry of Brazilian mtDNA lineages. *Am J Hum Genet*, 2000, 67, 444.

Anderson, PL; Aquilante, CL; Gardner, EM; Predhomme, J; McDaneld, P; Bushman, LR; Zheng, JH; et al. Atazanavir pharmacokinetics in genetically determined CYP3A5 expressors versus non-expressors. *J Antimicrob Chemother*, 2009, 64, 1071–1079.

Arab-Alameddine, M; Di Iulio, J; Buclin, T; Rotger, M; Lubomirov, R; Cavassini, M; Fayet, A; De´costerd, LA; et al. Pharmacogenetics-based population pharmacokinetic analysis of efavirenz in HIV-1-infected individuals. *Clin Pharmacol Ther*, 2009, 85, 485–494.

Arrieta-Bolaños, E; Madrigal, JA; Marsh, SG; Shaw, BE; Salazar-Sánchez, L. The frequency of HLA-B(*)57:01 and the risk of abacavir hypersensitivity reactions in the majority population of Costa Rica. *Hum Immunol.*, 2014, 75(11), 1092-6. doi: 10.1016/j.humimm.2014.09.011.

Arrieta-Bolaños, E; Maldonado-Torres, H; Dimitriu, O; Hoddinott, MA; Fowles, F; Shah, A; Orlich-Pérez, P; McWhinnie, AJ; Alfaro-Bourrouet, W; Buján-Boza, W; Little, AM; Salazar-Sánchez, L; Madrigal, JA. HLA-A, -B, -C, -DQB1, and -DRB1,3,4,5 allele and haplotype frequencies in the Costa Rica Central Valley Population and its relationship to worldwide populations. *Hum Immunol.*, 2011, 72(1), 80-6.

Barreiro, P; Fernández-Montero, JV; de Mendoza, C; Labarga, P; Soriano, V. Pharmacogenetics of antiretroviral therapy. *Expert Opin Drugs Metab Toxicol.*, 2014, 10(8), 1119-1130.

Berger, EA; Murphy, PM; y Farber, JM. Chemokine receptors as HIV-1 coreceptors: roles in viral entry, tropism, and disease. *Annu Rev Immunol*, 1999, 17, 657– 700.

Bernal, F; Vásquez, P; Giadalah, C; Rodríguez, L; Villagrán, A. Incidence of adverse drugs reactions in patients initiating or changing antiretroviral therapy. *Rev Chilena Infectol*, 2013, 30(5), 507 – 512.

Beutler, E; Gelbart, T; Demina, A. Racial variability in the UDP-glucuronosyltransferase 1 (UGT1A1) promoter: a balanced polymorphism for regulation of bilirubin metabolism? *Proc Natl Acad Sci USA*., 1998, 95, 8170–8174.

Bissio, E; Lopardo, GD. Incidence of hyperbilirubinemia and jaundice due to atazanavir in a cohort of Hispanic patients. *AIDS Res Hum Retroviruses*, 2013, 29(3), 415-7.

Cabrera, SE; Santos, D; Valverde, MP; Domínguez-Gil, A; Gonza´ lez, F; Luna, G; García, MJ. Influence of the cytochrome P450 2B6 genotype on population pharmacokinetics of efavirenz in human immunodeficiency virus patients. *Antimicrob Agents Chemother*, 2009, 53, 2791–2798.

Carr, DF; la Porte, CJ; Pirmohamed, M; Owen, A; Cortes, CP. Haplotype structure of CYP2B6 and association with plasma efavirenz concentrations in a Chilean HIV cohort. *J Antimicrob Chemother*, 2010, 65, 1889–1893.

Carriquiry, G; Fink, V; Robert, J; Giganti, M; Jayathilake, K; Blevins, M; Cahn, P; Grinsztejn, B; Wolff, M; Pape, J; Padgett, D; Sierra, J; Gotuzzo, E; Carey, C; Shepherd, B. Mortality and loss to follow-up among HIV-infected persons on long-term antiretroviral therapy in Latin America and the Caribbean *Journal of the International AIDS Society*, 2015, 18, 20016

Cavalli, S; Hirata, M; e Hirata, R. Detection of MboII polymorphism at the 5' promoter region of CYP3A4. *Clin Chem*., 2001, 47, 348-351.

Celi, AP; Greco, M; Martinez, E; Vargas, C; Belaunzaran, F; Mejia, F. Latin American HIV Workshop Study Group. Presentation to care with advanced HIV disease is still a problem in Latin America. Journal of the International. AIDS Society 2016, 19 (Suppl 1). P038 http://dx.doi.org/10.7448/IAS.19.2.21071

Cesar, C; Shepherd, BE; Jenkins, CA; Ghidinelli, M; Castro, JL; et al. Use of Third Line Antiretroviral Therapy in Latin America. *PLoS ONE*, 2014, 9(9), e106887.

Cohen, Chen, McCauley, Gamble, Hosseinipour, Kumarasamy et al. Antiretroviral Therapy for the Prevention of HIV-1 Transmission. *N Engl J Med* 2016; 375:830-839

Cortes, CP; Siccardi, M; Chaikan, A; Owen, A; Zhang, G; la Porte, CJ. Correlates of efavirenz exposure in Chilean patients affected with human immunodeficiency virus reveals a novel association with a polymorphism in the constitutive androstane receptor. *Ther Drug Monit*., 2013, 35(1), 78-83.

Court, MH. Interindividual variability in hepatic drug glucuronidation: studies into the role of age, sex, enzyme inducers, and genetic polymorphism using the human liver bank as a model system. *Drug Metab Rev*, 2010, 42, 209–224.

Cozzi-Lepri, A; Phillips, A; Clotet, B; Mocroft, A; Ruiz, L; Kirk, O; et al. For the EuroSIDA Study Group. Detection of HIV drug resistance during antiretroviral treatment and clinical progression in a large European cohort study. *AIDS*, 2008, 22, 2187 – 98.

Cressey, TR; y Lallemant, M. Pharmacogenetics of antiretroviral drugs for the treatment of HIV-infected patients: an update. *Infect Genet Evol*, 2007, 7, 333–342.

Crovella, S; Biller, L; Santos, S; Salustiano, A; Brandao, L; Guimaraes, R; Segat, L; Filho, J; Arraes, L. Frequency of HLA B*5701 allele carriers in abacavir treated-HIV infected patients and controls from northeastern Brazil. *CLINICS*, 2011, 66(8), 1485-1487.

Cullen, BR. Nuclear mRNA export: insights from virology. *Trends Biochem Sci*, 2003, 28, 419–424.

Cummins, NW; Neuhaus, J; Chub, H; Neaton, J; Wyenc, C; Rockstroh, J; Skiest, D; Boyd, M; Khoog, S; Rotger, M; Telenti, A; Weinshilbouma, R; Badley, A; for the INSIGHT Study, Group. Investigation of Efavirenz Discontinuation inMulti-ethnic Populations of HIV-positive Individuals by Genetic Analysis. *EBioMedicine*, 2015, 2, 706–712.

CYP allele nomenclature committee. The Human Cytochrome P450 (CYP) Allele Nomenclature Database: Allele nomenclature for Cytochrome P450 enzymes <http://www.cypalleles.ki.se/index.htm> (*accessed on October 12, 2016*).

Damronglerd, P; Chonlaphat, Sukasem; Wilawan, Thipmontree; Apichaya, Puangpetch; Sasisopin, Kiertiburanakul. A pharmacogenomic prospective randomized controlled trial of CYP2B6 polymorphisms and efavirenz dose adjustment among HI V-infected Thai patients: a pilot study. *Pharmacogenomics and Personalized Medicine*, 2015, 8, 155–162.

Davaalkham, J; Hayashida, T; Tsuchiya, K; Gatanaga, H; Nyamkhuu, D; Oka, S. Allele and genotype frequencies of cytochrome P450 2B6 gene in a Mongolian population. *Drug Metab Dispos*., 2009, 37(10), 1991-1993.

de Pablo, R; Beraun, Y; Nieto, A; Calzada, JE; Rementeria, MC; Sanz, L; Lopez-Nevot, MA; Martin, J. HLA class I and class II allele distribution in the Peruvian population. *Tissue Antigens*., 2000, 56, 507-14

Deeks, SG; Phillips, AN. Clinical Review: HIV infection, antiretroviral treatment, ageing, and non-AIDS related morbidity. *BMJ*, 2009, 338, a3172 – a3190.

Desta, Z; Saussele, T; Ward, B; Blievernicht, J; Li, L; Klein, K; Flockhart, DA; Zanger; UM. Impact of CYP2B6 polymorphism on hepatic efavirenz metabolism *in vitro*. *Pharmacogenomics*, 2007, 8, 547–558.

Dhoro, M; Zvada, S; Ngara, B; Nhachi, C; Kadzirange, G; Chonzi, P; Masimirembwa, C. CYP2B6*6, CYP2B6*18, Body weight and sex are predictors of efavirenz pharmacokinetics and treatment response: population pharmacokinetic modeling in an HIV/AIDS and TB cohort in Zimbabwe. *BMC Pharmacol Toxicol*., 2015, 16, 4.

Erickson, DA; Mather, G; Trager, WF; Levy, RH; Keirns, JJ. Characterization of the *in vitro* biotransformation of the HIV-1 reverse transcriptase inhibitor nevirapine by human hepatic cytochromes P-450. *Drug Metab Dispos*, 1999, 27, 1488–1495.

Estrela, RC; Ribeiro, FS; Barroso, PF; Tuyama, M; Gregório, SP; Dias-Neto, E; Struchiner, CJ; Suarez-Kurtz, G. ABCB1 polymorphisms and the concentrations of lopinavir and ritonavir in blood, semen and saliva of HIV-infected men under antiretroviral therapy. *Pharmacogenomics*., 2009, 10(2), 311-8.

Estrela, RC; Santoro, AB; Barroso, PF; Tuyama, M; Suarez-Kurtz, G. CYP3A5 genotype has no impact on plasma trough concentrations of lopinavir and ritonavir in HIV-infected subjects. *Clin Pharmacol Ther*., 2008, 84(2), 205-7

Evans, DT; Serra-Moreno, R; Singh, RK; y Guatelli, JC. BST-2/tetherin: a new component of the innate immune response to enveloped viruses. *Trends Microbiol*, 2010, 18, 388–396.

Evans, J; Swart, M; Soko, N; Wonkam, A; Huzair, F; Dandara, C. A Global Health Diagnostic for Personalized Medicine in Resource-Constrained World Settings: A Simple PCR-RFLP Method for Genotyping CYP2B6 g.15582C > T and Science and Policy Relevance for Optimal Use of Antiretroviral Drug Efavirenz OMICS *A Journal of Integrative Biology*, 2015, 19(6), 332-338.

Evans, W; Relling, M. Pharmacogenomics: Translating function genomics into rational therapeutics. *Science*., 1999, 286, 487-491.

Gatanaga, H; Hayashida, T; Tsuchiya, K; Yoshino, M; Kuwahara, T; Tsukada, H; Fujimoto, K; Sato, I; Ueda, M; Horiba, M; et al. Successful efavirenz dose reduction in HIV type 1-infected individuals with cytochrome P4502B6*6 and *26. *Clin Infect Dis*, 2007, 45, 1230–1237.

Gendzekhadze, K; Montagnani, S; Ogando, V; Balbas, O; Mendez-Castellano, H; Layrisse, Z. Colonia Tovar: the history of a semi-isolated Venezuelan population of German ancestry described by HLA class I genes. *Tissue Antigens*, 2003, 62(5), 401-7.

Gibson, G; Plant, N; Swales, K; Ayrton, A; y El-Sankary, W. Receptor dependent transcriptional activation of cytochrome P450 3A genes: induction mechanisms, species differences and inter-individual variation in man. *Xenobiotica*, 2002, 32, 165–206.

Guilherme, Suarez-Kurtz. Pharmacogenetics in the Brazilian population. *Frontiers in Pharmacology*, 2010, 1(118), 1-10

Gupta, A; Nadkarni, G; Yang, WT; Chandrasekhar, A; Gupte, N; Bisson, GP; Hosseinipour, et al. Early mortality in adults initiating antiretroviral therapy (ART) in low- and middle-income countries (LMIC): a systematic review and meta-analysis *PLoS One*, 2011, 6(12), e28691.

Haas, DW; Tarr, PE. Perspectives on pharmacogenomics of antiretroviral medications and HIV-associated comorbidities. *Curr Opin HIV AIDS*., 2015, 10(2), 116-22.

Haas, DW; Ribaudo, HJ; Kim, RB; Tierney, C; Wilkinson, GR; Gulick, RM; Clifford, DB; Hulgan, T; Marzolini, C; Acosta, EP. Pharmacogenetics of efavirenz and central nervous system side effects: an Adult AIDS Clinical Trials Group study. *AIDS*, 2004, 18, 2391–2400.

Hawkins, T. Understanding and managing the adverse effects of antiretroviral therapy. *Antiviral Res*., 2010, 85, 201- 209.

Hollenstein, K; Dawson, RJ; y Locher, KP. Structure and mechanism of ABC transporter proteins. *Curr. Opin. Struct. Biol*., 2007, 17 (4), 412–8.

Holzinger, ER.; Grady, B; Ritchie, MD; et al. Genomewide association study of plasma efavirenz pharmacokinetics in AIDS Clinical Trials Group protocols implicates several CYP2B6 variants. *Pharmacogenet Genom*, 2012, 12, 858–867.

Hughes, DA; Vilar, FJ; Ward, CC; Alfirevic, A; Park, BK; Pirmohamed, M. Cost-effectiveness analysis of HLA B*5701 genotyping in preventing abacavir hypersensitivity. *Pharmacogenetics*, 2004, 14, 335-342.

Hui, KH; Lee, SS; Lam, TN. Dose Optimization of Efavirenz Based on Individual CYP2B6 Polymorphisms in Chinese Patients Positive for HIV. CPT Pharmacometrics Syst. *Pharmacol*, 2016, 5, 182–191.

Jacob, RM; Johnstone, EC; Neville, MJ; Walton, RT. Identification of CYP2B6 sequence variants by use of multiplex PCR with allele-specific genotyping. *Clin Chem*., 2004, 50(8), 1372-7.

Josephson, F; Allqvist, A; Janabi, M; Sayi, J; Aklillu, E; Jande, M; Mahindi, M; Burhenne, J; Bottiger, Y; Gustafsson, LL; Haefeli, WE; Bertilsson, L. CYP3A5 genotype has an impact on the metabolism of the HIV protease inhibitor saquinavir. *Clin Pharmacol Ther*., 2007, 81(5), 708-12.

Kimchi-Sarfaty, C; Oh, JM; Kim, IW; Sauna, ZE; Calcagno, AM; Ambudkar, SV; y Gottesman, MM. A “silent” polymorphism in the MDR1 gene changes substrate specificity. *Science*, 2007, 315(5811), 525 - 528.

Kiser, JJ; Aquilante, CL; Anderson, PL; King, TM; Carten, ML; y Fletcher, CV. Clinical and genetic determinants of intracellular tenofovir diphosphate concentrations in HIV-infected patients. *J Acquir Immune Defic Syndr*, 2008, 47, 298–303.

Kwara, A; Lartey, M; Sagoe, KW; Kenu, E; Court, MH. CYP2B6, CYP2A6 and UGT2B7 genetic polymorphisms are predictors of efavirenz mid-dose concentration in HIV-infected patients. *AIDS*, 2009, 23, 2101–2106.

Lima, V; Harrigan, R; Bangsberg, D; Hogg, R; Gross, R; Yip, B; et al. The combined effect of modern highly active antiretroviral therapy regimens and adherence on mortality over time. *J Acquir Immune Defic Syndr*, 2009, 50 (5), 529 – 536.

Llibre, JM; Podzamczer, D. Effect of efavirenz versus nevirapine in antiretroviral-naive individuals in the HIV-CAUSAL Collaboration Cohort. *AIDS*, 2012, 26(16), 2117-2118.

Lowenhaupt, EA; Matson, K; Qureishi, B; Saitoh, A; Pugatch, D. Psychosis in a 12-year-old HIV-positive girl with an increased serum concentration of efavirenz. *Clin Infect Dis*, 2007, 45, e128–130.

Lubomirov, R; Colombo, S; di Iulio, J; Ledergerber, B; Martinez, R; Cavassini, M; Hirschel, B; Bernasconi, E; Elzi, L; Vernazza, P; et al. Association of pharmacogenetic markers with premature discontinuation of first-line anti-HIV therapy: an observational cohort study. *J Infect Dis*, 2011, 203, 246–257.

Maartens, G; Celum, C; Lewin, SR. HIV infection: epidemiology, pathogenesis, treatment, and prevention. *Lancet*, 2014, 384 (9939), 258-271.

Mahungu, T; Smith, C; Turner, F; Egan, D; Youle, M; Johnson, M; Khoo, S; Back, Dj; Owen, A. Cytochrome P450 2B6 516G>T is associated with plasma concentrations of nevirapine at both 200 mg twice daily and 400 mg once daily in an ethnically diverse population. *HIV Med*, 2009, 10, 310–317.

Martin, AM; Nolan, D; Gaudieri, S; Almeida, CA; Nolan, R; James, I; Carvalho, F; Phillips, E; Christiansen, FT; Purcell, AW; McCluskey, J; Mallal, S. Predisposition to abacavir hypersensitivity conferred by HLA-B*5701 and a haplotypic Hsp70-Hom variant. *Proc Natl Acad Sci USA*, 2004, 101, 4180-4185.

Martín, AS; Gómez, AI; García-Berrocal, B; Figueroa, SC; Sánchez, MC; Calvo Hernández, MV; Gonzalez-Buitrago, JM; Valverde Merino, MP; Tovar, CB; Martín, AF; Isidoro-García, M. Dose reduction of efavirenz: an observational study describing cost-effectiveness, pharmacokinetics and pharmacogenetics. *Pharmacogenomics*, 2014, 15(7), 997-1006.

Martinez-Laso, J; Siles, N; Moscoso, J; Zamora, J; Serrano-Vela, J; I.R-A-Cachafeiro, J; Castro, M; Serrano-Rios, M; Arnaiz-Villena, A. Origin of Bolivian Quechua Amerindians: their relationship with other American Indians and Asians according to HLA genes. *European Journal of Medical Genetics*, 2006, 49, 169–185.

Mathiesen, S; Justesen, US; Von Lüttichau, HR; Hansen, AB. Genotyping of CYP2B6 and therapeutic drug monitoring in an HIV-infected patient with high efavirenz plasma concentrations and severe CNS side-effects. *Scand J Infect Dis.*, 2006, 38(8), 733-735.

Michaud, V; Bar-Magen, T; Turgeon, J; Flockhart, D; Desta, Z; y Wainberg, MA. The Dual Role of Pharmacogenetics in HIV Treatment: Mutations and Polymorphisms Regulating Antiretroviral Drug Resistance and Disposition. *Pharmacol Rev.*, 2012, 64 (1), 803–833.

MINSAL (2013a), Serie Guías Clínicas AUGE "Sindrome de inmunodeficiencia adquirida VIH/SIDA".

MINSAL (2013b), Informe nacional: "Evolución VIH/SIDA, Chile 1984 - 2012". Departamento de Epidemiología División de Planificación Sanitaria Ministerio de Salud de Chile.

Molina, J; Andrade-Villanueva, J; Echevarria, J; Chetchotisakd, P; Corral, J; David, N; et al. For the CASTLE Study Team. Once-daily atazanavir/ritonavir versus twice-daily lopinavir/ritonavir, each in combination with tenofovir and emtricitabine, for management of antiretroviral- naive HIV-1-infected patients: 96 week efficacy and safety results of the CASTLE study. *J Acquir Immune Defic Syndr*, 2010, 53, 323 – 32.

Moragas, M; Belloso, WH; Baquedano, MS; Gutierrez, MI; Bissio, E; Larriba, JM; Fay, F; Aulicino, P; Gurevich, JM; Yaunguzian, MF; Maldonado, AC; Falistocco, C; Sen, L; Mangano, A. Prevalence of HLA-B*57:01 allele in Argentinean HIV-1 infected patients. *Tissue Antigens*., 2015, 86(1), 28-31.

Nieuwkerk, P; Oort, F. Self-reported adherence to antiretroviral therapy for HIV-1 infection and virologic treatment response: a meta-analysis. *J Acquir Immune Defic Syndr*, 2005, 38(4), 445 – 448.

OPS, Organización Panamericana de la Salud 2011. "Experiencias Exitosas en el Manejo de la Adherencia al Tratamiento Antirretroviral en Latinoamérica" Washington, D. C.

Ortiz de Montellano, PR. 2005. Cytochrome P450: Structure, Mechanism, and Biochemistry. Kluwer Academic/Plenum Publishers, New York.

Park, WB; Choe, PG; Song, KH; Jeon, JH; Park, SW; Kim, HB; Kim, NJ; Oh, MD; Choe, KW. Genetic factors influencing severe atazanavir-associated hyperbilirubinemia in a population with low UDP-glucuronosyltransferase 1A1*28 allele frequency. *Clin Infect Dis*, 2010, 51, 101–106.

Phillips, EJ; Mallal, SA. Pharmacogenetics and the potential for the individualization of antiretroviral therapy. *Curr Opin Infect Dis*, 2008, 21(1), 16 – 24.

Poggi, H; Vera, A; Lagos, M; Solari, S; Rodríguez, PL; Pérez, CM. HLA-B*5701 frequency in Chilean HIV-infected patients and in general population. *Braz J Infect Dis*., 2010, 14(5), 510-2.

Pozniak, A; Gallant, J; DeJesus, E; Arribas, J; Gazzard, B; Campo, R; et al. Tenofovir disoproxil fumarate, emtricitabine, and efavirenz versus fixed-dose zidovudine/ lamivudine and efavirenz in antiretroviral-naive patients: virologic, immunologic, and morphologic changes-a 96-week analysis. *J Acquir Immune Defic Syndr*, 2006, 43, 535 – 40.

Rey, D; Parga-Lozano, C; Moscoso, J; Areces, C; Enriquez-de-Salamanca, M; Fernández-Honrado, M; Abd-El-Fatah-Khalil, S; Alonso-Rubio, J; Arnaiz-Villena, A. HLA genetic profile of Mapuche (Araucanian) Amerindians from Chile. *Mol Biol Rep*, 2013, (7), 4257-67.

Rezk, N; Tidwell, RR; Kashuba, A. Simultaneous determination of six HIV nucleoside analogue reverse transcriptase inhibitors and nevirapine by liquid chromatography with ultraviolet absorbance detection. *Journal of Chromatography B*, 2003, 791, 137 – 147.

Richman, DD; Margolis, DM; Delaney, M; Greene, WC; Hazuda, D; Pomerantz, RJ. The challenge of finding a cure for HIV infection. *Science*, 2009, 323(5919), 1304-1307.

Roco, A; Quiñones, L; Agúndez, JA; García-Martín, E; Squicciarini, V; Miranda, C; Garay, J; Farfán, N; Saavedra, I; Cáceres, D; Ibarra, C; Varela, N. Frequencies of 23 functionally significant variant alleles related with metabolism of antineoplastic drugs in the chilean population: comparison with caucasian and asian populations. *Front Genet*., 2012, 3, 229.

Rosenberg ES, Altfeld M, Poon SH, et al. Immune control of HIV-1 after early treatment of acute infection. Nature. Sep 28 2000;407(6803):523-526

Ruiz, TM; da Costa, SM; Ribas, F; Luz, PR; Lima, SS; da Graça Bicalho, M. Human leukocyte antigen allelic groups and haplotypes in a brazilian sample of volunteer donors for bone marrow transplant in Curitiba, Paraná, Brazil. *Transplant Proc.*, 2005, 37(5), 2293-6.

Sankatsing, SU; Beijnen, JH; Schinkel, AH; Lange, JM; y Prins, JM. P-glycoprotein in human immunodeficiency virus type 1 infection and therapy. *Antimicrob Agents Chemother*, 2004, 48, 1073–1081.

Sierra, B; Alegre, R; Pérez, AB; García, G; Sturn-Ramirez, K; Obasanjo, O; Aguirre, E; Alvarez, M; Rodriguez-Roche, R; Valdés, L; Kanki, P; Guzmán, MG. HLA-A, -B, -C, and -DRB1 allele frequencies in Cuban individuals with antecedents of dengue 2 disease: advantages of the Cuban population for HLA studies of dengue virus infection. *Hum Immunol.*, 2007, 68(6), 531-40. Epub 2007 Mar 28.

Sinxadi, PZ; Leger, PD; McIlleron, H; et al. Pharmacogenetics of plasma efavirenz exposure in HIV-infected adultsand children in South Africa. *Br J Clin Pharmacol.*, 2015, 80(1), 146-56.

Sloan, RD; Kuhl, BD; Donahue, DA; Roland, A; Bar-Magen, T; Wainberg, MA. Transcription of preintegrated HIV-1 cDNA modulates cell surface expression of major histocompatibility complex class I via Nef. *J Virol*, 2011, 85, 2828–2836.

Ståhle, L; Moberg, L; Svensson, JO; So¨nnerborg, A. Efavirenz plasma concentrations in HIV-infected patients: inter- and intraindividual variability and clinical effects. *Ther Drug Monit*, 2004, 26, 267–270.

Takeuchi, K; Kobayashi, Y; Tamaki, S; Ishihara, T; Maruo, Y; Araki, J; Mifuji, R; Itani, T; Kuroda, M; Sato, H; et al. Genetic polymorphisms of bilirubin uridine diphosphate-glucuronosyltransferase gene in Japanese patients with Crigler-Najjar syndrome or Gilbert's syndrome as well as in healthy Japanese subjects. *J Gastroenterol Hepatol.*, 2004, 19, 1023–1028.

Tsuchiya, K; Gatanaga, H; Tachikawa, N; Teruya, K; Kikuchi, Y; Yoshino, M; Kuwahara, T; Shirasaka, T; Kimura, S; Oka, S. Homozygous CYP2B6*6 (Q172H and K262R) correlates with high plasma efavirenz concentrations in HIV-1 patients treated with standard efavirenz-containing regimens. *Biochem Biophys Res Commun*, 2004, 319, 1322–1326.

Turner, ML; Reed-Walker, K; King, JR; et al. Simultaneous determination of nine antiretroviral compounds in human plasma using liquid chromatography. *J Chromatogr B Analyt Technol Biomed Life Sci*, 2003, 784, 331–341.

Turriziani, O; Gianotti, N; Falasca, F; Boni, A; Vestri, AR; Zoccoli, A; Lazzarin, A; Antonelli, G. Expression levels of MDR1, MRP1, MRP4, and MRP5 in peripheral blood mononuclear cells from HIV infected patients failing antiretroviral therapy. *J Med Virol*, 2008, 80, 766–771.

UNAIDS (Joint United Nations Programme on HIV/AIDS) World AIDS day report. Switzerland , UNAIDS, 2016. http://www.unaids.org/en/resources/documents/2016/Global-AIDS-update-2016.

van Leth, F; Phanuphak, P; Ruxrungtham, K; Baraldi, E; Miller, S; Gazzard, B; et al. for the 2NN Study team Comparison of first-line antiretroviral therapy with regimens including nevirapine, efavirenz, or both drugs, plus stavudine and lamivudine: a randomised open-label trial, the 2NN Study. *Lancet*, 2004, 363, 1253 – 1263.

Williams, F; Meenagh, A; Darke, C; Acosta, A; Daar, AS; Gorodezky, C; Hammond, M; Nascimento, E; Middleton, D. Analysis of the distribution of HLA-B alleles in populations from five continents. *Hum Immunol.*, 2001, 62(6), 645-50.

World Health Organization, Consolidated guidelines on the use of antiretroviral drugs for treating and preventing HIV infection. Update June 2016

Wyen, C; Hendra, H; Vogel, M; Hoffmann, C; Knechten, H; Brockmeyer, NH; Bogner, JR; Rockstroh, J; Esser, S; Jaeger, H; et al. Impact of CYP2B6 983T>C polymorphism on non-nucleoside reverse transcriptase inhibitor plasma concentrations in HIV-infected patients. *J Antimicrob Chemother*, 2008, 61, 914–918.

Yimer, G; Amogne, W; Habtewold, A; Makonnen, E; Ueda, N; Suda, A; Worku, A; Haefeli, WE; Burhenne, J; Aderaye, G; Lindquist, L; Aklillu, E. High plasma efavirenz level and CYP2B6*6 are associated with efavirenz-based HAART-induced liver injury in the treatment of naïve HIV patients from Ethiopia: a prospective cohort study. *Pharmacogenomics J.*, 2012, 12(6), 499-506.

Zanger, UM; Klein, K. Pharmacogenetics of cytochrome P450 2B6 (CYP2B6): advances on polymorphisms, mechanisms, and clinical relevance. *Front Genet.*, 2013, 4(24), 1 - 12.

Zastre, JA; Chan, GN; Ronaldson, PT; Ramaswamy, M; Couraud, PO; Romero, IA; Weksler, B; Bendayan, M; Bendayan, R. Up-regulation of P-glycoprotein by HIV protease inhibitors in a human brain microvessel endothelial cell line. *J Neurosci Res*, 2009, 87, 1023–1036.

Zhu, M; Kaul, S; Nandy, P; Grasela, DM; Pfister, M. Model-based approach to characterize efavirenz autoinduction and concurrent enzyme induction with carbamazepine. *Antimicrob Agents Chemother*, 2009, 53, 2346–2353.

In: Pharmacogenomics in Latin America
Editor: Luis A. Quiñones
ISBN: 978-1-53611-031-9

Chapter 11

MOLECULAR BASES OF EPILEPTOGENESIS AND MULTIDRUG RESISTANCE IN REFRACTORY EPILEPSY: LATIN AMERICAN APPROACHES

Alberto J. Lazarowski*[1,2,*]*, PhD
and Liliana A. Czornyj*[2,3,†]*, MD
[1]INFIBIOC-School of Pharmacy and Biochemistry,
University of Buenos Aires,CABA, Argentina
[2]Fundación Investigar, CABA, Argentina
[3]Neurology Service, Children´s Hospital "Juan P Garrahan", CABA, Argentina

ABSTRACT

Brain overexpression of MDR-1 gene encoded P-glycoprotein (P-gp), has been described to play a central role in the pharmacoresistance of epilepsy. It is important to remember that in specific types of cells as normal neurons, P-gp is not expressed; however, their expression can be induced by repetitive seizures as well as status epilepticus. Interindividual differences of this inducible property can also be related with SNP polymorphisms on MDR-1 gene, others ABC-transporters, as well as CYP-enzymes, all affecting drug absorption, steady stay plasmatic AEDs concentrations as well as brain penetration of these drugs. Additionally, P-gp activation can induce membrane depolarization and it can be acting in the intrinsic mechanism of epileptogenesis when P-gp is expressed in neurons. Furthermore, P-gp can also produce the phosphatydylserine (PS) translocation from inner side to external side of the plasmatic membrane of stressed neurons and reducing the seizure threshold. This floppase activity cannot be inhibited by current therapeutics protocols with combined AEDs and so perhaps explaining the persistence of 30-40% of patients with pharmacoresistant epilepsy. According with these data, a speculative consideration is that epileptogenesis and/or pharmacoresistant epilepsy could be the clinical result of a wide spectrum of abnormal changes, producing a permanent lower seizure threshold produced by P-gp overexpression in neurons.

Keywords: epileptogenesis, MDR-1 gene, refractory epilepsy, Latin America, pharmacogenetics

* Corresponding Author E-mail: alazarowski@gmail.com.
† tominadia@hotmail.com.

INTRODUCTION

Epilepsy comprises a heterogeneous group of disorders that are characterized by recurrent unprovoked seizures of different etiologies. To date epilepsy is one of the most frequently nervous system diseases affecting children and youths (Kwong et al., 2003). Despite the long list of new antiepileptic drugs (AEDs) introduced for better treatment of epileptic patients, the percentage of drug-resistant cases, i.e., refractory epilepsy (RE) has not decrease. Furthermore, even using multidrug-based therapies, pharmacoresistant epilepsy remains untreatable in near 30-40% of the cases (Lazarowski et al., 2015).

One intriguing feature of drug resistant epilepsy is that this phenotype can be acquired secondary to high frequency seizure episodes (Loscher & Brandt, 2010). This particular phenotype, can be explained by the increased expression of P-glycoprotein (P-gp), encoded by the ABCB1/MDR-1 gene, which can be induced by seizures (Auzmendi et al., 2014). Patients who are unresponsive to a first and second AED treatment will often remain unresponsive to additional treatments, including new AEDs or multiple AED combinations, suggesting that multi-drug resistant (MDR) phenotype could be developed previously to AEDs exposure (Brodie et al., 2012).

The CC genotype of C3435T gene MDR-1 polymorphism was related to an excessive production of P-gp in the intestinal mucosa, affecting the drug plasma concentration (Hoffmeyer et al., 2000). Similar increased expression was also demonstrated with the same dependency within the blood-brain barrier (Siddiqui et al., 2003).

After these initial associations, several single nucleotide polymorphisms (SNPs) studies on ABCB1/MDR-1 gene, suggested that MDR phenotype might be genetically determined in RE patients in which a homozygous genotype of the C allele was more likely to yield multidrug-resistant phenotypes, compared to the T allele. This was further supported by evidence from functional studies (Marzolini et al., 2004; Kimchi-Sarfaty et al., 2007).

A meta-analysis of 57 studies involving 12407 patients (6083 drug-resistant and 6324 drug-responsive patients) with epilepsy, evaluated all three polymorphisms (C3435T, G2677T/A, and C1236T) of MDR-1/ABCB1 gene. In this study, a wide spectrum of minor allele frequencies across different ethnicities with a significantly decreased risk of AEDs resistance was only observed in Caucasian patients with T allele of C3435T variant, but not with the other two SNPs. In contrasts, all studies in Indians and Asians patients no significant association was observed with AEDs resistance (Li et al., 2015). However, no other studies with the same definition, in other ethnicities, could replicate this association, therefore, challenging the validity of the initial associations (Kim et al., 2006a and b; Kim et al., 2009; Lakhan et al., 2009; Tan et al., 2004). Furthermore, although the efflux transporter ABCG2 gene, which encodes for the breast cancer resistant protein (BCRP), contributes to the integrity of the blood brain barrier and has a considerable substrate overlap with P-glycoprotein, pharmacogenetic data in epilepsy is scarce and inconsistent (Kwan et al., 2011).

Perhaps, the underlying disease pathobiology in each epileptic syndrome could have an effect in determining the AED response, and thus, pharmacogenetics studies in epilepsies are not conclusive, because they have included all epilepsy syndromes considering only their response profile. These factors together with ethnic differences and variability in defining drug resistance among studies could have significantly contributed for the inconsistencies in the results (Balan et al., 2014).

On the other hand, cytochrome P450 enzymes primarily catalyze processes of oxidation of approximately 70% of the most often AEDs used, and two isoenzymes as CYP3A4 and CYP3A5, have the greatest importance in the metabolism of those drugs AEDs (Klotz, 2007). Therefore, the substantial heterogeneity of pharmacologic action exhibited by the same drug in a particular patient can be explained by expression/induction of drug metabolizing enzyme as well as transporters that efflux or limits the influx of the drug, are both encoded by inducible genes. Consequently, repetitive seizures, stress or the administration of different drugs could generate differentiated responses on each patient according to the polymorphic variants of said genes. And it could be expected to occur particularly in refractory epileptic cases as compared with responders.

In this regards, a long list of studies were examined to determine if there were any haplotypes as biomarker of risk for RE, and controversial results were reported (Wojtczak & Skretkowicz, 2009; Kwan et al., 2007; Emich-Widera et al., 2013; Haerian et al., 2010). It is clear that the likelihood of multidrug resistance has a multifactorial nature that includes the complexity of the events regulating transporters as well as the role of genetic variants in drug targets. In spite of these observations, the "transporter hypothesis" for pharmacoresistant phenotypes remains the most preferred choice for understanding drug resistance in epilepsy (Haerian et al., 2010).

MECHANISMS OF EPILEPSIES

The mechanism that leads to seizure arises from the excitability of synaptic terminals, depending on the amount of excitatory neurotransmitter released (e.g., glutamic acid or activation of glutamatergic receptors) as well as on an insufficient release of neurotransmitter inhibitor γ-aminobutyric acid (GABA). Consequently, excitability dependents on the final extent of membrane depolarization produced inducing spontaneous epileptic seizures. The imbalance between the excitatory (high) and the inhibitory (reduced) stimuli are the main mechanism of neuronal membrane depolarization and the onset of seizures. GABA is only synthesized in the nervous system from glutamic acid. Neuronal axons have a resting membrane potential of about -70 mV inside versus outside. Action potentials occur due to net positive inward of ion fluxes, resulting in local changes in the membrane potential. Membrane potentials vary with the activation of either ligand- or voltage-gated ion channels, which are affected by changes in either the membrane potential or intracellular ion concentrations. Under physiologic conditions, action potentials occur when a neuron is excited enough to overcome the so-called threshold of excitation and the membrane potential shoots from -70 to about +40 mV. After this excitation (depolarization) event, neuron hyperpolarizes again and membrane potential will decrease below resting potential, resuming resting potential once the neurotransmitters return to baseline. Undoubtedly, both acquired and heritable factors may favor neuronal membrane depolarization and initiate seizure discharge, and therefore the most common epilepsy syndromes can be polygenic and also include environmental influences (Tan et al., 2004).

According to the ILAE classification, in the so-called "symptomatic" epilepsies, a not-genetics cause can be easily considered as the responsible factor for the disease. However, about 1% of the general population develops recurrent seizures for no obvious reason and without the presence of any neurological abnormality. These are called idiopathic epilepsies, a complex disease with high heritability, but for which little are known about its genetic architecture (WHO, 2008; Heinzen et al., 2012). In this regard, an increased excitability of neuronal circuits genetically determined, provides an attractive explanation as to why otherwise normal individuals, can develop unprovoked seizures without an identifiable cause of onset. To assess progress in linking the molecular genetics of epilepsy to the clinic, the mechanisms associated with the range of genes now known to be related to epilepsy syndromes have been comprehensively surveyed (Reid et al., 2009; Singh et al., 2002).

Long lists of gene mutations were identified as directly associated with the etiology of several epileptic syndromes. However, despite the fact that the genetic etiology in generalized epilepsies is now widely accepted, the focal epilepsies are currently attributed to environmental factors such as damage at birth, infections, head trauma, or brain lesions (tumors or vascular damage) (Andermann et al., 2005).

Genetic Influence on Epileptogenesis

One increasingly accepted important concept suggests that there is a heritable, basal predisposition to epilepsy although the syndrome depends on external factors acquired prenatally or postnatally (Berkovic & Scheffer, 1999). Although the presence of a mutant allele should be sufficient to cause the manifestation of the epileptic phenotype, several studies show that the penetrance of these mutations usually are not complete, and the age of onset and severity of the phenotype can be variable among families. This suggests that the expression of genes involved in epilepsy can be modulated by additional, still unidentified genetic and/or environmental factors (Ottman, 2005). The effect of genetic influence on the epileptogenic process was initially investigated by Schauwecker and colleagues (Schauwecker, 2007). In this context, perhaps, epileptogenesis should be evaluated under similar considerations. Furthermore, the effect of genetic influence on epileptogenesis is supposed to be the strongest factor in idiopathic epilepsies, and combined effects of genetic and acquired factors on epileptogenesis was also suggested. For example, epileptogenic insults, particularly, status epilepticus (SE), can result in changes in both ligand-gated and ion-gated channels, that are associated with altered function, and this phenomenon, known as acquired channelopathy, has been described in the dendritic, somatic, and axonal channels (Ellerkmann et al., 2003; Berbard et al., 2004).

These observations are in concordance with other modifications in the normal function of neuronal network observed after repetitive seizures or SE. All of them are related with cellular alterations that include neurodegeneration, neurogenesis, axonal sprouting, axonal injury, dendritic remodeling, gliosis, invasion of inflammatory cells, angiogenesis, alterations in extracellular matrix, and acquired channelopathies. In all cases, up or down regulation of a wide spectrum of genes without preexistent mutations can be reversible or permanent changes where epigenetic regulatory mechanisms can also be involved (Pitkänen & Lukasiuk, 2009).

The first speculative consideration is that in epilepsy, epileptogenesis and/or pharmacoresistant epilepsy could be the clinical result of a wide spectrum of abnormal changes, producing a permanent lower seizure threshold. Furthermore, all these alterations could be both secondary to, as well as irrespective to the primary cellular, or molecular alterations, with or without preexistent related mutations.

What is epilepsy and what mechanism triggers epileptogenesis? The clinical diversity observed in epileptic seizure disorders is a reflection of the numerous cellular and network routes to seizure genesis. The pathophysiology underlying the epileptic process includes mechanisms involved in initiation of seizures (ictogenesis) as well as those involved in transforming a normal brain into a seizure-prone brain (epileptogenesis) (Fisher et al., 2005). However, this definition does not explain the biological bases of the epilepsy. More accepted is the current concept that epileptogenesis is a sum of complex cellular and molecular mechanisms produced during a latency period previous to the appearance of the first spontaneous seizure. This concept refers to a period that begins after the occurrence of traumatic brain injury insult (TBI), stroke, or even during the insult as during prolonged febrile seizure, SE, encephalitis, etc., and later resulting in an epileptic syndrome. Perhaps, we can say that at least in epilepsy, everything is genetics, including the trauma consequences.

Molecular mechanisms underlying during mentioned latency period or epileptogenesis, should be the result of events occurring on at the synaptic or neuronal network level. Few studies have been designed to specifically study this latency period on time period after the occurrence of the first seizures. In these studies, individual genes show different expression profiles and some genes are regulated throughout the latent phase and also after epilepsy diagnosis, whereas others are only transiently regulated (Becker et al., 2003; Andermann et al., 2005).

Because epileptogenesis includes both the latency period between the insult and occurrence of seizures and the progression of epilepsy, clusters of genes could show similar patterns of expression changes over time and observed as waves of orchestrated gene expression. One intriguing feature of these on-off-genetic regulations is related with the natural course of epileptogenesis that could be influenced by genetic predisposition, epigenetic mechanisms, external factor (infections, toxic, stress) as well as the AEDs use. A total of 124 genes, related with other 20 different functional properties have been described to be regulated in at least two studies. Furthermore, all epigenetic mechanisms that includes DNA and histone methylation, histone acetylation and histone phosphorylation, were also demonstrated to be active during epigenetic process (Pitkänen & Lukasiuk, 2011).

One important feature of the electric property of neuronal membranes is the continuous maintenance of lipid asymmetry that is accomplished by integral membrane transporters that specifically flip (out-to-in translocation), flop (in-to-out translocation) or scramble lipids across the bilayer. Lipid flippases are ATP-dependent membrane proteins as P4 ATPases, whereas lipid floppases are more related with ABC (ATP-binding cassette) transporters expression and activity.

ABC-transporter P-gp, BCRP or MRPs (Multidrug resistance-associated proteins), are nor expressed in normal, mature neurons, however they are overexpressed in neurons from both patients and experimental models of refractory epilepsy (Xiong et al., 2015; Sun et al., 2016; Czornyj & Lazarowski, 2014; Lazarowski et al., 2007; Mizutani et al., 2008). P-gp (ABCB1) not only is responsible for pleiotropic drug resistance in tumor cells, but it was also found to transport various phospholipid analogues, including phosphatidylcholine (PC) and phosphatidylethanolamine (PE), as well as the sphingolipid GlcCer from the cytoplasmic to the exoplasmic leaflet of the plasma membrane (Veldman et al., 2002). It is known that P-gp overexpression is related to pharmacoresistant to chemotherapeutics in cancer. Furthermore, cells induced to express P-gp either by drug stimulation or retroviral gene transduction with P-gp cDNA, are also resistant to cell death induced by a range of death stimuli such as Fas ligand, TNFα, UV irradiation and other factors that activate the caspase apoptotic cascade. Interestingly, overexpression of P-gp transporters in drug-resistant cells is accompanied by altered membrane content of cholesterol, SM, GlcCer and other glycosphingolipids (Bolhuis et al., 1996).

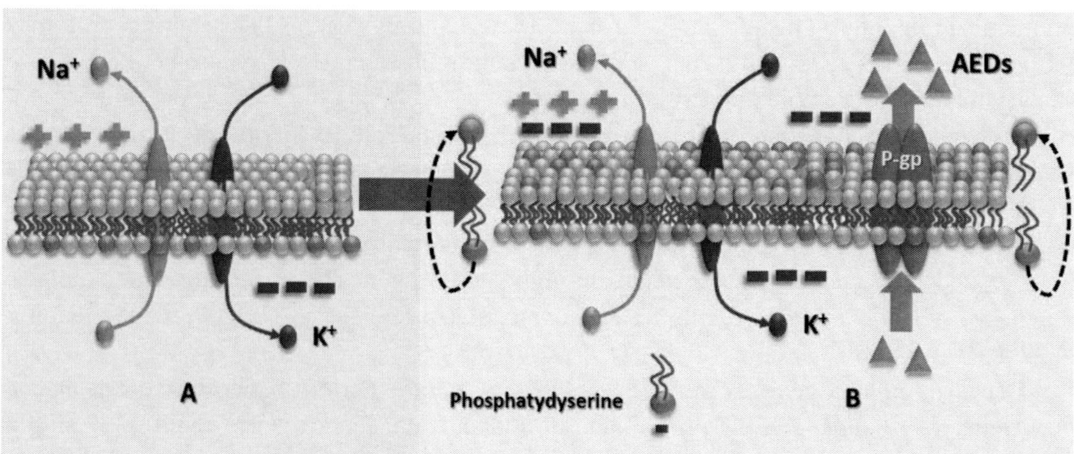

Figure 1. A: normal polarized membrane; B: P-gp expression induces a translocation of some phospholipids as phosphatydylserine, producing a more anionic charge outside of the membrane, and then a higher depolarization, irrespective of its normal activity as drug transporter.

The ABC-transporters, particularly P-gp, irrespective of the classical drug efflux, can also acts as a hydrophobic vacuum cleaner, where lipid substrates diffuse into the membrane bilayer and, subsequently, extruded from a central channel of the transporter into the extracellular space in an ATP-dependent process (Higgins & Gottesman, 1992). Additionally, the floppase model explains the translocation of lipids, most commonly phospholipids as phosphatidylserine (PS), from the inner to outer leaflet of biological membranes (López-García et al., 2014)). Progressive P-gp expression in neurons that previously as normal neurons do not express P-gp, can increase the amount of PS translocated to external face of the plasmatic membrane and increase he membrane depolarization (Figure 1B). Under these conditions, thresholds for new complete depolarization and new seizures will be facilitated.

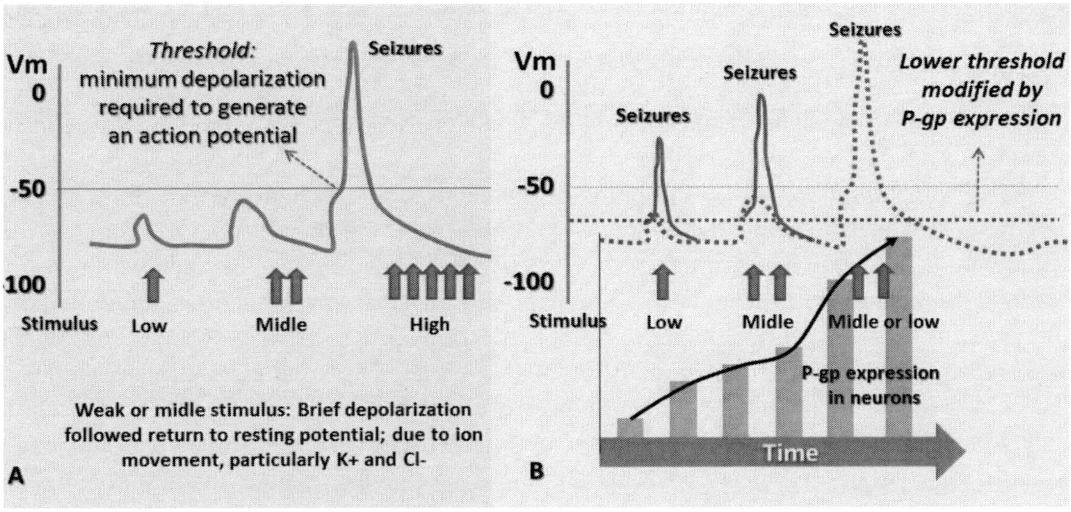

Figure 2. **A:** High level of stimulus will be needed to overcome the threshold and complete trigger the action potential of the membrane; **B:** progressive accumulation of stimulus, could induce an also progressive expression of P-gp, resulting in a reduced level of the threshold and increasing the susceptibility to new seizures.

The threshold for an action potential is reached when voltage-gated ion channels are activated, and depolarization that does not generate an action potential will be a subthreshold stimulus. Based on the all-or-none principle, some subthreshold stimulus can induce P-gp overexpression without depolarization of neurons. However, and according with the PS translocation, when enough amount of P-gp is expressed in neurons producing membrane pre-depolarize, the same subthreshold stimulus will produce a complete membrane depolarization, inducing new seizures (Figure 2).

Several brain injuries or diseases are directly related with a high risk for the development of epileptic syndromes. It is clear that not all patients under similar injuries will have epilepsy; however, the risk of this group is higher as compared with normal individuals. These situations exclude all epileptic cases with genetic etiology, as a long list of different alterations or mutations in ion channels, neurodevelopment malformations, metabolic disease, etc (Revised in Genetics of Epilepsy and Refractory Epilepsy. Lazarowski A & Czornyj L; Colloquium series on The GeneTiC Basis of human Disease; Editor Michael Dean, Ph.D., Head, Human Genetics Section, Senior Investigator, Laboratory of Experimental Immunology, National Cancer Institute, at Frederick).

PHARMACOGENETICS AND EPILEPSIA

Others factors related to pharmacogenetics can also contribute to inter-individual variability in drug response. Many AEDs are metabolized by a variety of enzymatic reactions, and the cytochrome P450 (CYP) family has attracted considerable attention. Some of the CYPs exist as genetic (allelic) variants, which may also affect the plasma concentrations or drug exposure. Regarding the metabolism of AEDs, the polymorphic CYP2C9 and CYP2C19 are of particular interest. There have been recent advances in discovering factors such as these, especially those underlying the risk of medication toxicity. The evidence about whether such polymorphisms affect the clinical action of AEDs indicated that CYP2D6, CYP2C9, CYP3A4, and CYP2D19 are clearly involved in the metabolism of most antiepileptic drugs, given the allele frequency in the population and the associated variability in the clinical response (Saldaña-Cruz et al., 2013).

Despite the observation of overlapping of several of these mechanisms, only a fraction, of the affected patients develops an epileptic syndrome from the same primary disease. Is this difference in susceptibility based on any genetic differences between them? Probably, different brain insults produced by brain hypoxia, vascular malformations, brain tumors, autoimmunity, brain inflammation, brain infections, hemorrhagic stroke, metabolic unbalance, inborn error of metabolism, brain trauma, etc., can induce secondary epileptic syndromes. All of them share the induction of expression of ABC-transporters, particularly P-gp, encoded by a gene which has multiple transcription factors. Consequently, perhaps, therapeutics focusing on blocking these mechanisms could avoid not only the pharmacoresistance, but also the epileptohgenesis.

According to these concepts, we not only suggest that therapeutics against function of P-gp will control pharmacoresistant epilepsy (Robey et al., 2013), but also therapeutics avoiding P-gp expression could control epileptogenesis (Lazarowski et al., 2015)

Although the P-gp efflux transport protein is overexpressed in resected tissue of patients with epilepsy, the presence of polymorphisms in MDR1/ABCB1 and MRP2/ABCC2 in patients with antiepileptic-drugs resistant epilepsy (ADR) is controversial.

Additionally, CYP polymorphisms could also explain several drug resistance phenotypes. As previously demonstrated for others therapeutic drugs and diseases (Acevedo et al., 2003; Cortés et al., 2013; Lardo et al., 2015; Buendía et al., 2015), in Latin American countries was demonstrated that combined polymorphisms of CYP and ABC-transporters could be more effective to identify drug resistant epileptic patients, who also showed persistent low levels of AEDs. An exploratory study on genotype-phenotype relationship, was developed to identify nucleotide changes and to search for new and reported mutations in patients with RE. After a rigorously selected population, 22 samples from drug-resistant patients with epilepsy and 7 samples from patients with good response to AEDs were selected (Escalante-Santiago et al., 2014). In this study, eleven exons in both above-mentioned genes were genotyped and the concentration of drugs in saliva and plasma was determined. The concentration of valproic acid in saliva was lower in refractory patients than in responders. In ABCB1, five reported SNPs and five unreported nucleotide changes were identified; rs2229109 (GA) and rs2032582 (AT and AG) were found only in the refractory patients. Of six SNPs associated with the ABCC2 that were found in the study population, rs3740066 (TT) and 66744T >A (TG) were found only in the ADR. The strongest risk factor in the ABCB1 gene was identified as the TA genotype of rs2032582, whereas for the ABCC2 gene the strongest risk factor was the T allele of rs3740066. The screening of SNPs in ACBC1 and ABCC2 indicates that the Mexican patients with epilepsy in this study display frequently reported ABCC1 polymorphisms; however, in subjects with a higher risk factor for drug resistance, new nucleotide changes were found in the ABCC2 gene. Thus, the population of Mexican patients with AED-resistant epilepsy (ADR) used in this study exhibits genetic variability with respect to those reported in other study populations; however, it is necessary to explore this polymorphism in a larger population of patients with pharmacoresistant epilepsy.

From the above, it follows that the combination of inheritable genetic factors (mutations and polymorphisms) together with external factors, result in processes that modify the normal balance of neuronal membrane potentials.

These changes may lead to non-epileptic isolated seizures that are commonly sensitive to AEDs, or generate permanent changes that trigger the development of epileptic syndromes and refractory epilepsies.

REFERENCES

Acevedo, C. A., Quiñones, L. A., Catalán, J., Cáceres, D. D., Fullá, J. A., Roco, A. M. (2014). Impact of CYP1A1, GSTM1, and GSTT1 polymorphisms in overall and specific prostate cancer survival. *Urol Oncol,* 32(3):280-90.

Andermann, F., Kobayashi, E., Andermann, E. (2005). Genetic focal epilepsies: state of the art and paths to the future. *Epilepsia*, 46 (Suppl 10):61–7.

Auzmendi, J., Merelli, A., Girardi, E., Orozco-Suarez, S., Rocha, L., Lazarowski, A. (2014). Progressive heart P-glycoprotein (P-gp) overexpression after experimental repetitive seizures (ERS) associated with fatal status epilepticus (FSE). Is it related with SUDEP? *Molecular & Cellular Epilepsy*, 1:e66(1-9).

Balan, S., Bharathan, S., P, Vellichiramal, N. N., Sathyan, S., Joseph, V., Radhakrishnan, K., Banerjee, M. (2014). Genetic Association Analysis of ATP Binding Cassette Protein Family Reveals a Novel Association of ABCB1 Genetic Variants with Epilepsy Risk, but Not with Drug-Resistance. *PLoS One,* 9(2):e89253.

Becker, A. J., Chen, J., Zien, A., Sochivko, D., Normann, S., Schramm, J., Elger, C. E., Wiestler, O. D., Blümcke, I. (2003). Correlated stage- and subfi eldassociated hippocampal gene expression patterns in experimental and human temporal lobe epilepsy. *Eur J Neurosci*, 18:2792–802.

Berkovic, S. F. and Scheffer, I. E. (1999). Genetics of the epilepsies. *Curr Opin Neurol*, 12:177–82.

Bernard, C., Anderson, A., Becker, A., Poolos, N. P., Beck, H., Johnston, D. (2004) Acquired dendritic channelopathy in temporal lobe epilepsy. *Science*, 305:532–5.

Bolhuis, H., van Veen, H.W., Molenaar, D., Poolman, B., Driessen, A.J. and Konings, W.N. (1996). Multidrug resistance in Lactococcus lactis: evidence for ATP-dependent drug extrusion from the inner leaflet of the cytoplasmic membrane. *EMBO J.*, 15:4239–4245.

Brodie, M., Barry, S., Bamagous, G., Norrie, J., Kwan, P. (2012). Patterns of treatment response in newly diagnosed epilepsy. N*eurology*, 78:1548-1554.

Buendía, J. A., Otamendi, E., Kravetz, M. C., Cairo, F., Ruf, A., de Davila, M., Powazniak, Y., Nafissi, J., Lazarowski, A., Bramuglia, G., Villamil, F. (2015). Combinational Effect of CYP3A5 and MDR-1 Polymorphisms on Tacrolimus Pharmacokinetics in Liver Transplant Patients. *Exp Clin Transplant.*, 13(5):441-8.

Cortes, C. P., Siccardi, M., Chaikan, A., Owen, A., Zhang, G., la Porte, C. J. (2013). Correlates of efavirenz exposure in Chilean patients affected with human immunodeficiency virus reveals a novel association with a polymorphism in the constitutive androstane receptor. *Ther Drug Monit*, 35(1):78-83.

Czornyj, L., Lazarowski, A. (2014). ABC-transporters as stem-cell markers in brain dysplasia/tumor epilepsies. *Front Biosci (Landmark Ed),*19:1425-35.

Ellerkmann, R. K., Remym S., Chenm J., Sochivkom D., Elgerm C., E., Urban, B. W., Becker, A., Beck, H. (2003) Molecular and functional changes in voltage-dependent Na^+ channels following pilocarpine-induced status epilepticus in rat dentate granule cells. *Neuroscience*, 119:323–33.

Emich-Widera, E., Likus, W., Kazek, B., Niemiec, P. B., Balcerzyk, A., Sieron, A. L., Zak, I. (2013). CYP3A5*3 and C3435T MDR1 polymorphisms in prognostication of drug-resistant epilepsy in children and adolescents. *BioMed Research International*, Article ID 526837:1-7.

Escalante-Santiago, D., Feria-Romero, I A., Ribas-Aparicio, R. M., Rayo-Mares, D., Fagiolino, P., Vázquez, M., Escamilla-Núñez, C., Grijalva-Otero, I., López-García, M. A., Orozco-Suárez, S. (2014). MDR-1 and MRP2 Gene Polymorphisms in Mexican Epileptic Pediatric Patients with Complex Partial Seizures. *Front Neurol.*, 95:184.

Fisher, R S., van Emde Boas, W., Blume, W., Elger, C., Genton, P., Lee, P., Engel, JJr. (2005). Epileptic seizures and epilepsy: definitions proposed by the International League Against Epilepsy (ILAE) and the International Bureau for Epilepsy (IBE). *Epilepsia*,46:470–2.

Haerian, B. S., Roslan, H., Raymond, A. A., Tan, C. T., Lim, K. S., Zulkifli, S. Z., Mohamed, E. H., Tan, H. J., Mohamed, Z. (2010). ABCB1C3435T polymorphism and the risk of resistance to antiepileptic drugs in epilepsy: a systematic review andmeta-analysis. *Seizure*, 19,6:339–346.

Heinzen, E. L., Depondt, C., Cavalleri, G. L., Ruzzo, E. K., Walley, N. M., Need, A. C., Ge, D., He, M., Cirulli, E. T., Zhao, Q., Cronin, K. D., Gumbs, C. E., Campbell, C. R., Hong, L. K., Maia, J. M., Shianna, K. V., McCormack, M., Radtke, R. A., O'Conner, G. D., Mikati, M. A., Gallentine, W. B., Husain, A. M., Sinha, S. R., Chinthapalli, K., Puranam, R. S., McNamara, J. O., Ottman, R., Sisodiya, S. M., Delanty, N., Goldstein, D. B. (2012). Exome sequencing followed by large-scale genotyping fails to identify single rare variants of large effect in idiopathic generalized epilepsy. *Am J Hum Genet,* 91:293–302.

Higgins, C.F. and Gottesman, M.M. (1992). Is the multidrug transporter a flippase? *Trends Biochem. Sci.* 17:18–21.

Hoffmeyer, S., Burk, O., von Richter, O., Arnold, H. P., Brockmöller, J., Johne, A., Cascorbi, I., Gerloff, T., Roots, I., Eichelbaum, M., Brinkmann, U. (2000). Functional polymorphisms of the human multidrug-resistance gene: multiple sequence variations and correlation of one allele with P-glycoprotein expression and activity in vivo. *Proceedings of the National Academy of Sciences* 97(7):3473-8.

Kim, D. W., Kim, M., Lee, S. K., Kang, R., Lee, S. Y. (2006a). Lack of association between C3435T nucleotide MDR1 genetic polymorphism and multidrug-resistant epilepsy. *Seizure*, 15:344–347.

Kim, D. W., Lee, S. K., Chu, K., Jang, I. J., Yu, K. S., Cho, J. Y., Kim, S. J. (2009). Lack of association between ABCB1, ABCG2, and ABCC2 genetic polymorphisms and multidrug resistance in partial epilepsy. *Epilepsy research,* 84:86–90.

Kim, Y. O., Kim, M. K., Woo, Y. J., Lee, M. C., Kim, J. H., Park, K. W., Kim, E. Y., Roh, Y. I., Kim, C. J. (2006b). Single nucleotide polymorphisms in the multidrug resistance 1 gene in Korean epileptics. *Seizure*, 15:67–72.

Kimchi-Sarfaty, C., Oh, J. M., Kim, I. W., Sauna, Z. E., Calcagno, A. M., Ambudkar, S. V., Gottesman, M. M. (2007). A "silent" polymorphism in the MDR1 gene changes substrate specificity. *Science*, 315:525–528.

Klotz, U. (2007). The role of pharmacogenetics in the metabolism of antiepileptic drugs: pharmacokinetic and therapeutic implications. *Clinical Pharmacokinetics,*46,4:271-279.

Kwan, P., Baum, L., Wong, V., Ng, P. W., Lui, C. H., Sin, N. C., Hui, A. C., Yu, E., Wong, L. K. (2007). Association between ABCB1 C3435T polymorphism and drug-resistant epilepsy in Han Chinese. *Epilepsy and Behavior*, 11,1:112–117.

Kwan, P., Wong, V., Ng, P. W., Lui, C. H., Sin, N. C., Poon, W. S., Ng, H. K., Wong, K. S., Baum, L. (2011).Gene-wide tagging study of the association between ABCC2, ABCC5 and ABCG2 genetic polymorphisms and multidrug resistance in epilepsy. *Pharmacogenomics*, 12:319–325.

Kwong, K. L., Sung, W. Y., Wong, S. N., So, K. T. (2003) Early predictors of medical intractability in childhood epilepsy," *Pediatric Neurology*, 29,1:46–52.

Lakhan, R., Misra, U. K., Kalita, J., Pradhan, S., Gogtay, N. J., Singh, M. K., Mittal, B. (2009). No association of ABCB1 polymorphisms with drug-refractory epilepsy in a north Indian population. *Epilepsy & Behavior*, 14: 78–82.

Lardo, M., Castro, M., Moiraghi, B., Rojas F., Borda, N., Rey, J. A., Lazarowski, A. (2015) MDR1/ABCB1 gene polymorphisms in patients with chronic myeloid leukemia. *Blood Res.*, 50(3):154-9.

Lazarowski, A., Czornyj, L., Lubienieki, F., Girardi, E., Vazquez, S., D'Giano, C. (2007). ABC transporters during epilepsy and mechanisms underlying multidrug resistance in refractory epilepsy. *Epilepsia*, 48 Suppl 5:140-9.

Lazarowski, A., Czornyj, L., Rocha L. (2015). The complexity of roles of P-glycoprotein in refractory epilepsy: pharmacoresistance, epileptogenesis, SUDEP and relapsing marker after surgical treatment. *ADMET & DMPK*; 3(2):110-121.

Li, H., Wang, B., Chang, C., Wu, M., Xu, Y., Jiang, Y. (2015) The Roles of Variants in Human Multidrug Resistance (MDR1) Gene and Their Haplotypes on Antiepileptic Drugs Response: A Meta-Analysis of 57 Studies. *PLoS One.*,10(3):e0122043.

Lopez-Garcia, M. A., Feria-Romero, I. A., Fernando-Serrano, H., Escalante-Santiago, D., Grijalva, I., Orozco-Suarez, S. (2014). Genetic polymorphisms associated with antiepileptic metabolism. *Front Biosci* (Elite Ed). 6:377-86.

Loscher, W., Brandt, C. (2010) High seizure frequency prior to antiepileptic treatment is a predictor of pharmacoresistant epilepsy in a rat model of temporal lobe epilepsy. *Epilepsia*, 51:89–97.

Marzolini, C., Paus, E., Buclin, T., Kim, R. B. (2004). Polymorphisms in Human MDR1 (P-glycoprotein): Recent Advances and Clinical Relevance&ast. *Clinical Pharmacology & Therapeutics*, 75: 13–33.

Mizutani, T., Masuda, M., Nakai, E., Furumiya, K., Togawa, H., Nakamura, Y., Kawai, Y., Nakahira, K., Shinkai, S., Takahashi, K. (2008). Genuine functions of P-glycoprotein (ABCB1). *Curr. Drug Metab,* 9:167–174.

Ottman, R. (2005). Analysis of genetically complex epilepsies. *Epilepsia*, 46 (Suppl 10):7–14.

Pitkänen, A., Lukasiuk, K. (2011). Mechanisms of epileptogenesis and potential treatment targets. *Lancet Neurol*, 10:173–86.

Pitkänen, A., Lukasiuk, K. (2009). Molecular and cellular basis of epileptogenesis in symptomatic epilepsy. *Epilepsy & Behavior*, 14:16–25.

Reid, C. A., Berkovic, S. F., Petrou, S. (2009). Mechanisms of human inherited epilepsies. *Prog Neurobiol*, 87:41–57.

Robey, R. W., Lazarowski, A., Bates, S. E. (2008). P-Glycoprotein—a Clinical Target in Drug-Refractory Epilepsy?. *Mol Pharmacol*, 73:1343–1346.

Saldaña-Cruz, A. M., Sánchez-Corona, J., Márquez de Santiago, D. A., García-Zapién, A. G., Flores-Martínez, S. E. (2013). Pharmacogenetics and antiepileptic drug metabolism: implication of genetic variants in cytochromes P450. *Rev Neurol.*, 56(9):471-9.

Schauwecker, P. E. (2007). Role of genetic influences in animal models of status. *Epilepsia*, 48 (Suppl. 8):21–3.

Siddiqui, A., Kerb, R., Weale, M. E., Brinkmann, U., Smith, A., Goldstein, D. B., Wood, N. W., Sisodiya, S. M. (2003) Association of multidrug resistance in epilepsy with a polymorphism in the drug transporter gene ABCB1. *NEJM,* 348:1442–1448.

Singh, R., Gardner, R.J., Crossland, K. M., Scheffer, I. E., Berkovic, S. F. (2002). Chromosomal abnormalities and epilepsy: a review for clinicians and gene hunters. *Epilepsia*,43:127–40.

Sun, Y., Luo, X., Yang, K., Sun, X., Li, X., Zhang, C., Ma, S., Liu, Y., Yin, J. (2016). Neural overexpression of multidrug resistance-associated protein 1 and refractory epilepsy: a meta-analysis of nine studies. *J. Int J Neurosci.*,126(4):308-17.

Tan, N. C., Heron, S. E., Scheffer, I. E., Pelekanos, J. T., McMahon, J. M., Vears, D. F., Mulley, J. C., Berkovic, S. F. (2004). Failure to confirm association of a polymorphism in ABCB1 with multidrug-resistant epilepsy. *Neurology*, 63: 1090–1092.

Tan, N. C., Mulley, J. C., Berkovic, S. F. (2004). Genetic association studies in epilepsy: the truth is out there. *Epilepsia*;45:1429–42.

Veldman, R. J., Klappe, K., Hinrichs, J., Hummel, I., van der Schaaf, G., Sietsma, H., Kok, J. W. (2002). Altered sphingolipid metabolism in multidrug-resistant ovarian cancer cells is due to uncoupling of glycolipid biosynthesis in the Golgi apparatus. *FASEB J,* 16: 1111–1113.

WHO, *World Health Organization Epilepsy,* (2009). Fact Sheet No. 999. WHO.

Wojtczak, A. and Skretkowicz, J. (2009). Clinical significance of some genetic polymorphisms of cytochrome P-450: family CYP1 and subfamilies CYP2A, CYP2B and CYP2C. *Polski Merkuriusz Lekarski,*26,153: 248–252.

Xiong, J., Mao, D. A., Liu, L. Q. (2015). Research Progress on the Role of ABC Transporters in the Drug Resistance Mechanism of Intractable Epilepsy. Biomed Res Int., 2015:194541.

In: Pharmacogenomics in Latin America
Editor: Luis A. Quiñones
ISBN: 978-1-53611-031-9

Chapter 12

PHARMACOEPIGENOMICS OF CANCER: OPPORTUNITIES IN LATIN AMERICA

Germán R. Perez*[*]*, PhD
Facultad de Ciencias Bioquímicas y Farmacéuticas,
Universidad Nacional de Rosario.
Gammalab, Grupo Gamma SA, Argentina

ABSTRACT

Epigenetics is the study of a set of metastable states, somatically hereditary, of gene expression with no alterations in the DNA sequence. Epigenetic changes include DNA methylation, histone modifications and RNA-mediated silencing. Altering any of these epigenetic mechanisms leads to inappropriate gene expression, and the development of cancer and other epigenetic diseases. The most studied epigenetic mechanism that influences gene expression is DNA methylation.

On the other hand, preventive medicine, the application of preventive measures to establish the criteria that allows each person to receive appropriate treatment can use biomarkers to detect people with high-risk diseases, and implement appropriate early detection programs. This preventive medicine and also personalized medicine is based, to a great extent, in pharmacogenomics but also on pharmacoepigenomic tools.

While Pharmacogenomic studies are growing in Latin America and several papers are recently published the biography on pharmacoepigenetic studies is still scarce.

Keywords: pharmacoepigenomics, Latin America, cancer, SNPs, epigenetics

INTRODUCTION

The development of cancer proceeds through multiple mechanisms (Hanahan and Weinberg 2000, Hirschey, DeBerardinis et al. 2015). The accumulation of alterations that

[*] Corresponding Author E-mail: grperez@igamma.com.

affect the structure and function of several genes can cause cells progression to malignancy (Herceg and Hainaut 2007, Smith, Guyton et al. 2015). Somatic mutations are produced and accumulated at a higher rate in cancer cells than in normal cells (Saletta, Dalla Pozza et al. 2015). These mutations comprised a series of structural changes in DNA that include minor changes in the nucleotide sequence like single nucleotide polymorphisms (SNP), as well as large chromosomal rearrangements (deletions or duplications) (Haraksingh and Snyder 2013, Pang, Migita et al. 2013, Poot and Haaf 2015). Availability of genomic SNP maps have raised expectations for the application of pharmacogenetics to optimize therapies for individual patients (Pang, MacDonald et al. 2010).

Epigenetics is the study of a set of metastable states, somatically hereditary, of gene expression with no alterations in the DNA sequence (Zoghbi and Beaudet 2016). Thus, epigenetic phenomena can be defined as changes in the genetic material, particularly in the genomic DNA and chromatin, altering the regulation of gene expression so that somatically inherited and sometimes by germline, unchanged in the DNA sequence (Kargul and Laurent 2009, Avgustinova and Benitah 2016). Therefore, it is not a mutation.

Epigenetic changes include DNA methylation, histone modifications and RNA-mediated silencing (Cedar and Bergman 2009, Hernando-Herraez, Garcia-Perez et al. 2015). These are essential mechanisms for the stable propagation of gene activities from one cell generation to the next (Furrow and Feldman 2014). Altering any of these three epigenetic mechanisms leads to inappropriate gene expression, and the development of cancer and other epigenetic diseases (Verma, Maruvada et al. 2004, Sharp, Stathaki et al. 2011, Eggermann, Perez de Nanclares et al. 2015).

The most studied epigenetic mechanism that influences gene expression is DNA methylation (Hernando-Herraez, Garcia-Perez et al. 2015, Schubeler 2015, Tillo, Mukerjee et al. 2016). This post-replicative DNA modification occurs primarily in the 5-position of cytosine rings that are found in CpG dinucleotides (Kurdyukov and Bullock 2016) (Jaenisch and Bird 2003). Eighty percent of CpG dinucleotides are usually dispersed in repetitive sequences of genome, and are called CpG islands (Schubeler 2015). These CpG islands, with a variable length of 0.5 to 3 kb, occur every 100 kb in the genome, and are located in the 5' region of nearly half of all human genes, including the promoter region, untranslated region, and exon 1 (Ziller, Muller et al. 2011).

In neoplastic processes, two forms of aberrant DNA methylation are observed: i) total loss of 5-methyl-cytosine (global hypomethylation) and ii) gene promoter-associated (CpG island-specific) hypermethylation (Issa 2004, Luczak and Jagodzinski 2006, Kurkjian, Kummar et al. 2008, Paska and Hudler 2015). A *CpG island* is defined as a region of DNA with more than 200 base pairs (typically of 300 – 3,000 bp) with a GC content ≥50% (Yan, Herman et al. 2016). There are approximately 28 million CpG sites in the genome, and only 7% reside within CpG islands, while most of them are out (Fazzari and Greally 2004).

The Methylation

Hypermethylation of CpG islands inactivates tumor suppressor genes and activates oncogenes (Waterfall, Killian et al. 2014). A group of enzymes called DNA methyltransferases (DNMTs) methylate and maintains genome methylation patterns, which are of vital importance in various biological processes, including development, genomic imprinting and tumorigenesis (Jin and Robertson 2013, Subramaniam, Thombre et al. 2014). Two DNMTs types can be distinguished considering its basic functions: i) DNMT1 is the main responsible for the post-replicative methylation (maintenance of DNA methylation, Figure 1B) (Robert, Morin et al. 2003, Lin and Wang 2014), and ii) DNMT3A and 3B are responsible for methylation of new CpG sites (*de novo* methylation, Figure 1A) (Jair, Bachman et al. 2006, Rajendran, Shanmuganandam et al. 2011, Lin and Wang 2014).

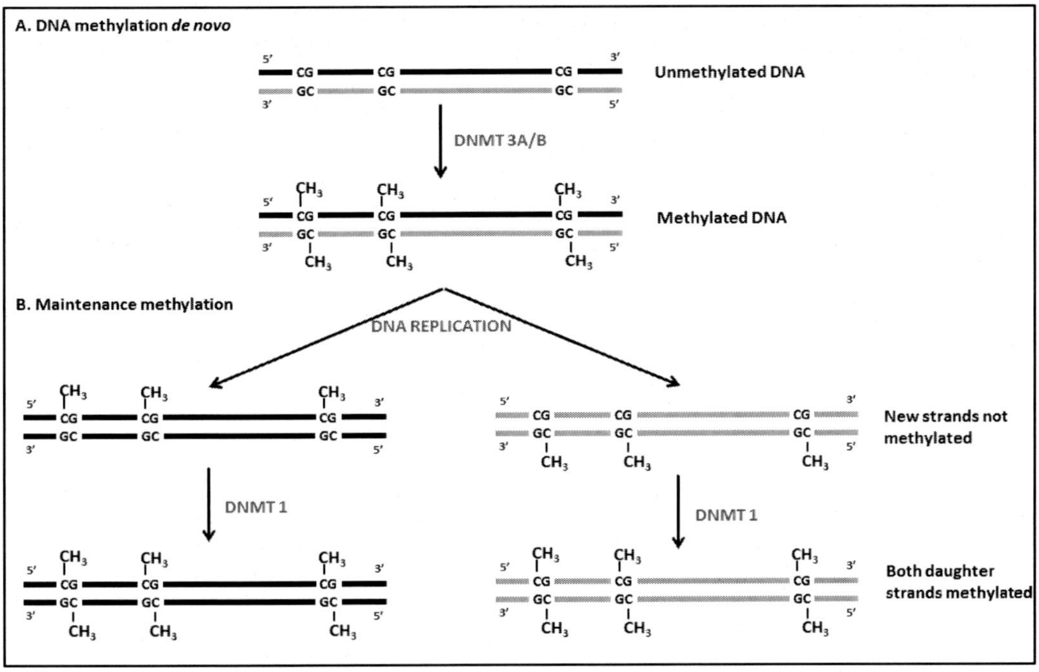

Figure 1. DNA methylation. Covalent addition of a methyl group to the cytosine in DNA de novo by DNMT3A/B (A) and maintained after DNA replication by DNMT1 (B).

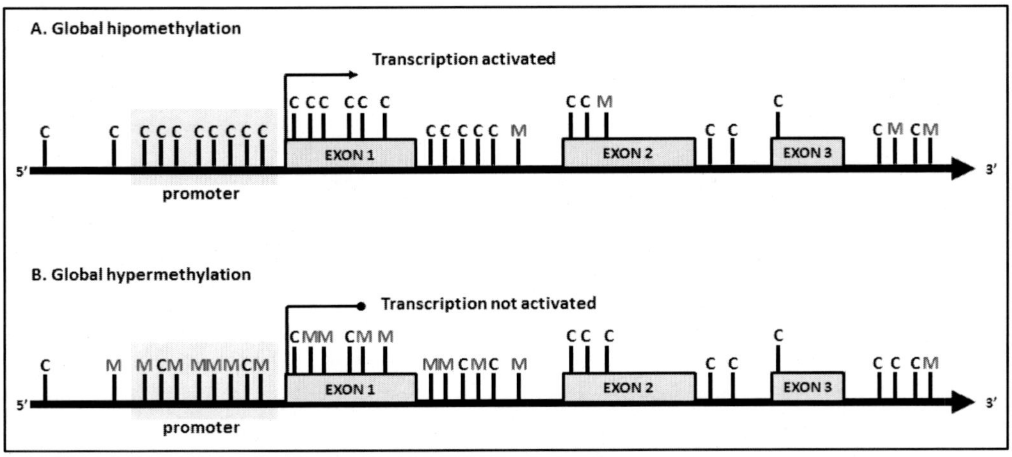

Figure 2. Cell changes in DNA methylation. (A) In global hypomethylation, CpG islands of active promoters are not methylated, thus allowing transcriptional activation. (B) In global hypermethylation, CpG islands of gene promoters are methylated and transcription is not activated.

Moreover, hypomethylation can contribute to carcinogenesis by different mechanisms, depending on whether it occurs globally throughout the genome or in specific genes (Kisseljova and Kisseljov 2005, Funaki, Nakamura et al. 2015, Lee and Wiemels 2016). Although the precise implications of global hypomethylation is under debate (activation of cellular proto-oncogenes, induction of chromosome instability), gene promoter-associated hypermethylation is clearly associated with gene inactivation (Toyota and Issa 2000, Herceg and Hainaut 2007). Thus, DNA methylation can promote the neoplastic process by local hypermethylation, resulting in silencing of tumor suppressor genes (Figura 2B), or causing activation of cellular oncogenes by global hypomethylation (Figura 2A) (Feinberg and Tycko 2004, Herceg and Hainaut 2007, Moarii, Boeva et al. 2015).

PREDICTIVE AND PERSONALIZE MEDICINE

In recent decades, health policies has given special attention to preventive medicine, in order to increase the performance of health systems (Akhmetov and Bubnov 2015). Preventive medicine can be defined as the application of sanitary measures to prevent the disease. However, the application of preventive measures to "all" the population to prevent "everything" is impossible, both scientifically and economically. *Predictive medicine* comes to establish the criteria that allows each person to receive appropriate preventive measures (Dietel 2007, Simon 2011). Therefore, the goal is to identify biomarkers to detect people with high-risk diseases, and implement appropriate early detection programs (Sadee and Dai 2005). On the other hand, *precision medicine* refers to medical treatment and prevention strategies based on individual variability due to molecular causes (Ashley 2015, Barlas 2015).

While *Pharmacogenetics* studies the actions and interactions between drugs in each individual based on their genes, i.e., the different responses that each person would have to the same medicine, *Pharmacogenomics* studies the effects of drugs regarding gene expression in general (Harper and Topol 2012). *Personalized medicine* uses these concepts to determine how the presence of variations in the genome (DNA nucleotide sequence or epigenetic patterns) predicts the risk of toxicity or therapeutic failure if a drug is delivered to a specific individual: "*the right medicine at the right dose for a particular patient*" (Agrawal and Khan 2007, Katsnelson 2013).

EPIGENETIC BIOMARKERS IN CANCER

The discovery and use of epigenetic biomarkers can be extremely beneficial in the early detection and prevention of cancer (Bakulski and Fallin 2014, Verma 2015). A significant number of cancer-related genes were associated with high levels of methylation in the otherwise unmethylated promoter region (Akhavan-Niaki and Samadani 2013, Gokul and Khosla 2013, Ng and Yu 2015). While it is unclear, whether methylation is an initiating event or a secondary event in gene silencing, there is no doubt it plays a key role in the process of tumorigenesis (Gokul and Khosla 2013). Methylation levels in these genes can be detected and used as a biomarker for early diagnosis and prognosis of the neoplastic process (Kumar and Verma 2009, Choi and Lee 2013, Chen, Lee et al. 2015).

Several studies report increased levels of cell-free DNA in plasma or serum from cancer patients (Francis and Stein 2015). In addition to genetic changes, epigenetic alterations in circulating DNA from different types of tumors were detected, and such changes have opened new possibilities in cancer detection and risk assessment (Warton and Samimi 2015). The clinical sensitivity in detection of human cancer associated biomarkers in body fluids would increase by using multiple epigenetic markers (Heitzer, Ulz et al. 2015, Ulz, Auer et al. 2016).

While in recent years, the epigenetic cancer have focused primarily on changes in DNA methylation, there have been only a few studies on specific histone modifications as potential biomarkers. The histone modifications include: i) methylation in lysine and arginine residues, ii) lysine residues acetylation, iii) ubiquitination and SUMOylation of lysines and iv) phosphorylation of serine and threonine (Santos-Rosa and Caldas 2005). Lysine residues acetylation and methylation are the most characterized epigenetic modifications, key transcriptional activation/repression mechanisms. Histone methyltransferases enzymes (HMT), histone demethylases (HDM), histone acetyltransferase (HAT) and histone deacetylase (HDAC), regulate these processes (Gibbons 2005).

Histone modifications affect chromatin structure and influence gene expression by modifying the accessibility of DNA transcriptional machinery. For example, methylation of specific lysine residues near the amino-terminal ends of histones are crucial for the formation of the functional domains of chromatin (euchromatin and heterochromatin) (Waldmann and Schneider 2013). Since epigenetic modifications are not randomly distributed in the interphase nucleus, these changes probably influence the regulation of nuclear processes such as replication, transcription, DNA repair and chromosome condensation (Bannister and Kouzarides 2011).

In human cancers, epigenetic changes are more frequent than mutations (Sadikovic, Al-Romaih et al. 2008). While it is known that these alterations play an important role in cancer development, the weight of epigenetic modifications in personalized medicine has not been studied extensively (Tang, Xiong et al. 2014, Rasool, Malik et al. 2015, Yan, Herman et al. 2016).

Biomarkers identification to predict chemotherapy response is part of personalized medicine. Methylation patterns may be useful in assessing clinical outcomes or response to chemotherapeutic agents. Diverse DNA methylation profiles have been identified as specific biological markers of drug response in different types of tumors (Tang, Xiong et al. 2014, Hamm and Costa 2015).

The first report of a genetic alteration associated with sensitivity to a chemotherapeutic drug was the presence of Methyltransferase O^6-methylguanine-DNA (MGMT) gene methylation in patients with major response to chemotherapy with alkylating agents (Esteller, Garcia-Foncillas et al. 2000).

MGMT is an ubiquitous, highly conserved DNA repair enzyme that removes mutagenic adducts of O^6-guanine in DNA and this enzyme epigenetic silencing has been reported in a wide variety of tumors (Danam, Qian et al. 1999). MGMT quickly reverses the alkylation, including the methylation at the O^6 position of guanine by transfer of the alkyl group to the active site of the enzyme. Although O^6-alkylation is not the primary lesion induced by alkylating agents, it is the most cytotoxic (Gerson 2004). If the cell lacks MGMT protein O^6-alkylguanine accumulates in the DNA, which after the incorrectly association with thymidine, triggers the genes repair system activation (Gerson 2004). Therefore, cells deficient repair systems are highly resistant to alkylating agents, even in the absence of MGMT (Cankovic, Nikiforova et al. 2013).

The MGMT gene is located on chromosome 10q26 (Natarajan, Vermeulen et al. 1992). Its promoter contains the constitutive regulatory elements such as the TATA box and Cat box present in other genes, and also has a CpG island (Harris, Potter et al. 1991).

The region required for maximum activity of the promoter is at the 5' end of the gene (from -953 to +202 bp; transcription initiation site +1 bp) and comprise: i) a minimal promoter, ii) a promoter region MGMT enhancer-binding protein (meBP), and iii) a number of binding sites of the transcription factor, such as SP1 and P1 (Cankovic, Nikiforova et al. 2013).

The CpG island is located in the 5' region of the MGMT gene (-552 to +289 bp) and includes 97 CpG repeats, which are predominantly unmethylated in normal tissues. Methyl-CpG binding proteins, such as methyl-CpG-binding protein 2 (meCP2) and methyl-CpG-binding domain protein 2 (mBD2) bind to aberrantly methylated sequences, resulting in deterioration of the structure chromatin. This prevents binding of transcription factors, which causes gene silencing. Two gene regions susceptible to high levels of methylation has been identified. The region containing the enhancer element appears to be the most critical for the loss of expression of MGMT gene (Nakagawachi, Soejima et al. 2003).

MGMT gene expression levels vary considerably between different organs, with relatively higher levels in the liver and lower levels in the brain (Riemenschneider, Hegi et al. 2010). Tumors usually exhibit higher levels of expression compared to the healthy original tissue (Wesseling, van den Bent et al. 2015).

The first observation on the predictive value of MGMT protein levels was by immunofluorescence microscopy in patients with malignant gliomas over 10 years ago. Patients with low levels of MGMT protein showed a better response to treatment with carmustine (a nitrogen mustard β-chloro-nitrosourea compound used as an alkylating agent) than those who had high levels of protein (Garside, Pitt et al. 2007). Similarly, low levels of MGMT protein predicted longer survival in patients with gliomas treated prophylactically with temozolomide (TMZ), or in patients newly diagnosed with inoperable glioblastoma treated with neoadjuvant TMZ (Weller, Stupp et al. 2010).

TMZ is an alkylating agent used in treatment of some brain cancers, such as second-line treatment for astrocytoma and first-line treatment for glioblastoma multiforme (Johannessen and Bjerkvig 2012). The therapeutic benefit of TMZ depends on its ability to alkylate/ methylate DNA, which usually occurs at the N^7 or O^6 position of guanine residues (Figure 3A). TMZ damages DNA and triggers the death of tumor cells. However, some tumor cells are able to repair this type of DNA damage and thus decrease the therapeutic efficacy of the drug, through the expression of the MGMT protein (Jiang, Wei et al. 2011). Decreasing MGMT protein levels can be attributed to epigenetic silencing mediated by promoter methylation of MGMT gene (Figure 3B) (Hegi, Diserens et al. 2004, Brandes, Franceschi et al. 2009).

Because a correlation with survival has been demonstrated, in glioma patients treated with nitrosoureas or TMZ, the methylation status of the MGMT promoter would be a suitable biomarker to assess prognosis or to predict the benefit of using an alkylating agent with radiotherapy (Hegi, Diserens et al. 2004, Fiorica, Berretta et al. 2010, Cankovic, Nikiforova et al. 2013).

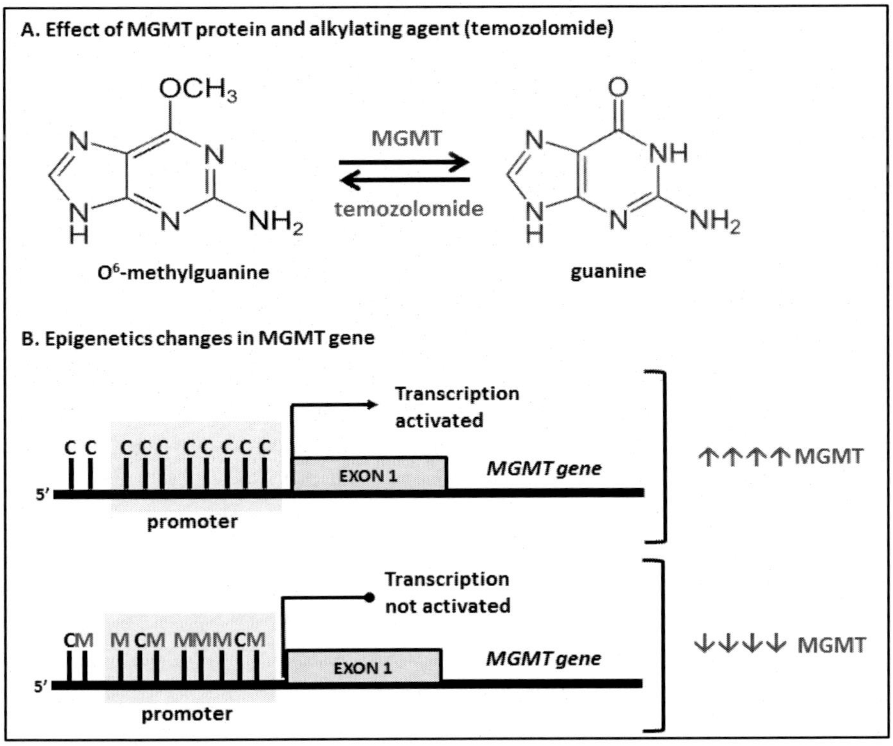

Figure 3. Epigenetic inactivation of MGMT and sensitivity to alkylating agents. (A) Damaged O^6-guanine by TMZ is repaired by MGMT. (B) Tumor cells with MGMT methylation are sensitive to TMZ due to the absence of O^6-methylguanine repair activity.

Telomerase is a specialized reverse transcriptase that extends telomere to compensate for its shortening during DNA replication (Liu 1999). In humans, telomerase comprises a protein complex and includes: i) a reverse transcriptase subunit (hTERT), ii) an RNA template (hTR) and iii) a telomerase-associated protein (hTEP1) (Liu 1999). hTERT is expressed in 80-90% of human tumors, but not in most normal tissues and somatic cells (Gladych, Wojtyla et al. 2011). Therefore, hTERT may be a biomarker applicable to early diagnosis and molecular classification of tumors, and the prognostic and therapeutic development for cancer (Poole, Andrews et al. 2001). Telomerase activation is tightly regulated at the transcriptional level (Gladych, Wojtyla et al. 2011). Several studies have indicated that the transcription of hTERT is the rate-limiting step in the expression of telomerase (Guilleret and Benhattar 2003).

5-Aza-2'-deoxycytidine (decitabine, DAC), a DNA methylation inhibitor, is used in the treatment of myelodysplastic syndromes, such as acute myeloid leukemia (AML) (Pettigrew, Armstrong et al. 2012). It is a 2'-deoxycytidine nucleoside analogue that selectively inhibits DNA methyltransferases and produce hypomethylation of gene promoters, which can cause a reactivation of tumor suppressor genes, induction of cell differentiation or cell senescence, followed by programmed cell death.

Clonal expansion in AML contributes to the progressive shortening of telomeres in cells, causing chromosomal abnormalities and genetic instability. Telomerase is activated and stabilizes critically short telomeres. This prevents cellular senescence and allow greater proliferation of the tumor cell. There have been observations of increased hTERT mRNA levels in AML patients, indicating a posttranscriptional regulation of hTERT gene, probably by epigenetic regulation by DNA methylation (Pettigrew, Armstrong et al. 2012). Moreover, several studies reported hypermethylation in tumor cells and hypomethylation in normal cells, suggesting that methylation could block the binding of transcription factors that repress hTERT gene expression. Studies in cell lines, demonstrated that treatment with DAC reduces expression of hTERT and telomerase activity, probably by direct demethylating the promoter.

The sustained higher hTERT expression levels trigger continuous activation of telomerase, which could contribute to the immortalization of glioma cells and their resistance to therapeutic measures (Reitman, Pirozzi et al. 2013).

Recently, the promoter region of the hTERT encoding gene has been characterized (Cong, Wen et al. 1999). Two mutations in the gene promoter, -124C>T (C228T) and -146T > C (C250T), have been identified as major somatic alterations (Figure 4) (Mosrati, Malmstrom et al. 2015). The presence of these mutations result in increased gene expression by creating *de novo* binding sites for T-cell transcription factors. In addition, they have been associated with increased mRNA expression and telomerase activity in various tumors (Wang, Kjellin et al. 2016, Wu, Li et al. 2016). For example, individuals with these mutations have increased cutaneous melanoma susceptibility (Huang, Hodis et al. 2013). However, high levels of hTERT mRNA were detected even in cases when hTERT promoter mutations where absent (Chen, Han et al. 2014).

These mutations have proven to be particularly common in most glioblastomas and oligodendrogliomas, and in 20-30% of medulloblastomas and other central nervous system tumors (Arita, Narita et al. 2013). Mutations hTERC promoter could be one of the causes of mortality in elderly patients, because it would lead to the persistence of high transcriptional activity of the gene even under TMZ treatment (Castelo-Branco, Choufani et al. 2013).

For medulloblastomas, the hTERT promoter mutations occur mainly in the subset of adult patients, despite a predominantly pediatric tumor (Remke, Ramaswamy et al. 2013). Similarly, these mutations are common among adult's glioblastomas, and almost never occur in pediatric glioblastomas (Castelo-Branco, Choufani et al. 2013). The absence of mutations in hTERT promoter in pediatric tumors has led to hypothesize a different origin of these tumors in pediatric patients (Koelsche, Sahm et al. 2013). Thus, pediatric tumors might arise from cells in which telomerase has been activated and, therefore, it is not necessary to acquire C228T and C250T mutations in the hTERT promoter telomerase deregulation (Castelo-Branco, Choufani et al. 2013, Reitman, Pirozzi et al. 2013).

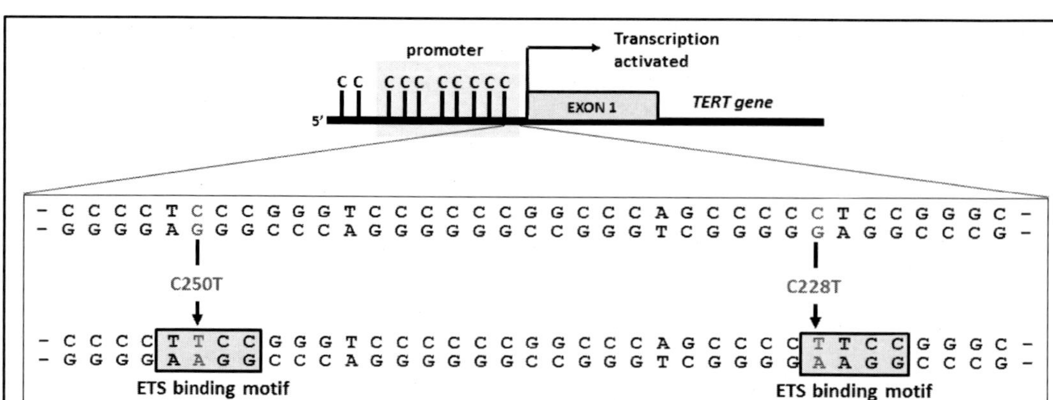

Figure 4. Mutations in the promoter region of the hTERT.

The hTERT gene promoter has a large CpG island and therefore might be under DNA methylation regulation (Guilleret and Benhattar 2003). Promoter hypermethylation has been associated with the loss of transcription, being an alternative mode of gene inactivation during cancer development (Shin, Kang et al. 2003). Methylation profiles for the hTERT gene promoter was recently tested in a variety of cell lines and tumor tissues.

Hypermethylation of CpG islands in gene promoters is associated with gene silencing, but that is not always the case (Guilleret and Benhattar 2004). For instance, hTERT promoter´s CpG islands hypermethylation causes activation of cancer related genes (Guilleret, Yan et al. 2002).

Studies in adult patients with glioblastomas have shown increased hTERT mRNA expression in the absence of mutations within the hTERT promoter. This increase may be explained by the hTERT promoter hypermethylation. In fact, it has been found an association between the hTERT promoter methylation and increased hTERT expression in pediatric brain tumors. This would indicate that methylation, and not mutation, of the hTERT promoter is to account for up-regulating hTERT in certain tumors.

While the promoter hypermethylation of the MGMT gene predicts response to radiotherapy and chemotherapy, is not applicable to all patients. Furthermore, MGMT methylation status may change from newly diagnosed with respect to a recurrent glioblastoma tumor (Zhang, Chan et al. 2015). Therefore, identifying new prognostic biomarkers for glioblastoma is very important. While the biological basis and ~~the~~ mechanisms by which overexpression of hTERT leads to cancer remain unclear, a greater understanding of them could lead to the development of clinically useful biomarkers.

Future studies of hTERT gene promoter methylation profile could provide evidence of their importance in the detection of individuals at increased risk of tumor development or recurrence, in order to optimize treatment and reduce complications associated with current therapy (Chen, Han et al. 2014).

Mitosis is a cellular process that leads to segregation of genetic material doubled in two genetically identical daughter cells. Errors in this process could lead to chromosomal instability or mutation and finally spread to cellular transformation. There are several checkpoints in the cell cycle to prevent the spread of cells with damaged genome (Sanbhnani and Yeong 2012). The protein encoded by CHFR gene (located in 12q24.33) acts as a checkpoint of cell cycle M phase (Sanbhnani and Yeong 2012). CHFR causes cell cycle arrest at the G2 phase to allow repair of damaged DNA.

CHFR is an ubiquitin-kinase and one of the target proteins is polo-like kinase 1 (Plk1) (Privette and Petty 2008). Plk1 is a serine / threonine kinase involved in the phosphorylation of Cdc25, thereby regulating the activity of cyclin-CDK B1 (Shtivelman 2003). The phosphorylation and activation of PLK1 are set by the Aurora kinase A (Yu, Minter-Dykhouse et al. 2005). Through ubiquitination and degradation of proteins PLK1 and Aurora A, CHFR is able of inhibiting the formation of cyclin-CDK B1 and thus promote the arrest of cellular cycle (van Vugt and Medema 2005).

The analysis in the CHFR gene coding sequence in small-cell carcinoma allowed the identification of three missense mutations that were associated with mitotic checkpoint defects. However, these mutations were only observed in a few patients. Furthermore, loss of the chromosomal region containing the CHFR gene (12q24.33) occurs more frequently in cancer and is associated with decreased gene expression.

Several studies in multiple cancer tissues (colorectal, hepatocellular, pancreatic, lung, myeloma, leukemia, head and neck) have demonstrated downregulation of the expression of CHFR, in some cases, by CpG island hypermethylation in CHFR promoter region, which span −905 to +783 bp relative to the transcription start site (Sakai, Hibi et al. 2005, Morioka, Hibi et al. 2006, Yanokura, Banno et al. 2007).

Multiple studies have shown that the CHFR promoter methylation profile can be detected in primary cancers as well as in blood, stool and peritoneal fluid of cancer patients (Privette and Petty 2008).

Taxanes are a group of anticancer drugs that inhibit cell growth by stopping cell division. These drugs are inhibitors of microtubule depolymerisation in mitotic cells.

The association between the expression and decreased sensitivity to microtubule inhibitors (docetaxel or paclitaxel) was first demonstrated in gastric cancer cell lines. Since not all patients respond to this therapy, the CHFR gene promoter methylation status could be an important determinant of therapy response. While this potential association remains under discussion for gastric cancer, stronger evidence has been reported in other cancers. This relationship has been reported in colon tumor cells, stomach and endometrium, among others. It has been observed that cells with CHFR normal expression are arrested in the G2 phase to repair damaged DNA and, therefore, are resistant to taxanes. However, cells with low CHFR expression levels (by CHFR promoter hypermethylation) are not able to detect DNA damage and exhibit a high sensitivity to the drug. Therefore, hypermethylation of the gene promoter could be use as CHFR molecular biomarker sensitivity to taxanes (Banno, Yanokura et al. 2007, Derks, Cleven et al. 2014).

During apoptosis and necrosis and cell proliferation, the cell DNA is released or actively secreted into the circulating blood. Levels of free circulating DNA (fcDNA) are elevated in the serum of some cancer patients (Heitzer, Ulz et al. 2015). The presence of tumor fcDNA in cancer patients stimulated the search for biomarkers in blood for early diagnosis of cancer. However, the detection and correlation of tumor free circulating DNA as a cancer biomarker has been difficult, mainly due to the high variability in serum and increased significantly in trauma, inflammation, stroke, and strenuous exercise. The characterization of specific mutations in tumor fcDNA enabled the development of tests for early diagnosis of cancer. Tumors often have aberrant DNA methylation profiles, which can be detected in the tumor fcDNA (Warton and Samimi 2015).

However, the successful implementation of these biomarkers in clinical practice requires highly sensitive and specific tests, since tumor fcDNA concentration may represent 0.1% of total circulating DNA. This has been observed particularly in the early stages of cancer.

There are three biomarkers based on DNA methylation: TMEFF2 (transmembrane protein with EGF like and two follistatin like domains 2), NGFR (Nerve Growth Factor Receptor) and SEPT9 (Septin 9).

Septins are a group of highly conserved GTP-binding proteins and have been implicated in the localization of cellular processes at cell division site (Mostowy and Cossart 2012). The SEPT9 gene is located on chromosome 17q25.3, it produces 18 different transcripts (based on multiple transcription start sites) encoding 15 polypeptides (McIlhatton, Burrows et al. 2001). Recent studies indicate a close relationship to carcinogenesis in breast cancer, colon, ovary, head and neck, leukemia and lymphoma (Scott, Hyland et al. 2005, McDade, Hall et al. 2007). Expression of the V4 transcript of SEPT9 in several tumor cell lines is absent or decreased and can be reactivated by treatment with 5-azacytidine (Li, Song et al. 2014). In addition, DNA hypermethylation in the V2 transcript promoter region of SEPT9 is characteristic in colon cancer carcinogenesis (Payne 2010). Several studies on the role of SEPT9 in carcinogenesis suggested that the presence of specific DNA methylation patterns in tissues may be an important mechanism responsible for the differential regulation of SEPT9 isoform expression (Song and Li 2015).

The main changes in the methylation pattern of SEPT9 V2 transcript in tumor tissues was observed only in one of the CpG islands, CpG island 3 (CGI3) (Wasserkort, Kalmar et al. 2013). This region contains the gene promoter and includes the ATG start code. Adenoma and CRC exhibit different methylation patterns and could reflect the progression to cell malignancy in colon mucosa (Molnar, Toth et al. 2015). Hypermethylation in the CGI3 may suppress the normal SEPT9 V2 transcript expression, which, in turn, disrupts the formation of structured filaments and key cellular functions (Wasserkort, Kalmar et al. 2013).

The SEPT9 assay could be applied not only in colorectal cancer detection and screening, but also in monitorization and evaluation of therapy (Li, Song et al. 2014). Some studies indicate that SEPT9 methylation levels are closely related to the development of CRC (Toth, Wasserkort et al. 2014). However, it is necessary to define whether this correlation can be used as an indicator of recurrence or metastasis and if would be useful to predict response or resistance to chemotherapy (Li, Song et al. 2014).

PHARMACOEPIGENETIC STUDIES IN LATIN AMERICA

Latin American biography on pharmacoepigenetic studies is scarce. Only a few authors have been published. Bruno et al. reported six patients presenting aggressive pituitary tumors with intention-to-treat with TMZ (Bruno, Juarez-Allen et al. 2015). In this study, no expression of MGMT was observed by immunohistochemistry in surgical specimens. It has been reported that a low expression or the absence of this enzyme strongly correlates with the response to TMZ. However, two patients who completed the minimum treatment period showed a satisfactory response even though no expression of MGMT protein were detected. Molecular assays could provide more accurate data on epigenetic silencing by MGMT gene promoter methylation.

Castro et al. studied the biological effect of the administration of TMZ in three glioma cell lines by analyzing the relationship between MGMT protein expression levels and treatment resistance and DNA repair (Castro, Cayado-Gutierrez et al. 2015). The study results agreed with previous reports: low expression of MGMT leads to a better TMZ treatment response.

Various groups have studied the promoter methylation profile of several genes in different types of tumors. They performed studies on the status of MGMT gene methylation in neoplastic processes: lung cancer (Pulling, Divine et al. 2003, Guzman, Depix et al. 2012), melanoma (Torres, Luo et al. 2013), gastric cancer (Bernal, Aguayo et al. 2008), gastric leiomyoma (Branham, Pellicer et al. 2014), Gallbladder carcinoma (Garcia, Manterola et al. 2009), breast carcinomas (Branham, Marzese et al. 2012), etc. However, the response to specific treatment for these diseases and their relationship with the MGMT gene methylation status was not studied.

Gigek et al. investigated the promoter methylation status and hTERT protein expression in gastric cancer and normal mucosa samples (Gigek, Leal et al. 2009). In this study, hTERT expression was associated with gastric cancer and the promotor hypermethylation was significantly higher in tumours than in normal mucosa, but was not associated with a higher frequency of hTERT expression. These results may have an impact on the anti-telomerase strategy for cancer therapy.

Conclusion

Our knowledge of epigenetics in normal and neoplastic cellular processes increased significantly in recent years. However, epigenetic mechanisms related to therapy with different drugs requires more clinical research.

While the effect of some epigenetic changes in drug metabolism is known and some epigenetic drugs are being used clinically, the mechanisms of histone Modifications and RNA-mediated silencing need further development.

New personalized therapies based on these epigenetic processes will surely be available in the coming decades in clinical practice.

This will depend on whether we reduce the knowledge gap that currently exists between epigenetics and drug metabolism. Probably the development of new tools for studying the epigenome will collaborate to bring closer both research fields. The few scientific studies presented in this paper demonstrate the need to increase our knowledge in the pharmacoepigenomics area.

References

Agrawal, S. and F. Khan (2007). "Human genetic variation and personalized medicine." *Indian J Physiol Pharmacol* 51(1): 7-28.

Akhavan-Niaki, H. and A. A. Samadani (2013). "DNA methylation and cancer development: molecular mechanism." *Cell Biochem Biophys* 67(2): 501-513.

Akhmetov, I. and R. V. Bubnov (2015). "Assessing value of innovative molecular diagnostic tests in the concept of predictive, preventive, and personalized medicine." *EPMA J* 6: 19.

Arita, H., Y. Narita, S. Fukushima, K. Tateishi, Y. Matsushita, A. Yoshida, Y. Miyakita, M. Ohno, V. P. Collins, N. Kawahara, S. Shibui and K. Ichimura (2013). "Upregulating mutations in the TERT promoter commonly occur in adult malignant gliomas and are strongly associated with total 1p19q loss." *Acta Neuropathol* 126(2): 267-276.

Ashley, E. A. (2015). "The precision medicine initiative: a new national effort." *JAMA* 313(21): 2119-2120.

Avgustinova, A. and S. A. Benitah (2016). "The epigenetics of tumour initiation: cancer stem cells and their chromatin." *Curr Opin Genet Dev* 36: 8-15.

Bakulski, K. M. and M. D. Fallin (2014). "Epigenetic epidemiology: promises for public health research." *Environ Mol Mutagen* 55(3): 171-183.

Bannister, A. J. and T. Kouzarides (2011). "Regulation of chromatin by histone modifications." *Cell Res* 21(3): 381-395.

Banno, K., M. Yanokura, M. Kawaguchi, Y. Kuwabara, J. Akiyoshi, Y. Kobayashi, T. Iwata, A. Hirasawa, T. Fujii, N. Susumu, K. Tsukazaki and D. Aoki (2007). "Epigenetic inactivation of the CHFR gene in cervical cancer contributes to sensitivity to taxanes." *Int J Oncol* 31(4): 713-720.

Barlas, S. (2015). "Precision medicine initiative aims for a new generation of diagnostics and treatments: but is the promise of genetic targeting overinflated?" *P T* 40(5): 340-352.

Bernal, C., F. Aguayo, C. Villarroel, M. Vargas, I. Diaz, F. J. Ossandon, E. Santibanez, M. Palma, E. Aravena, C. Barrientos and A. H. Corvalan (2008). "Reprimo as a potential biomarker for early detection in gastric cancer." *Clin Cancer Res* 14(19): 6264-6269.

Brandes, A. A., E. Franceschi, A. Tosoni, F. Benevento, L. Scopece, V. Mazzocchi, A. Bacci, R. Agati, F. Calbucci and M. Ermani (2009). "Temozolomide concomitant and adjuvant to radiotherapy in elderly patients with glioblastoma: correlation with MGMT promoter methylation status." *Cancer* 115(15): 3512-3518.

Branham, M. T., D. M. Marzese, S. R. Laurito, F. E. Gago, J. I. Orozco, O. M. Tello, L. M. Vargas-Roig and M. Roque (2012). "Methylation profile of triple-negative breast carcinomas." *Oncogenesis* 1: e17.

Branham, M. T., M. Pellicer, E. Campoy, M. Palma, A. Correa and M. Roque (2014). "Epigenetic alterations in a gastric leiomyoma." *Case Rep Gastrointest Med* 2014: 371638.

Bruno, O. D., L. Juarez-Allen, S. B. Christiansen, M. Manavela, K. Danilowicz, C. Vigovich and R. M. Gomez (2015). "Temozolomide Therapy for Aggressive Pituitary Tumors: Results in a Small Series of Patients from Argentina." *Int J Endocrinol* 2015: 587893.

Cankovic, M., M. N. Nikiforova, M. Snuderl, A. M. Adesina, N. Lindeman, P. Y. Wen and E. Q. Lee (2013). "The role of MGMT testing in clinical practice: a report of the association for molecular pathology." *J Mol Diagn* 15(5): 539-555.

Castelo-Branco, P., S. Choufani, S. Mack, D. Gallagher, C. Zhang, T. Lipman, N. Zhukova, E. J. Walker, D. Martin, D. Merino, J. D. Wasserman, C. Elizabeth, N. Alon, L. Zhang, V. Hovestadt, M. Kool, D. T. Jones, G. Zadeh, S. Croul, C. Hawkins, J. Hitzler, J. C. Wang, S. Baruchel, P. B. Dirks, D. Malkin, S. Pfister, M. D. Taylor, R. Weksberg and U. Tabori (2013). "Methylation of the TERT promoter and risk stratification of childhood brain tumours: an integrative genomic and molecular study." *Lancet Oncol* 14(6): 534-542.

Castro, G. N., N. Cayado-Gutierrez, F. C. Zoppino, M. A. Fanelli, F. D. Cuello-Carrion, M. Sottile, S. B. Nadin and D. R. Ciocca (2015). "Effects of temozolomide (TMZ) on the expression and interaction of heat shock proteins (HSPs) and DNA repair proteins in human malignant glioma cells." *Cell Stress Chaperones* 20(2): 253-265.

Cedar, H. and Y. Bergman (2009). "Linking DNA methylation and histone modification: patterns and paradigms." *Nat Rev Genet* 10(5): 295-304.

Cong, Y. S., J. Wen and S. Bacchetti (1999). "The human telomerase catalytic subunit hTERT: organization of the gene and characterization of the promoter." *Hum Mol Genet* 8(1): 137-142.

Chen, C., S. Han, L. Meng, Z. Li, X. Zhang and A. Wu (2014). "TERT promoter mutations lead to high transcriptional activity under hypoxia and temozolomide treatment and predict poor prognosis in gliomas." *PLoS One* 9(6): e100297.

Chen, C. C., K. D. Lee, M. Y. Pai, P. Y. Chu, C. C. Hsu, C. C. Chiu, L. T. Chen, J. Y. Chang, S. H. Hsiao and Y. W. Leu (2015). "Changes in DNA methylation are associated with the development of drug resistance in cervical cancer cells." *Cancer Cell Int* 15: 98.

Choi, J. D. and J. S. Lee (2013). "Interplay between Epigenetics and Genetics in Cancer." *Genomics Inform* 11(4): 164-173.

Danam, R. P., X. C. Qian, S. R. Howell and T. P. Brent (1999). "Methylation of selected CpGs in the human O6-methylguanine-DNA methyltransferase promoter region as a marker of gene silencing." *Mol Carcinog* 24(2): 85-89.

Derks, S., A. H. Cleven, V. Melotte, K. M. Smits, J. C. Brandes, N. Azad, W. van Criekinge, A. P. de Bruine, J. G. Herman and M. van Engeland (2014). "Emerging evidence for CHFR as a cancer biomarker: from tumor biology to precision medicine." *Cancer Metastasis Rev* 33(1): 161-171.

Dietel, M. (2007). "Predictive medicine: incipient reality or fata morgana?" *J Pathol* 212(4): 353-355.

Eggermann, T., G. Perez de Nanclares, E. R. Maher, I. K. Temple, Z. Tumer, D. Monk, D. J. Mackay, K. Gronskov, A. Riccio, A. Linglart and I. Netchine (2015). "Imprinting disorders: a group of congenital disorders with overlapping patterns of molecular changes affecting imprinted loci." *Clin Epigenetics* 7: 123.

Esteller, M., J. Garcia-Foncillas, E. Andion, S. N. Goodman, O. F. Hidalgo, V. Vanaclocha, S. B. Baylin and J. G. Herman (2000). "Inactivation of the DNA-repair gene MGMT and the clinical response of gliomas to alkylating agents." *N Engl J Med* 343(19): 1350-1354.

Fazzari, M. J. and J. M. Greally (2004). "Epigenomics: beyond CpG islands." *Nat Rev Genet* 5(6): 446-455.

Feinberg, A. P. and B. Tycko (2004). "The history of cancer epigenetics." *Nat Rev Cancer* 4(2): 143-153.

Fiorica, F., M. Berretta, C. Colosimo, A. Stefanelli, S. Ursino, E. Zanet, T. Palmucci, D. Maugeri, M. Malaguarnera, S. Palmucci, M. Grasso, U. Tirelli and F. Cartei (2010). "Glioblastoma in elderly patients: safety and efficacy of adjuvant radiotherapy with concomitant temozolomide." *Arch Gerontol Geriatr* 51(1): 31-35.

Francis, G. and S. Stein (2015). "Circulating Cell-Free Tumour DNA in the Management of Cancer." *Int J Mol Sci* 16(6): 14122-14142.

Funaki, S., T. Nakamura, T. Nakatani, H. Umehara, H. Nakashima, M. Okumura, K. Oboki, K. Matsumoto, H. Saito and T. Nakano (2015). "Global DNA hypomethylation coupled to cellular transformation and metastatic ability." *FEBS Lett* 589(24 Pt B): 4053-4060.

Furrow, R. E. and M. W. Feldman (2014). "Genetic variation and the evolution of epigenetic regulation." *Evolution* 68(3): 673-683.

Garcia, P., C. Manterola, J. C. Araya, M. Villaseca, P. Guzman, A. Sanhueza, M. Thomas, H. Alvarez and J. C. Roa (2009). "Promoter methylation profile in preneoplastic and neoplastic gallbladder lesions." *Mol Carcinog* 48(1): 79-89.

Garside, R., M. Pitt, R. Anderson, G. Rogers, M. Dyer, S. Mealing, M. Somerville, A. Price and K. Stein (2007). "The effectiveness and cost-effectiveness of carmustine implants and temozolomide for the treatment of newly diagnosed high-grade glioma: a systematic review and economic evaluation." *Health Technol Assess* 11(45): iii-iv, ix-221.

Gerson, S. L. (2004). "MGMT: its role in cancer aetiology and cancer therapeutics." *Nat Rev Cancer* 4(4): 296-307.

Gibbons, R. J. (2005). "Histone modifying and chromatin remodelling enzymes in cancer and dysplastic syndromes." *Hum Mol Genet* 14 Spec No 1: R85-92.

Gigek, C. O., M. F. Leal, P. N. Silva, L. C. Lisboa, E. M. Lima, D. Q. Calcagno, P. P. Assumpcao, R. R. Burbano and A. Smith Mde (2009). "hTERT methylation and expression in gastric cancer." *Biomarkers* 14(8): 630-636.

Gladych, M., A. Wojtyla and B. Rubis (2011). "Human telomerase expression regulation." *Biochem Cell Biol* 89(4): 359-376.

Gokul, G. and S. Khosla (2013). "DNA methylation and cancer." *Subcell_Biochem* 61: 597-625.

Guilleret, I. and J. Benhattar (2003). "Demethylation of the human telomerase catalytic subunit (hTERT) gene promoter reduced hTERT expression and telomerase activity and shortened telomeres." *Exp Cell Res* 289(2): 326-334.

Guilleret, I. and J. Benhattar (2004). "Unusual distribution of DNA methylation within the hTERT CpG island in tissues and cell lines." *Biochem Biophys Res Commun* 325(3): 1037-1043.

Guilleret, I., P. Yan, F. Grange, R. Braunschweig, F. T. Bosman and J. Benhattar (2002). "Hypermethylation of the human telomerase catalytic subunit (hTERT) gene correlates with telomerase activity." *Int J Cancer* 101(4): 335-341.

Guzman, L., M. S. Depix, A. M. Salinas, R. Roldan, F. Aguayo, A. Silva and R. Vinet (2012). "Analysis of aberrant methylation on promoter sequences of tumor suppressor genes and total DNA in sputum samples: a promising tool for early detection of COPD and lung cancer in smokers." *Diagn Pathol* 7: 87.

Hamm, C. A. and F. F. Costa (2015). "Epigenomes as therapeutic targets." *Pharmacol Ther* 151: 72-86.

Hanahan, D. and R. A. Weinberg (2000). "The hallmarks of cancer." *Cell* 100(1): 57-70.

Haraksingh, R. R. and M. P. Snyder (2013). "Impacts of variation in the human genome on gene regulation." *J Mol Biol* 425(21): 3970-3977.

Harper, A. R. and E. J. Topol (2012). "Pharmacogenomics in clinical practice and drug development." *Nat Biotechnol* 30(11): 1117-1124.

Harris, L. C., P. M. Potter, K. Tano, S. Shiota, S. Mitra and T. P. Brent (1991). "Characterization of the promoter region of the human O6-methylguanine-DNA methyltransferase gene." *Nucleic Acids Res* 19(22): 6163-6167.

Hegi, M. E., A. C. Diserens, S. Godard, P. Y. Dietrich, L. Regli, S. Ostermann, P. Otten, G. Van Melle, N. de Tribolet and R. Stupp (2004). "Clinical trial substantiates the predictive value of O-6-methylguanine-DNA methyltransferase promoter methylation in glioblastoma patients treated with temozolomide." *Clin Cancer Res* 10(6): 1871-1874.

Heitzer, E., P. Ulz and J. B. Geigl (2015). "Circulating tumor DNA as a liquid biopsy for cancer." *Clin Chem* 61(1): 112-123.

Herceg, Z. and P. Hainaut (2007). "Genetic and epigenetic alterations as biomarkers for cancer detection, diagnosis and prognosis." *Mol Oncol* 1(1): 26-41.

Hernando-Herraez, I., R. Garcia-Perez, A. J. Sharp and T. Marques-Bonet (2015). "DNA Methylation: Insights into Human Evolution." *PLoS Genet* 11(12): e1005661.

Hirschey, M. D., R. J. DeBerardinis, A. M. Diehl, J. E. Drew, C. Frezza, M. F. Green, L. W. Jones, Y. H. Ko, A. Le, M. A. Lea, J. W. Locasale, V. D. Longo, C. A. Lyssiotis, E. McDonnell, M. Mehrmohamadi, G. Michelotti, V. Muralidhar, M. P. Murphy, P. L. Pedersen, B. Poore, L. Raffaghello, J. C. Rathmell, S. Sivanand, M. G. Vander Heiden,

K. E. Wellen and T. Target Validation (2015). "Dysregulated metabolism contributes to oncogenesis." *Semin Cancer Biol* 35 Suppl: S129-150.

Huang, F. W., E. Hodis, M. J. Xu, G. V. Kryukov, L. Chin and L. A. Garraway (2013). "Highly recurrent TERT promoter mutations in human melanoma." *Science* 339(6122): 957-959.

Issa, J. P. (2004). "CpG island methylator phenotype in cancer." *Nat Rev_Cancer* 4(12): 988-993.

Jaenisch, R. and A. Bird (2003). "Epigenetic regulation of gene expression: how the genome integrates intrinsic and environmental signals." *Nat Genet* 33 Suppl: 245-254.

Jair, K. W., K. E. Bachman, H. Suzuki, A. H. Ting, I. Rhee, R. W. Yen, S. B. Baylin and K. E. Schuebel (2006). "De novo CpG island methylation in human cancer cells." *Cancer Res* 66(2): 682-692.

Jiang, G., Z. P. Wei, D. S. Pei, Y. Xin, Y. Q. Liu and J. N. Zheng (2011). "A novel approach to overcome temozolomide resistance in glioma and melanoma: Inactivation of MGMT by gene therapy." *Biochem Biophys_Res Commun* 406(3): 311-314.

Jin, B. and K. D. Robertson (2013). "DNA methyltransferases, DNA damage repair, and cancer." *Adv Exp Med Biol* 754: 3-29.

Johannessen, T. C. and R. Bjerkvig (2012). "Molecular mechanisms of temozolomide resistance in glioblastoma multiforme." *Expert Rev Anticancer Ther* 12(5): 635-642.

Kargul, J. and G. J. Laurent (2009). "Epigenetics and human disease." *Int J_Biochem Cell Biol* 41(1): 1.

Katsnelson, A. (2013). "Momentum grows to make 'personalized' medicine more 'precise.'" *Nat Med* 19(3): 249.

Kisseljova, N. P. and F. L. Kisseljov (2005). "DNA demethylation and carcinogenesis." *Biochemistry (Mosc)* 70(7): 743-752.

Koelsche, C., F. Sahm, D. Capper, D. Reuss, D. Sturm, D. T. Jones, M. Kool, P. A. Northcott, B. Wiestler, K. Bohmer, J. Meyer, C. Mawrin, C. Hartmann, M. Mittelbronn, M. Platten, B. Brokinkel, M. Seiz, C. Herold-Mende, A. Unterberg, J. Schittenhelm, M. Weller, S. Pfister, W. Wick, A. Korshunov and A. von Deimling (2013). "Distribution of TERT promoter mutations in pediatric and adult tumors of the nervous system." *Acta Neuropathol* 126(6): 907-915.

Kumar, D. and M. Verma (2009). "Methods in cancer epigenetics and epidemiology." *Methods Mol Biol* 471: 273-288.

Kurdyukov, S. and M. Bullock (2016). "DNA Methylation Analysis: Choosing the Right Method." *Biology (Basel)* 5(1).

Kurkjian, C., S. Kummar and A. J. Murgo (2008). "DNA methylation: its role in cancer development and therapy." *Curr Probl Cancer* 32(5): 187-235.

Lee, S. T. and J. L. Wiemels (2016). "Genome-wide CpG island methylation and intergenic demethylation propensities vary among different tumor sites." *Nucleic Acids Res* 44(3): 1105-1117.

Li, Y., L. Song, Y. Gong and B. He (2014). "Detection of colorectal cancer by DNA methylation biomarker SEPT9: past, present and future." *Biomark Med* 8(5): 755-769.

Lin, R. K. and Y. C. Wang (2014). "Dysregulated transcriptional and post-translational control of DNA methyltransferases in cancer." *Cell Biosci* 4: 46.

Liu, J. P. (1999). "Studies of the molecular mechanisms in the regulation of telomerase activity." *FASEB J* 13(15): 2091-2104.

Luczak, M. W. and P. P. Jagodzinski (2006). "The role of DNA methylation in cancer development." *Folia Histochem Cytobiol* 44(3): 143-154.

McDade, S. S., P. A. Hall and S. E. Russell (2007). "Translational control of SEPT9 isoforms is perturbed in disease." *Hum Mol Genet* 16(7): 742-752.

McIlhatton, M. A., J. F. Burrows, P. G. Donaghy, S. Chanduloy, P. G. Johnston and S. E. Russell (2001). "Genomic organization, complex splicing pattern and expression of a human septin gene on chromosome 17q25.3." *Oncogene* 20(41): 5930-5939.

Moarii, M., V. Boeva, J. P. Vert and F. Reyal (2015). "Changes in correlation between promoter methylation and gene expression in cancer." *BMC Genomics* 16(1): 873.

Molnar, B., K. Toth, B. K. Bartak and Z. Tulassay (2015). "Plasma methylated septin 9: a colorectal cancer screening marker." *Expert Rev Mol Diagn* 15(2): 171-184.

Morioka, Y., K. Hibi, M. Sakai, M. Koike, M. Fujiwara, Y. Kodera, K. Ito and A. Nakao (2006). "Aberrant methylation of the CHFR gene in digestive tract cancer." *Anticancer Res* 26(3A): 1791-1795.

Mosrati, M. A., A. Malmstrom, M. Lysiak, A. Krysztofiak, M. Hallbeck, P. Milos, A. L. Hallbeck, C. Bratthall, M. Strandeus, M. Stenmark-Askmalm and P. Soderkvist (2015). "TERT promoter mutations and polymorphisms as prognostic factors in primary glioblastoma." *Oncotarget* 6(18): 16663-16673.

Mostowy, S. and P. Cossart (2012). "Septins: the fourth component of the cytoskeleton." *Nat Rev Mol Cell Biol* 13(3): 183-194.

Nakagawachi, T., H. Soejima, T. Urano, W. Zhao, K. Higashimoto, Y. Satoh, S. Matsukura, S. Kudo, Y. Kitajima, H. Harada, K. Furukawa, H. Matsuzaki, M. Emi, Y. Nakabeppu, K. Miyazaki, M. Sekiguchi and T. Mukai (2003). "Silencing effect of CpG island hypermethylation and histone modifications on O6-methylguanine-DNA methyltransferase (MGMT) gene expression in human cancer." *Oncogene* 22(55): 8835-8844.

Natarajan, A. T., S. Vermeulen, F. Darroudi, M. B. Valentine, T. P. Brent, S. Mitra and K. Tano (1992). "Chromosomal localization of human O6-methylguanine-DNA methyltransferase (MGMT) gene by in situ hybridization." *Mutagenesis* 7(1): 83-85.

Ng, J. M. and J. Yu (2015). "Promoter hypermethylation of tumour suppressor genes as potential biomarkers in colorectal cancer." *Int J Mol Sci* 16(2): 2472-2496.

Pang, A. W., J. R. MacDonald, D. Pinto, J. Wei, M. A. Rafiq, D. F. Conrad, H. Park, M. E. Hurles, C. Lee, J. C. Venter, E. F. Kirkness, S. Levy, L. Feuk and S. W. Scherer (2010). "Towards a comprehensive structural variation map of an individual human genome." *Genome Biol* 11(5): R52.

Pang, A. W., O. Migita, J. R. Macdonald, L. Feuk and S. W. Scherer (2013). "Mechanisms of formation of structural variation in a fully sequenced human genome." *Hum Mutat* 34(2): 345-354.

Paska, A. V. and P. Hudler (2015). "Aberrant methylation patterns in cancer: a clinical view." *Biochem Med (Zagreb)* 25(2): 161-176.

Payne, S. R. (2010). "From discovery to the clinic: the novel DNA methylation biomarker (m)SEPT9 for the detection of colorectal cancer in blood." *Epigenomics* 2(4): 575-585.

Pettigrew, K. A., R. N. Armstrong, H. A. Colyer, S. D. Zhang, I. M. Rea, R. E. Jones, D. M. Baird and K. I. Mills (2012). "Differential TERT promoter methylation and response to 5-aza-2'-deoxycytidine in acute myeloid leukemia cell lines: TERT expression, telomerase activity, telomere length, and cell death." *Genes Chromosomes Cancer* 51(8): 768-780.

Poole, J. C., L. G. Andrews and T. O. Tollefsbol (2001). "Activity, function, and gene regulation of the catalytic subunit of telomerase (hTERT)." *Gene* 269(1-2): 1-12.

Poot, M. and T. Haaf (2015). "Mechanisms of Origin, Phenotypic Effects and Diagnostic Implications of Complex Chromosome Rearrangements." *Mol Syndromol* 6(3): 110-134.

Privette, L. M. and E. M. Petty (2008). "CHFR: A Novel Mitotic Checkpoint Protein and Regulator of Tumorigenesis." *Transl Oncol* 1(2): 57-64.

Pulling, L. C., K. K. Divine, D. M. Klinge, F. D. Gilliland, T. Kang, A. G. Schwartz, T. J. Bocklage and S. A. Belinsky (2003). "Promoter hypermethylation of the O6-methylguanine-DNA methyltransferase gene: more common in lung adenocarcinomas from never-smokers than smokers and associated with tumor progression." *Cancer Res* 63(16): 4842-4848.

Rajendran, G., K. Shanmuganandam, A. Bendre, D. Muzumdar, A. Goel and A. Shiras (2011). "Epigenetic regulation of DNA methyltransferases: DNMT1 and DNMT3B in gliomas." *J Neurooncol* 104(2): 483-494.

Rasool, M., A. Malik, M. I. Naseer, A. Manan, S. Ansari, I. Begum, M. H. Qazi, P. Pushparaj, A. M. Abuzenadah, M. H. Al-Qahtani, M. A. Kamal and S. Gan (2015). "The role of epigenetics in personalized medicine: challenges and opportunities." *BMC Med Genomics* 8 Suppl 1: S5.

Reitman, Z. J., C. J. Pirozzi and H. Yan (2013). "Promoting a new brain tumor mutation: TERT promoter mutations in CNS tumors." *Acta Neuropathol* 126(6): 789-792.

Remke, M., V. Ramaswamy, J. Peacock, D. J. Shih, C. Koelsche, P. A. Northcott, N. Hill, F. M. Cavalli, M. Kool, X. Wang, S. C. Mack, M. Barszczyk, A. S. Morrissy, X. Wu, S. Agnihotri, B. Luu, D. T. Jones, L. Garzia, A. M. Dubuc, N. Zhukova, R. Vanner, J. M. Kros, P. J. French, E. G. Van Meir, R. Vibhakar, K. Zitterbart, J. A. Chan, L. Bognar, A. Klekner, B. Lach, S. Jung, A. G. Saad, L. M. Liau, S. Albrecht, M. Zollo, M. K. Cooper, R. C. Thompson, O. O. Delattre, F. Bourdeaut, F. F. Doz, M. Garami, P. Hauser, C. G. Carlotti, T. E. Van Meter, L. Massimi, D. Fults, S. L. Pomeroy, T. Kumabe, Y. S. Ra, J. R. Leonard, S. K. Elbabaa, J. Mora, J. B. Rubin, Y. J. Cho, R. E. McLendon, D. D. Bigner, C. G. Eberhart, M. Fouladi, R. J. Wechsler-Reya, C. C. Faria, S. E. Croul, A. Huang, E. Bouffet, C. E. Hawkins, P. B. Dirks, W. A. Weiss, U. Schuller, I. F. Pollack, S. Rutkowski, D. Meyronet, A. Jouvet, M. Fevre-Montange, N. Jabado, M. Perek-Polnik, W. A. Grajkowska, S. K. Kim, J. T. Rutka, D. Malkin, U. Tabori, S. M. Pfister, A. Korshunov, A. von Deimling and M. D. Taylor (2013). "TERT promoter mutations are highly recurrent in SHH subgroup medulloblastoma." *Acta Neuropathol* 126(6): 917-929.

Riemenschneider, M. J., M. E. Hegi and G. Reifenberger (2010). "MGMT promoter methylation in malignant gliomas." *Target Oncol* 5(3): 161-165.

Robert, M. F., S. Morin, N. Beaulieu, F. Gauthier, I. C. Chute, A. Barsalou and A. R. MacLeod (2003). "DNMT1 is required to maintain CpG methylation and aberrant gene silencing in human cancer cells." *Nat_Genet* 33(1): 61-65.

Sadee, W. and Z. Dai (2005). "Pharmacogenetics/genomics and personalized medicine." *Hum Mol Genet* 14 Spec No. 2: R207-214.

Sadikovic, B., K. Al-Romaih, J. A. Squire and M. Zielenska (2008). "Cause and consequences of genetic and epigenetic alterations in human cancer." *Curr Genomics* 9(6): 394-408.

Sakai, M., K. Hibi, N. Kanazumi, S. Nomoto, S. Inoue, S. Takeda and A. Nakao (2005). "Aberrant methylation of the CHFR gene in advanced hepatocellular carcinoma." *Hepatogastroenterology* 52(66): 1854-1857.

Saletta, F., L. Dalla Pozza and J. A. Byrne (2015). "Genetic causes of cancer predisposition in children and adolescents." *Transl Pediatr* 4(2): 67-75.

Sanbhnani, S. and F. M. Yeong (2012). "CHFR: a key checkpoint component implicated in a wide range of cancers." *Cell Mol Life Sci* 69(10): 1669-1687.

Santos-Rosa, H. and C. Caldas (2005). "Chromatin modifier enzymes, the histone code and cancer." *Eur J Cancer* 41(16): 2381-2402.

Scott, M., P. L. Hyland, G. McGregor, K. J. Hillan, S. E. Russell and P. A. Hall (2005). "Multimodality expression profiling shows SEPT9 to be overexpressed in a wide range of human tumours." *Oncogene* 24(29): 4688-4700.

Schubeler, D. (2015). "Function and information content of DNA methylation." *Nature* 517(7534): 321-326.

Sharp, A. J., E. Stathaki, E. Migliavacca, M. Brahmachary, S. B. Montgomery, Y. Dupre and S. E. Antonarakis (2011). "DNA methylation profiles of human active and inactive X chromosomes." *Genome Res* 21(10): 1592-1600.

Shin, K. H., M. K. Kang, E. Dicterow and N. H. Park (2003). "Hypermethylation of the hTERT promoter inhibits the expression of telomerase activity in normal oral fibroblasts and senescent normal oral keratinocytes." *Br J Cancer* 89(8): 1473-1478.

Shtivelman, E. (2003). "Promotion of mitosis by activated protein kinase B after DNA damage involves polo-like kinase 1 and checkpoint protein CHFR." *Mol Cancer Res* 1(13): 959-969.

Simon, R. (2011). "Genomic biomarkers in predictive medicine: an interim analysis." *EMBO Mol Med* 3(8): 429-435.

Smith, M. T., K. Z. Guyton, C. F. Gibbons, J. M. Fritz, C. J. Portier, I. Rusyn, D. M. DeMarini, J. C. Caldwell, R. J. Kavlock, P. Lambert, S. S. Hecht, J. R. Bucher, B. W. Stewart, R. Baan, V. J. Cogliano and K. Straif (2015). "Key Characteristics of Carcinogens as a Basis for Organizing Data on Mechanisms of Carcinogenesis." *Environ Health Perspect*.

Song, L. and Y. Li (2015). "SEPT9: A Specific Circulating Biomarker for Colorectal Cancer." *Adv Clin Chem* 72: 171-204.

Subramaniam, D., R. Thombre, A. Dhar and S. Anant (2014). "DNA methyltransferases: a novel target for prevention and therapy." *Front Oncol* 4: 80.

Tang, J., Y. Xiong, H. H. Zhou and X. P. Chen (2014). "DNA methylation and personalized medicine." *J Clin Pharm Ther* 39(6): 621-627.

Tillo, D., S. Mukerjee and C. Vinson (2016). "Inheritance of Cytosine Methylation." *J Cell Physiol*.

Torres, S. M., L. Luo, J. Lilyquist, C. A. Stidley, K. Flores, K. A. White, E. Erdei, M. Gonzales, S. Paine, R. I. Vogel, D. Lazovich and M. Berwick (2013). "DNA repair variants, indoor tanning, and risk of melanoma." *Pigment Cell Melanoma Res* 26(5): 677-684.

Toth, K., R. Wasserkort, F. Sipos, A. Kalmar, B. Wichmann, K. Leiszter, G. Valcz, M. Juhasz, P. Miheller, A. V. Patai, Z. Tulassay and B. Molnar (2014). "Detection of methylated septin 9 in tissue and plasma of colorectal patients with neoplasia and the relationship to the amount of circulating cell-free DNA." *PLoS One* 9(12): e115415.

Toyota, M. and J. P. Issa (2000). "The role of DNA hypermethylation in human neoplasia." *Electrophoresis* 21(2): 329-333.

Ulz, P., M. Auer and E. Heitzer (2016). "Detection of Circulating Tumor DNA in the Blood of Cancer Patients: An Important Tool in Cancer Chemoprevention." *Methods Mol Biol* 1379: 45-68.

van Vugt, M. A. and R. H. Medema (2005). "Getting in and out of mitosis with Polo-like kinase-1." *Oncogene* 24(17): 2844-2859.

Verma, M. (2015). "Cancer epigenetics: risk assessment, diagnosis, treatment, and prognosis. Preface." *Methods Mol Biol* 1238: v-vi.

Verma, M., P. Maruvada and S. Srivastava (2004). "Epigenetics and cancer." *Crit Rev Clin Lab Sci* 41(5-6): 585-607.

Waldmann, T. and R. Schneider (2013). "Targeting histone modifications--epigenetics in cancer." *Curr Opin Cell Biol* 25(2): 184-189.

Wang, N., H. Kjellin, A. Sofiadis, O. Fotouhi, C. C. Juhlin, M. Backdahl, J. Zedenius, D. Xu, J. Lehtio and C. Larsson (2016). "Genetic and epigenetic background and protein expression profiles in relation to telomerase activation in medullary thyroid carcinoma." *Oncotarget.*

Warton, K. and G. Samimi (2015). "Methylation of cell-free circulating DNA in the diagnosis of cancer." *Front Mol Biosci* 2: 13.

Wasserkort, R., A. Kalmar, G. Valcz, S. Spisak, M. Krispin, K. Toth, Z. Tulassay, A. Z. Sledziewski and B. Molnar (2013). "Aberrant septin 9 DNA methylation in colorectal cancer is restricted to a single CpG island." *BMC Cancer* 13: 398.

Waterfall, J. J., J. K. Killian and P. S. Meltzer (2014). "The role of mutation of metabolism-related genes in genomic hypermethylation." *Biochem_Biophys Res Commun* 455(1-2): 16-23.

Weller, M., R. Stupp, G. Reifenberger, A. A. Brandes, M. J. van den Bent, W. Wick and M. E. Hegi (2010). "MGMT promoter methylation in malignant gliomas: ready for personalized medicine?" *Nat Rev Neurol* 6(1): 39-51.

Wesseling, P., M. van den Bent and A. Perry (2015). "Oligodendroglioma: pathology, molecular mechanisms and markers." *Acta Neuropathol* 129(6): 809-827.

Wu, Y., G. Li, D. He, F. Yang, G. He, L. He, H. Zhang, Y. Deng, M. Fan, L. Shen, D. Zhou and Z. Zhang (2016). "Telomerase reverse transcriptase methylation predicts lymph node metastasis and prognosis in patients with gastric cancer." *Onco Targets Ther* 9: 279-286.

Yan, W., J. G. Herman and M. Guo (2016). "Epigenome-based personalized medicine in human cancer." *Epigenomics* 8(1): 119-133.

Yanokura, M., K. Banno, M. Kawaguchi, N. Hirao, A. Hirasawa, N. Susumu, K. Tsukazaki and D. Aoki (2007). "Relationship of aberrant DNA hypermethylation of CHFR with sensitivity to taxanes in endometrial cancer." *Oncol Rep* 17(1): 41-48.

Yu, X., K. Minter-Dykhouse, L. Malureanu, W. M. Zhao, D. Zhang, C. J. Merkle, I. M. Ward, H. Saya, G. Fang, J. van Deursen and J. Chen (2005). "Chfr is required for tumor suppression and Aurora A regulation." *Nat Genet* 37(4): 401-406.

Zhang, Z. Y., A. K. Chan, X. J. Ding, Z. Y. Qin, C. S. Hong, L. C. Chen, X. Zhang, F. P. Zhao, Y. Wang, Y. Wang, L. F. Zhou, Z. Zhuang, H. K. Ng, H. Yan, Y. Yao and Y. Mao (2015). "TERT promoter mutations contribute to IDH mutations in predicting differential responses to adjuvant therapies in WHO grade II and III diffuse gliomas." *Oncotarget* 6(28): 24871-24883.

Ziller, M. J., F. Muller, J. Liao, Y. Zhang, H. Gu, C. Bock, P. Boyle, C. B. Epstein, B. E. Bernstein, T. Lengauer, A. Gnirke and A. Meissner (2011). "Genomic distribution and inter-sample variation of non-CpG methylation across human cell types." *PLoS Genet* 7(12): e1002389.

Zoghbi, H. Y. and A. L. Beaudet (2016). "Epigenetics and Human Disease." *Cold Spring Harb Perspect Biol* 8(2).

In: Pharmacogenomics in Latin America
Editor: Luis A. Quiñones
ISBN: 978-1-53611-031-9

Chapter 13

FUTURE DIRECTIONS: CHALLENGES, OPPORTUNITIES AND LIMITATIONS

Maria A. Redal[1,*], MD and Luis A. Quiñones[2,†], PhD

[1]Institute of Physiopathology and Clinical Biochemistry, Faculty of Pharmacy and Biochemistry, University of Buenos Aires,
CDM Center of Molecular Diagnostic, Argentina

[2]Laboratory of Chemical Carcinogenesis and Pharmacogenetics, Department of Basic-Clinical Oncology (DOBC), Faculty of Medicine, University of Chile, Santiago, Chile

ABSTRACT

The ultimate goal of pharmacogenomic research is to predict individual's responses to drug therapy and subsequently adapt pharmacotherapeutic strategies. Therefore, the current challenge for personalized therapy is to define genetic profiles to predict the response to drugs and the progression of the diseases. However, despite the enormous amount of known information about the genetic basis of variable response to drugs, it has little influence on its application to the current clinical practice, particularly in Latin American region where there is a great genetic admixture. Thus, the present chapter pursues to contribute with a general vision of the future of the area to overcome the proper limitations of this region.

Keywords: pharmacogenomics, pharmacogenetics, pharmagenes, Latin America, ethnicity

INTRODUCTION

Since the completion of the human genome project and its potential ability to change the whole practice of medicine today, great expectations and enthusiasm regarding possible applications were positioned in the scientific community. Together, several millions of SNPs

* Corresponding Author E-mail. marianared@hotmail.com.

† lquinone@med.uchile.cl.

have been identified [SNP Consortium, 2016) and the effects of each specific SNPs are continuously under study (GWAS, 2016). However, human genome defined human similarity, not differences or intra and inter-variability. Thus, actually many researchers believe that pharmacogenomics can be one of the first successes in the study of individual differences, at least in relation to drug response.

The ultimate goal of pharmacogenomic research is to predict individual's responses to drug therapy and subsequently to adapt pharmacotherapeutic strategies. In this regard, it is estimated that gene polymorphisms account for 20% to 95% of the variability in therapeutic response and toxicity, depending on the drug (Evans & Mcleod, 2003). In this respect, of all the known drugs involved in adverse reactions about 80% are metabolized by polymorphic enzymes (Phillips et al., 2001) being CYP enzymes the more relevant ones (Table 1). Since 2004, several drugs refer to pharmacogenomic studies in the labeling information, some of them considered sufficient to guide treatment decisions (Zineh et al., 2004). An interesting advance was when, in 2005, FDA issued a guidance document for the industry about the referral data for genotyping drug metabolizing enzymes (*Guidance for Industry: Pharmacogenomic Data Submissions, March 2005*). In the same year the FDA approved the marketing of the first laboratory test system based on cytochrome P450 genotypes (Amplichip CYP450 test, 2005), which allows the use of genetic information to select appropriate doses of drugs and drugs for a wide variety of common conditions. However, in Latin America the test seems to have suboptimal results, which could be due to ethnic differences between Latin Americans and other human populations.

Table 1. Allelic variants of CYP enzymes (adapted from http://www.cypalleles.ki.se/)

Enzyme	Gene	Allelic Variant
CYP1A1	*CYP1A1*	*1,*2A,*2B,*2C,*3,*4, *5, *6, *7, *8, *9,*10, *11, *12,*13.
CYP1A2	*CYP1A2*	*1A, *1B, *1C, *1D, *1E, *1F, *1G, *1H, *1J,*1K, *1L*1M*1N,*1P, *1Q, *1R, *1S, *1T, *1U, *1V, *1W, *2, *2, *3, *4, *5, *6, *7, *8, *9, *10, *11, *12, *13, *14, *15, *16, *17, *18, *19,*20, *21.
CYP1B1	*CYP1B1*	**1, *2, *3, *4, *5, *6, *7,*8, *9, *10,*11, *12, *13, *14, *15, *16, *17, *18, *19, *20,*21,*22,*23, *24,*25, *26.
CYP2A6	*CYP2A6*	*1A, *1B1, *1B2, *1B3, *1B4, *1B5, *1B6, *1B7, *1B8, *1B9, *1B10, *1B11, *1B12, *1B13, *1B14, *1B15, *1B16, *1B17, *1C,*1D,*1E, *1F, *1G, *1H, *1J, *1K, *1L, *1X2A, *1X2B, *2, *3, *4A, *4B, *4C, *4D, *4F, *4G, *4H, *5,*6, *7, *8, *9A, *9B, *10,*11,*12A, *12B, *12C,*13, *14,*15, *16, *17, *18A, *18B, *18C, *19, *20, *21, *22,*23, *24A, *24B, *25, *26, *27, *28A,*28B, *29, *30, *31A, *31B, *32,*33, *34, *35A, *35B, *36, *37, *38, *39, *40, *41, *42, *43, *44, *45
CYP2A13	*CYP2A13*	*1A, *1B, *1C, *1D, *1E,*1F, *1G, *1H, *1J, *1K, *1L, *2A, *2B, *3, *4, *5, *6, *7, *8, *9, *10.
CYP2B6	*CYP2B6*	*1A, *1B, *1C, *1D, *1E, *1F, *1G, *1H, *1J, *1K, *1L,*1M, *1N, *2A, *2B, *3,*4A, *4B, *4C, *4D, *5A, *5B,*5C,*6A,*6B, *6C, *7A, *7B, *8, *9, *10, *11A, *11B, *13A, *13B, *14, *15A, *15B, *16, *17A, *17B, *18, *19, *20, *21, *22, *23, *24, *25, *26, *27, *28, *29, *30, *31, *32, *33, *34
CYP2C8	*CYP2C8*	*1A, *1B, *1C, *2, *3, *4, *5, *6, *7, *8, *9, *10, *11, *12, *13, *14.
CYP2C9	*CYP2C9*	*1A, *1B, *1C, *1D, *2A, *2B, 2C, *3A, *3B, *4, *5, *6, *7, *8, *9, *10, *11A, *11B, *12, *13, *14, *15, *16,*17, *18, *19, *20, *21, *22, *23, *24, *25, *26, *27, *28, *29, *30, *31, *32, *33, *34, *35, *36, *37, *38, *39, *40, *41, *42, *43, *44, *45, *46, *47, *48, *49, *50, *51, *52, *53, *54, *55, *56, *57, *58, *59, *60.
CYP2C19	*CYP2C19*	*1A, *1B,*1C, *2A, *2B, *2C, *2D, *2E, *2F, *2G, *2H, *2J, *3A, *3B, *3C, *4A, *4B, *5A, *5B, *6, *7, *8, *9, *10, *11, *12, *13, *14, *15, *16, *17, *18, *19, *20, *21, *22, *23, *24, *25, *26, *27, *28, *29, *30, *31, *32, *33, *34.

Table 1. (Continued)

Enzyme	Gene	Allelic Variant
CYP2D6	*CYP2D6*	*1A, *1B,*1C, *1D, *1XN, *2A, *2B, *2C, *2D, *2E, *2F, *2G, *2H, *2J, *2K, *2L, *2M, *2XN, *3A, *3B, *4A, *4B, *4C, *4D, *4F, *4G, *4H,*4J, *4K, *4L, *4M, *4N, *4P, *4X2, *5, *6A,*6B, *6C, *6D, *7, *8, *9, *10A,*10B, *10C, *10D, *10X2, *11, *12, *13, *14A,*14B, *15, *16, *17, *17XN, *18, *19, *20, *21A, *21B,*22, *23, *24, *25, *26, *27, *28, *29, *30, *31, *32, *33, *34, *35A, *35B, *35X2, *36, *37, *38, *39, *40, *41, *42, *43, *44, *45A, *45B, *46, *47, *48, *49, *50, *51, *52, *53, *54, *55, *56[a], *56B, *57, *58, *59, *60, *61, *62, *63, *64, *65, *66, *67, *68A, *68B, *69, *70, *71, *72, *73, *74, *75, *76, *77, *78, *79, *80, *81, *82, *83, *84, *85, *86, *87, *88, *89, *90, *91, *92, *93, *94A, *94B, *95, *96, *97, *98, *99, *100 *101, *102, *103, *104, *105.
CYP2E1	*CYP2E1*	*1A, *1B,*1C, *1CX2 *1D, *2, *3, *4, *5A, *5B, *6, *7A, *7B, *7C,
CYP2F1	*CYP2F1*	*1, *2A, *2B, *3, *4, *5A, *5B, *6
CYP2J2	*CYP2J2*	*1, *2, *3, *4, *5, *6, *7,*8, *9, *10.
CYP2R1	*CYP2R1*	*1, *2.
CYP2S1	*CYP2S1*	*1A, *1B, *1C, *1D, *1E,*1F, *1G, *1H, *2, *3, *4, *5A, *5B
CYP2W1	*CYP2W1*	*1A, *1B, *2, *3, *4, *5, *6.
CYP3A4	*CYP3A4*	*1A,*1B,*1C,*1D,*1F,*1G,*1H,*1J,*1K,*1L,*1M,*1N,*1P,*1Q,*1R,*1S,*1T,*2,*3,*4,*5,*6,*7,*8,*9,*10,*11,*12,*13,*14,*15A,*15B,*16A,*16B,*17,*18A,*18B,*19,*20,*21,*22,*23,*24,*25,*26
CYP3A5	*CYP3A5*	*1A, *1B, *1C, *1D, *1E, *2, *3A, *3B, *3C, *3D, *3E,*3F, *3G, *3H, *3I, *3J, *3K, *3L, *4, *5, *6, *7, *8, *9, *10, *11.
CYP3A7	*CYP3A7*	*1A, *1B, *1C, *1D, *2, *3.
CYP3A43	*CYP3A43*	*1A, *1B, *2A, *2B, *3.
CYP4A11	*CYP4A11*	*1
CYP4A22	*CYP4A22*	*1, *2, *3A, *3B, *3C, *3D, *3E, *4, *5, *6, *7, *8, *9, *10, *11, *12A, *12B. *13A, *13B, *14, *15
CYP4B1	*CYP4B1*	*1, *2A, *2B, *3, *4, *5, *6, *7.
CYP4F2	*CYP4F2*	*1, *2, *3.
CYP5A1	*CYP5A1*	*1A, *1B, *1C, *1D, *2, *3, *4, *5, *6, *7,*8, *9
CYP8A1	*CYP8A1*	*1A, *1B, *1C, *1D, *1E, *1F, *1G, *1H, *1J, *1K, *1L, *2, *3, *4.
CYP19A1	*CYP19A1*	*1, *2, *3, *4, *5
CYP21A2	*CYP21A2*	*1A, *1B, *2, *3, *4, *5, *6, *7, 8, *9, *10,*11, *12, *13, *14, *15, *16, *17, *18, *19, *20A, *20B, *20C, *20D, *20E, *20F, *20G,*20H, *20J, *20K, *20L, *20M, *20N, *20P, *20Q, *20R, *20S, *20T, *20U, *20V, *21, *22, *23, *24, *25, *26, *27, *28, *29, *30, *31, *32, *33, *34, *35, *36, *37, *38, *39, *40, *41, *42, *43, *44, *45, *46, *47, *48, *49, *50, *51, *52, *53, *54, *55, *56, *57, *58, *59, *60, *61, *62, *63, *64, *65, *66, *67, *68, *69, *70, *71, *72, *73, *74, *75, *76, *77, *78, *79, *80, *81, *82, *83, *84, *85, *86, *87, *88, *89, *90, *91, *92, *93, *94, *95, *96, *97, *98, *99, *100 *101, *102, *103, *104, *105, *106, *107, *108, *109, *110, *111, *112, *113, *114, *115, *116, *117, *118, *119, *120, *121, *122, *123, *124, *125, *126, *127, *128, *129, *130, *131, *132, *133, *134, *135, *136, *137, *138, *139, *140, *141, *142, *143, *144, *145, *146, *147, *148, *149, *150, *151, *152, *153, *154, *155, *156, *157, *158, *159, *160, *161, *162, *163, *164, *165, *166, *167, *168, *169, *170, *171, *172, *173, *174, *175, *176, *177, *178, *179, *180, *181.
CYP26A1	*CYP26A1*	*1, *2, *3, *4.

Nowadays some authors estimate that in the next 10 years, an important percentage of the new approved drugs will include a pharmacogenomic study. It is currently clear, considering that FDA from 2013 have recommended almost 200 pharmacogenomic biomarkers for drug monitoring, in order to improve prescription dosage including antivirals, antibiotics, psychiatry drugs, analgesic and anticancer agents (FDA, 2016). In some cases this information has been incorporated into the dataset long after the drug was approved by regulatory agencies. In other cases, pharmacogenomic data has been obtained during the process of drug development and has been taken into account for approval. Until now no Latin American regulatory authority have included pharmacogenomics criteria for approval of drugs.

Therefore, the current challenge for personalized therapy is to define genetic profiles to predict the response to drugs and the progression of the diseases (Agúndez et al., 2012a y b; Gardiner et al., 2006; Huang et al., 2006; Gurwitz & Lunshof, 2009; Gladding et al., 2013; Huang & Temple, 2008). Information to address this challenge can only be obtained from case-control and prospective studies with a pharmacogenomics basis, particularly in mixed and complex populations as Latin America (Quiñones et al., 2014).

LIMITATIONS OF PHARMACOGENOMIC CLINICAL APPLICATION

However, despite the enormous amount of known information about the genetic basis of variable response to drugs, it has little influence on its application to the current clinical practice, particularly in Latin American region. Thus, acceptance of pharmacogenomic studies in medical practice will be gradual and probably slower as required whether no strong efforts be performed through outreach and training activities. All over the world, several issues have prevented rapid implementation of pharmacogenomics, such as, a) lack of readily available clinical laboratories which can perform these tests quickly and cost-effectively, b) shortage of health care professionals who can interpret the test data and associated clinical pharmacology and c) doubts whether insurance companies will pay for the study. In addition, many ethical questions pose continuing challenges. However, the number of drugs approved with a reference to the genetic study in labeling information is increasing.

Of course pharmacogenomics has several limitations to its application in clinical practice to be considered, some of them have been analyzed previously by Agúndez et al., (2012a) and Quiñones et al., (2014). Briefly, these limitations include the lack of sufficient evidence for cost–efficiency, the need for the identification of new biomarkers for drug toxicity and response, technical limitations and ethnicity questions. Together, we know that inter-individual variability to drug response exists, even in individuals with identical pharmacogenomic profile, giving rise to the idea that pharmacogenomics is only one of the several factors to be considered in dose adjustment. Therefore algorithms including anthropometric, lifestyle and environmental factors appear to be the best approach.

It is accepted that the result of cost-efficiency of genetic testing depends primarily on the therapeutic window of drug and the magnitude of the inter-individual variability in its response (Webster et al., 2004). In this regard, the selection of scenarios with a greatest potential impact is a crucial issue to the gradual acceptance of the pharmacogenomics tests and its eventual economic support by public health systems in Latin America.

Another restriction for the use of pharmacogenomics is the insufficient information about pharmagenes in Latin American populations, which prevents direct extrapolation of the dosage of drugs with clinical studies performed in other ethnic groups. Therefore, ethnicity appears to be an important issue in Latin America. In this sense, in order to have a first approach, particularly in American Hispanic populations, we have previously discussed the implications of interethnic and intraethnic genetic variability (García-Martin et al., 2006; Borovia et al., 2009; Restrepo et al., 2011, Roco et al., 2012, Flores-Gutierrez et al., 2016). In this respect, it is clear that there is a need for developing more and well designed studies in Latin American populations to better address the issue that the introduction of pharmacogenomics in clinical practice. These studies should include ethnic comparison of pharmacogenomic profiles, the impact of polymorphism on phenotype, gene expression and regulation, metabolic profiles of patients and pharmacoepigenetic research with a given drug and relevant environmental factors that influence drug response.

Moreover, as in other areas of science, it has been questioned the value of the associations reported between genetic and different clinical outcomes depending on the size of the effect variants. Many pharmacogenomic studies give RR values of about 1.5, which undoubtedly affects the statistical power of the results reported (Ioannides J., 2003). In this regard it is essential to promote replication of pharmacogenomic evaluations in different populations, in bigger enough samples to reduce the possibility of type I errors.

On the other hand, in the phases of drug development, the current emphasis is placed on obtaining population results, and there is minimal information obtained about individual differences in therapeutic response throughout the premarket stage. Beyond the development of population sub-studies with a particular demographic group, recently FDA has begun requiring information about specific metabolic pathways involved in pharmacokinetic processes for final approval of new drugs (PharmGKB, 2016; Relling & Hoffman, 2007)).

Certainly, although clinical trials are the best proof of evidence in current clinical practice, limitations on the individual extrapolation allow questioning its *sine qua non* use as a preliminary step to sanitary acceptance, and thus a recommendation of a pharmacogenomic study should be mandatory.

Effective integration of pharmacogenomics information in medical practice will also require a significant educational effort aimed at health professionals. At the moment, pharmacogenomics curriculum content in undergraduate medical education is minimal, like offering postgraduate courses or seminars. Familiarity with genetic analysis is a clear determinant of their routine application (Feero et al., 2009).

Some authors have warned about the need to protect the different communities, particularly some ethnic groups, of potential secondary discriminatory actions as result of pharmacogenomic studies (Weijer & Miller, 2004). While maintaining confidentiality is an essential aspect as with handling any sensitive data of patients, the implications of pharmacogenomics knowledge should be primarily individual rather than population (Noah L., 2002).

CONCLUSION

Clinical practice guidelines and protocols may help to overtake the major groups of barriers to pharmacogenetic implementation (Quiñones et al., 2014) (Figure 1). Moreover, we believe that governmental support and promotion for the use of pharmacogenomics biomarkers in the countries of this region will greatly influence help to overcome barriers.

The healthcare professionals (prescribers, insurers and regulators) will want to know if there is a substantial impact of pharmacogenomics on the safety and efficacy of the drug on an individual. Of course, before use in the clinical routine selected pharmagenes must demonstrate, in retrospective and prospective studies, a value sufficient to have good cost-effectiveness.

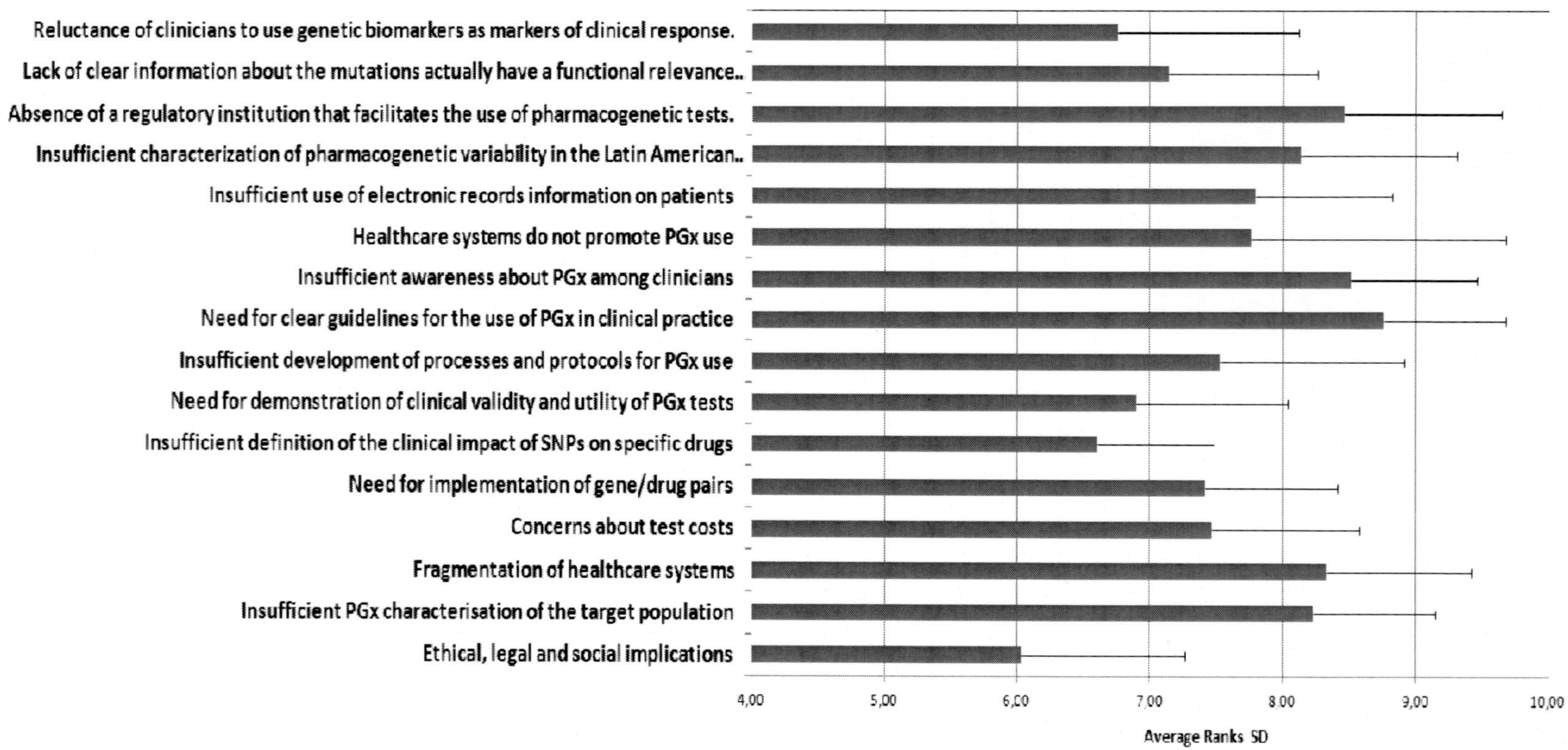

Figure 1. Highest-ranking barriers for implementing the use of pharmacogenomics testing, based on a survey in Latin America and the Caribbean Scientific and Clinical Researchers. Data related to average importance (on a scale of 1–10) are plotted along the x-axis. (Extracted from *Curr Drug Metab*. 2014 Feb;15(2):202-8).

Pharmacology of the future intends to conduct individualized pharmacotherapeutic treatment for the manifestation of a disease and the appropriate dose for the therapeutic effect in a given patient, minimizing the risk of adverse reactions. Therefore the main idea is the accomplishment of the five "R" for drug therapy "the Right dose of the Right drug for the Right indication in the Right patient at the Right time". For instance, nowadays the individualized treatments are a pressing need. The current formula of standard pharmacotherapy is not ideal according to the great variability between patients.

The rapidly evolving field of pharmacogenomics holds great promise for assisting the selection of patient-individualized treatment regimens and dosages. A vast number of single nucleotide polymorphisms have been discovered in genes thought to be involved in the regulation of drug metabolism; however, relatively few studies have been conducted that establish a link between genotype, efficacy and safety of drugs.

The new paradigm of individualized therapy should combine molecular (genetic) information, not genetic, demographic and clinical observation to determine the best treatment for a patient in the selection of drugs and dosage, in order to optimize the pharmacotherapeutic response of patients.

In short, integration of pharmacogenomics in clinical practice needs training of healthcare professionals and citizens, moreover legal and regulatory guidelines and safeguards will be needed. The answers to the question of which patient should receive which drug and dose will be not easy, but we believe that the approach offered by pharmacogenomics should be incorporated into the decision-making process. A more rational use of expensive treatment drugs together with actions to minimize patient toxic events and its consequences, would dramatically reduce medical costs, as an added benefit.

REFERENCES

Agúndez JA, Abad-Santos F, Aldea A, Alonso-Navarro H, Bernal ML, Borobia AM, Borrás E, Carballo M, Carvajal A, García-Muñiz JD, Gervasini G, Jiménez-Jiménez FJ, Lucena MI, Martínez C, Sacristán JA, Salado I, Sinués B, Vicente J, García-Martín E. Toward a clinical practice guide in pharmacogenomics testing for functional polymorphisms of drug-metabolizing enzymes. Gene/drug pairs and barriers perceived in Spain. *Front. Genet.* 2012a, 3:273.

Agúndez JA, Del Barrio J, Padró T, Stephens C, Farré M, Andrade RJ, Badimon L, García-Martín E, Vilahur G, Lucena MI. Trends in qualifying biomarkers in drug safety. Consensus of the 2011 meeting of the Spanish Society of Clinical Pharmacology, *Front. Pharmacol.* 2012b, 3:2.

AmpliChip CYP450 Test. The Medical Letter Inc. *Med. Lett. Drugs. Ther.* 2005; 47: 71–2.

Borobia AM, López-Parra AM, Tabarés B, Ramirez E, Baeza C, Arroyo-Pardo E, Carcas AJ. CYP2C9 polymorphism in five autochthonous population of the same geographic area (Spanish Pyrenees). *Pharmacol. Res.* 2009, 59, 107–111.

Evans WE, Mcleod HL. Pharmacogenomics-drug disposition, drug targets, and side effects. *N. Engl. J. Med.* 2003, 348, 538-549.

FDA, U.S. Food and Drug Administration, Center for Drug Evaluation and research. Guidance for Industry: International Conference on Harmonisation document ICH-E4,

Dose-response information to support drug registration http://www.fda.gov/cder/guidance/iche4.pdf (November 1994) Accessed in June 20 2016.

Feero WG, Guttmacher AE, Collins FS. The genome gets personal-almost. *JAMA* 2009; 2991351-2.

Flores-Gutierrez S., Rodríguez-Larralde A., Vívenes de Lugo M. & Castro de Guerra D. Distribution of polymorphisms in the CYP2C9 gene and CYP2C19/CYP2C9 haplotypes among Venezuelan populations. *Annals of Human Biology* (Ahead of Print).

Food and Drug Administration-USA (FDA). Table of Pharmacogenomic Biomarkers in Drug Labels. Available on http://www.fda.gov/drugs/scienceresearch/researchareas/pharmacogenetics/ucm083378.htm (accessed: August 25, 2016).

Garcia-Martin E, Martinez C, Ladero JM and Agúndez JA. Interethnic and intraethnic variability of CYP2C8 and CYP2C9 polymorphisms in healthy individuals. *Mol. Diagn. Ther.* 2006, 10, 29–40.

Gardiner SJ, Begg EJ. Pharmacogenetics, drug-metabolizing enzymes, and clinical practice. *Pharmacol. Rev.* 2006, 58, 521-90.

Gladding PA. Clinical applications of pharmacogenetics: Present and near future. *Cleve Clin. J. Med.* 2013, 80(8):477-82.

Gurwitz D, Lunshof JE. Personalized pharmacotherapy: genotypes, biomarkers, and beyond. *Clin. Pharmacol. Ther.* 2009, 85(2), 142.

GWAS. Genome Wide Association Studies. 2008. http://gwas.nih.gov/ (accessed: August 25, 2016).

Huang SM, Goodsaid F, Rahman A, Frueh F. Application of pharmaco-genetics in clinical pharmacology. *Toxicol. Mechanisms and Methods* 2006, 16, 89-99.

Huang SM, Temple R. Is this the drug or dose for you?: Impact and consideration of ethnic factors in global drug development, regulatory review and clinical practice. *Clin Pharmacol Ther* 2008; 84:287-94.

Ioannides JP. Genetic associations: False or true? Trends Mol Med 2003; 9:135-8.

Noah L. The coming pharmacogenomics revolution: tailoring drugs to fit patients` genetic profiles. *Jurimetrics* 2002; 43:1-28.

PharmGKB. The Pharmacogenomic Knowledge Base. Avalaible on https://www.pharmgkb.org (accessed: September 11, 2016)

Phillips KA, Veenstra DL, Oren E, Lee JK, Sadee W. Potential role of pharmacogenomics in reducing adverse drug reactions: a systematic review. *JAMA* 2001, 286(18), 2270-9.

Relling MV, Hoffman JM. Should pharmacogenomic studies be required for new drug approval? *Clin Pharmacol Ther* 2007; 82:425-8.

Restrepo JG, Martínez C, García-Agúndez A, Gaviria E, Laguna JJ, García-Martín E, Agúndez JA. Cytochrome P450 CYP2B6 genotypes and haplotypes in a Colombian population: identification of novel variant CYP2B6 alleles. *Pharmacogenet. Genomics* 2011, 21, 773–778.

Roco A, Quiñones L, Agúndez JA, García-Martín E, Squicciarini V, Miranda C, Garay J, Farfán N, Saavedra I, Cáceres D, Ibarra C, Varela N. Allele frequencies of 23 functionally significant variant alleles related with metabolism of antineoplastic drugs in the Chilean population: comparison with Caucasian and Asian populations. *Front. Genetics* 2012, 3(art 229): 1 – 9.

SNP Single Nucleotide Polymorphism consortium, http://snp.cshl.org/ (accessed: August 25, 2016).

The Human Cytochrome P450 (CYP) Allele Nomenclature Database. Available on http://www.cypalleles.ki.se. (Accessed: September 11, 2016).

Webster A, Martin P, Lewis G, et al. Integrating pharmacogenetics into society: in search of a model. *Nature Rev* 2004; 5:663-9.

Weijer C, Miller PB. Protecting communities in pharmacogenetic and pharmacogenomic research. Pharmacogenomics J 2004; 4:9-16.

Zineh I, Gerhard T, Aquilante CL, et al. Availability of pharmacogenomics-based prescribing information in drug package inserts for currently approved drugs. *Pharmacogenomics J.* 2004, 4(6), 354-8.

EDITOR'S CONTACT INFORMATION

Dr. Luis A. Quiñones
Professor,
Faculty of Medicine. University of Chile
Carlos Schachtebeck 299, lnterior Quinta Normal
Santiago, Chile
Email: lquinone@med.uchile.cl
Telephone: (562) 29770741-744

INDEX

#

A

B

C

D

F

G

H

I

J

K

L

M

N

O

P

Q

R

S

T

U

V

W

X

Y

Z

γ